Alternative & Mystical Healing Therapies

Alternative & Mystical Healing Therapies

Are They Medically Sound & Spiritually Safe??

Edwin A. Noyes M.D., MPH

Copyright © 2015 by Edwin A. Noyes M.D., MPH.

Library of Congress Control Number:		2015916201
ISBN:	Hardcover	978-1-5144-1174-2
	Softcover	978-1-5144-1173-5
	eBook	978-1-5144-1172-8

All rights reserved. No part of this book may be reproduced or transmitted in any form or by any means, electronic or mechanical, including photocopying, recording, or by any information storage and retrieval system, without permission in writing from the copyright owner.

Any people depicted in stock imagery provided by Thinkstock are models, and such images are being used for illustrative purposes only. Certain stock imagery © Thinkstock.

CITATION

NKJV
Scripture quotations marked NKJV are taken from the New King James Version. Copyright © 1982 by Thomas Nelson, Incorporated. Used by permission. All rights reserved.

Contact author
Edwin A. Noyes M.D. MPH
Ph. 503-357-6571
Edwina.noyes@gmail.com and/or spiritsdeception@aol.com

Diagram of Occultism and One World Government used by permission of Gary Kah

Print information available on the last page.

Rev. date: 08/17/2018

To order additional copies of this book, contact:
Xlibris
1-888-795-4274
www.Xlibris.com
Orders@Xlibris.com

Contents

0. Introduction xiii
1. Winds Of Change 1
2. Two Great Spiritualistic Deceptions 6
3. Babylonian Spiritualistic Mysteries In Health And Healing From Eden To Babylon ... 16
4. Universal Energy 34
5. Babylonian Spiritualistic Mysteries In The Christian Civilization 41
6. Meditation: Ayurveda The Ancient Healing Tradition Of India 52
7. Mindfulness Meditation 75
8. Yoga-Yoga Exercises And Cleansing: Ayurveda: The Ancient Healing Tradition Of India ... 81
9. Acupuncture And Chinese Traditional Medicine 113
10. Visualization And Guided Imagery 146
11. Reflexology And Other Energy-Balancing Therapies 165
12. Reiki: Craniosacral Therapies 193
13. Mystical Herbology 204
14. Crystal Healing, Talismans, Amulets 224
15. Homeopathy 243
16. Divination As A Diagnostic Tool 260
17. Those Who Practice Magic Arts 282
18. Hypnosis 295
19. Biofeedback 305
20. A Critique Of Vibrational Medicine: The Handbook Of Subtle-Energy Therapies, Third Edition ... 317
21. Babylonian Spiritualistic Mysteries: Compatible With The Atonement? 325

Glossary 331
Index 367

Endorsements

It's Not Quite All Hokus-Pokus

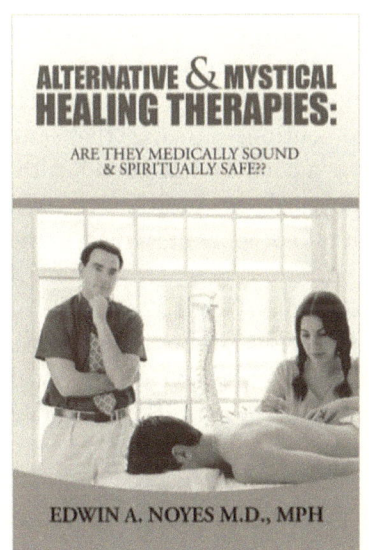

With one close relative of mine involved with yoga, two others with acupuncture, and still remembering my mother administering 'cupping' on my dad's back when he had a doozer of a cold, I wanted to see what the medical profession had to say about these and other alternative and mystical healing therapies. Edwin Noyes' book was just the ticket. Not only does it explain in detail what the mainline medical practitioners believe with respect to such therapies, but also describes the results of research carried out with regards to each type.

But Noyes went one step further as far as I was concerned. Writing as a Christian, he interweaves his understanding of what God and the Bible have to say on mystical healing therapies, carefully pointing out the dangers for the Christian believer.

Noyes is a balanced writer, pointing out that there are alternative & mystical therapies that actually do work, if not for everybody, for some. So, yes, there is power in many of these alternatives to scientific medical treatment. What worries Noyes and should worry us is the source of that power. Taking us back to the very beginning, this former U.S. Army physician and surgeon explains how evil does not want to defeat good in direct combat, but rather achieves its goal by convincing us to blend the "good" in such a way with itself so that the evil is often not even recognized and lingers around to create havoc for mankind.

The book is also very historical in nature introducing us to three world centers and periods of medical influence. Also, specific categories of therapy are described starting with their origin, the growth of their influence, as well as their modern age status and acceptance by the world including segments of the medical profession.

It turns out, as the author very successfully shows, that the "New Age" treatments are anything but new. Rather, they are a return to the "Ancient Age" of Eastern mysticism and beliefs held during the period prior to sound medical science and research. Most of the ancient Eastern religions and their origins play a prominent part in today's alternative 'healing' therapies. Noyes also gives us evidence in writing of how the promoters of such therapies, in order to succeed in the West, keep quiet about their link to their religious or mystical sources and proudly claim they don't have to refer to them. They know the spiritual effect will impact a participant over time without his knowing it. And before one knows, the idea that we all are, or can be, gods, will entice us to continue pursuing that state of perfect balance that each therapy claims as a condition of good health. For example, as you study and focus on the physical yoga position, you will eventually be ready to investigate the spiritual component, which is the "entire essence of the subject".

The list of therapies and practices covered is long. Noyes also focuses of the various requirements for magnetism, energy flows, thought processes, etc. required by most of them. He examines each and shares documented evidence which points to the fact that almost all are not effective as real alternative healing remedies – most having the same or less impact than placebos.

What surprises him is how many of these (yoga being the prime example, but there are others) are thriving in the Christian church; some with the blessing of some well-known pastors. Outside the Church, he takes on and exposes the likes of Deepak Chopra and Dr. Oz. He reserves even greater arguments for acupuncture, reflexology, and visualization techniques that are used widely today; the latter often in corporate business settings.

I remember several decades ago being in hospital with pericarditis (an infection and inflammation of the lining around the heart) and going through some pretty rough nights. One of the nurses practiced (without my consent) what was quite common in those days – the Therapeutic Touch therapy. Some of you may remember it or experienced it. Noyes explains it well. I can assure you, that is not what healed me.

And just when you thought the things you were allowing in your life may have escaped Noyes' criticism, up come sections on herbology and flower therapy, crystals, homeopathy, divination, hypnosis, and biofeedback.

Let me conclude with one quote near the end of the book:

> *"This book does not present the idea that these methods do not work. The purpose of the book is to help us in answering the questions 'Who makes it work?' and "What power is behind it?"'*

You'll need to come to your own conclusion. But the book will stay on my reference shelf as an excellent tool to turn to for details about anything any one of my children, grandchildren, friends, or clients throw at me in support of why they swear by these alternative and mystical healing therapies.

- By Ken B. Godevenos, President, Accord Resolutions Services Inc., Toronto, Ontario, May 13, 2016. www.accordconsulting.com

Eastern and New Age mystical symbolism and practices have pervaded Western culture now for a few decades. Little did I realize, though, how tightly connected the spiritual aspect to the practices are to the varying healing methods. As a Christian believer I wondered if the healing power inherent in these rituals is indeed from God when the philosophies of the sources are contrary to what we have received in Scripture.

In our modern era where the general population is increasingly skeptical of the wide use (and perhaps overuse) of pharmaceuticals, the market is large for the common consumer to search out effective alternatives to our ills. Many physicians are mixing drug therapy with the ancient methods. Dr. Noyes shares his years of research in, *Alternative and Mystical Healing Therapies: Are They Medical Sound and Spiritually Safe:??*and this informative volume addresses the metaphysical side to widely-accepted, ancient, mystical healing techniques. Never have I seen such a convenient handbook on the subject and greatly appreciate it."

Gail Steel, Accounts/ Subscriptions
Christian Book Store

Endorsement Statement for
Alternative and Mystical Healing Therapies: Are They Medically Sound and Spiritually Safe?

Millions of sincere people in need of healing turn to alternative and mystical therapies. I was one of them. Very few are aware of the quackery, spiritual deception and danger that lurks hidden behind these seemingly promising methodologies. Dr. Ed Noyes' carefully-researched book is a profound warning to all who have an ear to hear.

Will Baron, author of *Deceived by the New Age*

I had the pleasure and good fortune of meeting Dr. Edwin Noyes a number of years ago in Atlanta, Georgia. We sat together and shared our ministries, and have since come to highly respect one another. Our ministries are, in a way very similar; mine, being more specific and focusing on the use of spiritualism incorporated in the use of specific teachings that many Protestant churches have adopted. Dr. Noyes, on the other hand has done a far more exhaustive study on the various types of spiritualistic methods used through many different healing avenues, all dangerously deceptive, and ultimately leading to the disaster of the spiritual life.

Dr. Noyes asked me to share a little of my past experience. Prior to my own conversion, I searched for years through many of those "avenues" mentioned above; spirit mediums, Sylva Mind Control, Edgar Cayce Society, and on and on, reading and studying the various methods that use the supernatural, since this is what was occurring in my life. Not having a biblical back ground at the time, I did not know of the warnings that existed in scripture, so my search led me through the various religions and philosophies that incorporated what I knew and was sure of – the supernatural. I knew it was real.

I dabbled in many of the uses of the supernatural from automatic writing to astral projection and psychic phenomena, even to the extent of being trained as a spirit medium. This is where God finally intervened. For years I had been praying every day for two things I could not seem to find, yet desired more than anything else – to understand the reason we exist, and how to gain victory over those things in my life I knew were sinful. God led in a way that would not allow victory until He finally led me to the only solution, the power of our Lord and Savior, Jesus Christ.

After about a year of being disciples of the well-known guru, Sri Chinmoy, spiritual leader for the United Nations in New York, God finally led Rosalie and me out of the quagmire of the occult and Eastern Religions into His light. Disheartened once again, both of us desperately and totally surrendered to God, pleading for Him to lead us to the truth because we were unable to find it on our own. This was a true surrender on our part, one in which we were ready to surrender all dabbling with the supernatural, which allowed God to pull us out of that trap; a trap that many never escape from. Thank God for what He did for us as He providentially had me get a new job, and need to move – right next door to the minister who studied with us for the next year, leading us into a saving relationship with Lord. We were baptized and eventually called into the ministry, where we served the Lord for the last 40 years.

I want to add a fact about these deceptions God delivered us from. We erroneously believed that we had the power to extract the truth from the mixture of truth and error that we were exposed to. We were wrong and learned that when you engage these powers deceiving you, you are constantly under their control and cannot discern truth from error. This is extremely important to understand because many who advocate these methods believe in this false and incorrect dynamic, falling for this error in thinking. I share this testimony so others who may be caught in this trap will see that if we are willing to flee from the deceptive teachings of spiritualism, something very difficult for some, God can and will deliver us, and that we need to understand that God would not have us practice separating the truth from the error in these teachings, for as long as we continue to listen to these false and deceptive theories, our minds will continue to be under the influence of the evil powers that espouse them. Like it or not, for this reason, we should not continue to study or listen, but need to altogether flee from every aspect of these teachings.

Getting back to Dr. Noyes book, I want to point out what an excellent and unique work he does of unfolding how demonic supernatural power is what is behind most methods and techniques of not only the healing arts, but all other supernatural traps used by the powers of darkness, from martial arts to mind control, yoga and all the modern arts involving energy manipulation. He exposes how it is the belief in pantheism that lies at the heart of most of these deceptions, also expertly outlining the use of these powers throughout history, from the earlier eastern religions all the way down to the world we live in today. He reveals the almost universal deception, the idea that each of us is simply a projection of – and actually consist of, "God" one of the most dangerous and invasive of these theories. If we make this revolutionary false discovery, that we are "God," the natural conclusion is that all we need do to have infinite supernatural power at our fingertips, is exercise that power that is naturally within each of us. This "God" within us is often referred to in the occult religions and philosophies as the "Universal Subconscious Mind," and is the basis of all the deception Dr. Noyes is able to expose, and in which he has done an excellent work in the writing of *Alternative & Mystical Healing Therapies: Are They Medically Sound and/or Spiritually Safe?*

I would recommend this book to all whose lives touch in any way, or have any connection with those who are influenced by the use of energy above and beyond what comes naturally through methods that are not supernatural or fully understood. Those working in the healing arts, such as massage therapists, chiropractors, physical therapists, or any who use arts that manipulate energy in the new techniques that are being devised daily, need to have this book in their library, and that is - in my opinion, without exception. Thank you Dr. Noyes for the time you dedicated to give the world a warning desperately needed.

Pastor Rick Howard

0

INTRODUCTION

In 1980, a book *The Aquarian Conspiracy* made its debut upon the American scene. It quickly became a hit, especially with a special group of people with similar beliefs and worldview, yet they were little known to each other. Author Marilyn Ferguson was the publisher of a bimonthly journal—*Brain/Mind Bulletin* (circulation 10,000) which encompassed research, theory, innovation relating to learning, health, psychiatry, psychology, states of consciousness, dreams, meditation, and similar related subjects. Her position as editor and publisher brought her into contact with voluminous information that had not previously been collected and brought together to be shared with those interested.

She had contact with people from many various professions and vocations. As she received, filtered, analyzed, and published information in her bimonthly bulletin, a mental picture began to slowly form in her mind as she observed a change, a transformation taking place in the core belief system of many people. This change was occurring in individuals and in society at large. It was slow at first, starting in the sixties but picked up momentum in an accelerating manner with each decade. The movement was without hierarchal leadership, organization, or funding. It seemed to be arising everywhere spontaneously by small networking individuals and groups. This change was seen in medicine, education, social sciences, hard science, and even the government.

This change appeared to follow the aftermath of the social activism of the 1960s and 1970s and was moving toward a "historical synthesis," i.e., a social transformation coming from a personal transformation—a "heart change" and then forming into a worldwide society change. With the publishing of *The Aquarian Conspiracy*, the massed information Marilyn had collected, now organized and placed out into the open for all to see, stimulated with even greater speed and widespread acceptance and promulgation of these changes of worldview and transformation.

I am sure the reader by this time is asking what is changing in individuals and society as a whole. Answer: a change in a person's *core belief system—one's worldview!* Such as where did we come from? What are we doing here? What is the future? A change from a Western worldview formed mostly from Judeo-Christian concepts of our origin, purpose, and destiny toward an Eastern pantheistic perspective of "divinity within"— "the godhood of man."

Ferguson proceeded to bring out into the open the methods by which transformation within an individual is initiated and then more fully developed. *Health and healing* is a dominant avenue, and a vast array of techniques has been developed to "heal body and mind." The Christian believes that choosing to follow the Eastern pantheistic pathway separates him from his Savior, Jesus Christ the Divine Son of God. Pantheistic healing techniques are presented with an exceedingly deceptive philosophy and explanation as to how they are believed to effect healing. To accept Satan's counterfeit healing modalities gives him homage and worship.

The purpose of this book is to present information which facilitates making an intelligent choice as to whether or not the reader would choose to participate in a particular healing therapy. Many different methods of healing are promoted as being of true value but are founded on pagan doctrines originating from a counterfeit of the Biblical story of creation. This book further explains why these different therapies that carry occult or pagan principles in the explanation as to their power to heal cannot be separated from their attachment to such religions.

On the back side of the cover of this book, *Alternative and Mystical Healing Therapies: Are They Medically Sound and Spiritually Safe?* are lists of some popular quasi-healing methodologies that have come into our culture in the past thirty-five to forty years. Some of them are of ancient origin and are only new to us. The concern I present in this text has more to do with the *spiritual danger* imposed from accepting and using those techniques than from a strictly medical concern. In short, it is my contention that accepting the concepts promoted in the explanation for the *power* behind their healing capabilities might well separate us from eternal life.

Since publishing the book *Spiritualistic Deceptions in Health and Healing* in August 2007, I have encountered individuals who have asked me why I had not written on certain other practices in health and healing that they also considered affiliated with *spiritualism*. This word *spiritualism*, as presented throughout this text, is defined much more widely than the act of communication with the deceased. Its base definition comes from the statement made by the serpent in the Garden, "You will become wise like God," actually become a god, a concept that mankind possesses divinity within throughout life and progresses toward "godhood." Also that by various physical and mental methods of "manipulating the *divine within*," healing is believed to be effected.

It has been more than ten years since I started writing the book, *Spiritualistic Deceptions in Health and Healing*, and eight years since its publication. These years have given me time to contemplate the above stated requests and the effectiveness of the book in bringing an understanding of spiritualism's encroachment into the healing arts. During this time, use of alternative and complementary medicine has rapidly increased and been accepted, as if it were part and parcel of general medicine. Less and less do people have concern as to whether there may be any reason that one should question the value or spiritual safety in accepting and using a particular healing method, that at one time was considered suspect.

Many different methods of healing are being promoted as of true value but are founded in pagan doctrines originating from a counterfeit story of creation wherein man possesses "divinity within." This book further explains why these different therapies that carry occult or pagan principles in the explanations of their power to heal cannot be separated from their attachment to those religions and, one's use of, could present to the Christian spiritual danger.

Edwin A. Noyes, MD, MPH

1

WINDS OF CHANGE

April 6, 1971, *The Ping Heard Round the World* occurred. The American ping-pong team, while competing in the World Table Tennis Championship held in Japan, received a surprise invitation from the Republic of China for an all-expense paid visit to their country. When the team stepped across a bridge from Hong Kong to China on April 10, the era of Ping-pong diplomacy" was initiated.

On April 14, Premier Chou En-lai, at a banquet in the Great Hall, invited American journalists to visit China, closed to foreign visitors since 1949. Ping-pong diplomacy signaled change. July 15 of the same year, the American government announced that President Nixon would be going to China for an official state visit the following year. The winds of change were blowing.

Reporters from America did visit China, and their stories were read with great interest. Stories of a different kind of anesthetic for surgery caught the attention of Americans more than most other aspects of the China reporting. The stories of a man undergoing an appendectomy and, of another person, chest surgery while awake seemed like science fiction. It was the first time most Americans had heard the word *acupuncture*. Glowing stories of what it could do initiated a great desire for further investigation. How surprising it was to hear that it had been around for millennia, and yet the "art" was not generally known in America.

Other changes had been occurring in America for several years. Students on college campuses appearances were different. Instead of nicely dressed young people, the trend was to wear Farmer Brown overalls. Cultural values changed. Music interests changed from melodious to the "beat." The Beatles from England descended on the scene and were followed by many copycat groups. Drug use increased. Smoking marijuana became popular, as did Eastern religions. The Beatles made popular practicing transcendental meditation in place of using psychedelic drugs because they could obtain a "high" without drugs. The famous Woodstock festival of 1969 was an open expression of changing cultural values and practices. Across the country, we saw missionaries of the Eastern religions such as Hare Krishna and followers of gurus such as Hindu Rajneesh Bhagwan Shree, Maharishi Mahesh Yogi, and Paramahansa Yogananda.

Early in this changing cultural norm of society, transcendental meditation followers quickly became widespread, followed by yoga and natural childbirth classes. We soon began to hear of many other methods of health and healing, such as aromatherapy, essential oils, applied kinesiology, iridology, and magnet therapy, etc.

Another societal change was the declining number of people believing in a Biblical six-day creation. Evolution, as the answer for origins, had been around for a long time, but it was not a universal belief among Christians. The answer that the pagan gave for his origin began to be a contender in answering the question, "Where did we come from?" Pagan theology also crept in through a movement that suddenly appeared in the mid-1970s—the New Age Movement. Its theology was that of theosophy teachings derived from Vedanta Hinduism, Buddhism, and Western occultism, which included belief in reincarnation.

Beginning in the mid to late 1970s, new medical therapies started to emerge along with the New Age Movement. Advertisements of seminars and conferences promoting and teaching such methods as yoga, transcendental meditation, acupuncture, therapeutic touch, and many other treatment modalities were sent to doctors' offices. These methods of treatment became very popular with nonprofessionals, and teaching seminars were conducted for the public. Many people with no real training in medical science obtained certificates of expertise and became practitioners in these various treatment approaches. As time progressed, there was an ever increasing awareness of these alternative methods. Also, there was rapid growth in the variety of healing disciplines offered to the public, often by chiropractors, naturopaths, and sometimes nurses and nonmedically trained people.

In the 1980s, medical doctors became more aware of these different treatment methods that were becoming increasingly popular, and patients told their doctors of trying these methods. Medical offices received invitations announcing seminars and teaching sessions for the various new nontraditional medical treatments. One such invitation came to my office from a Catholic hospital in Tucson, Arizona, announcing a three-day seminar; the instructors for the meetings were *traditional medicine men* (shamans) from the Navajo Indian Reservation and other reservations. I still have that invitation.

Few doctors accepted these methods at first. Newer medical graduates were more likely to accept them because of the worldview many of them held as to man's origin. These methods were, to a great extent, the result of the New Age Movement and the theosophy (pagan theology) taught.

The winds of change continue to blow, and now we see a much greater interest in the new (yet ancient) therapeutic methods. Their use can now be found to some degree in many hospitals; even many medical schools have adopted and are experimenting with various alternative healing disciplines. Medical clinics are forming across the nation integrating the conventional medical practice with the nonconventional style of treatment.

Many insurance companies include alternative health coverage in their policies. The coverage often covers acupuncture, chiropractors, massage and somatic therapies, etc. Some workplaces promote and finance attendance at fitness centers, athletic clubs, health spas, and other wellness centers that are featuring meditation, yoga, yoga exercises, tai chi, and martial arts of various types.

I read books written by Christian authors exposing these new medical therapies as being spiritistic. As I developed a much greater understanding of the worldviews of those using and promoting these methods of medical care, I realized that belief in and use of these healing methods was a result of their *worldview/pagan theology—nature worship*.

Satan attempts to thwart any blessing God gives to man. Early in the history of the world, he designed a system of health and healing to counterfeit God's methods. That same counterfeit system exists today just as it has through ages past.

> "There is a way that seems right unto a man, but the end is the way of death" (Proverbs 14:12).

The purpose of this book is to unmask today's popular spiritistic counterfeit system of health and healing.

> And have no fellowship with the unfruitful works of darkness, but rather expose them (Ephesians 5:11).

"Lest Satan should take advantage of us: For we are not ignorant of his devices" (II Corinthians 2:11).

The spiritualistic invasion of present-day medical care must be recognized for what it is—not a marvelous new approach to health and healing but ancient methods repainted in silver and gold.

A *worldview* refers to our understanding and belief as to our origin, purpose, and future, as well as to the power that gave us life. In the Christian's worldview, man was created and is sustained by a Creator God who is a personal Being. Life, health, and happiness come from being in harmony with His laws of the physical world as well as the spiritual realm. Man disobeyed God's law and lost eternal life in paradise. Man can regain eternal life by believing in the merits of His shed blood to cover our sins and following after the *Divine Son of God, Jesus Christ*.

Modern neo-evolutionary theory was introduced approximately one hundred sixty years ago. According to this worldview, we are here as a result of a long, natural process of random selection and chance, and there is no future after death. The evolutionist has no answer as to how or from where the *spark of life* came.

What was the worldview of the non-Christian regarding his origin prior to the theory of evolution? We will look to the explanation of creation in pagan religions to find this answer. Many of the treatment methods in the pagan concept for healing are *not* dependent upon the physical laws recognized in science. There is a looking to a "vital force" or special "energy" supposedly permeating the universe from which all substance is said to have originated. Life is believed to repeat itself in different bodies and creatures. The goal in life is to escape from this cycle of reincarnation and enter into the spirit life of nirvana.

How is it that ancient healing practices find their way into modern scientific medicine? Did this change come after random selection, controlled, double-blind scientific tests conducted to evaluate these procedures before accepting them? Was there solid evidence of value as shown by statistical evaluation? No! None whatsoever!

Why then have these new methodologies been accepted? They are not explained or understood under the recognized laws of science. They have not been shown to make a difference in disorders such as tuberculosis, cancer, diabetes, heart disease, gallstones, fractures, endocrine malfunctions, or other such organic disorders. Those parts of the world that used these practices for health care for thousands of years have a dismal record of health. These methods appear to have their influence mainly on disorders where there are great subjective symptoms such as pain, nausea, stress, and various musculoskeletal discomforts.

The best explanation for the questions I have asked above is that an acceptance of and changing belief in one's worldview has allowed the acceptance of unproven and nonscientific methods. A worldview is formed by answering the questions: Where did I come from? Why am I here? Where am I going? The Christian's worldview is:

> Man was formed from the dust of the ground and the Creator God breathed into him the breath of life and man became a living soul (living being NKJ, Genesis 2:7). Man was created for God's glory (Isaiah 43:7), and placed in paradise. Then man, by believing and trusting the serpent in the tree instead of God, lost paradise and eternal life (Genesis 2 and 3).
>
> We are invited to believe in the merits of the shed blood of the Divine Son of God, repent, and by faith accept the merits of His shed blood, receive eternal life and live in paradise of the earth made new (John 14:1–3; Revelation 21, 22).

The above outline of our creation, redemption, and restoration is to be contrasted with the story of the origin of the universe, earth, and man from the pagan and nature worshiper's worldview. First, before we explore the pagan's story of creation, let us explore in the next chapter a little more of the story of man's loss of life in paradise and the effort of the great adversary to distract us from accepting the invitation from Jesus Christ to regain our lost inheritance.

2

Two Great Spiritualistic Deceptions

The subject of the Biblical story of a great spiritualistic deception at the beginning of earth's history in the Garden of Eden and a great worldwide spiritualistic deception that is to occur at the end of time is the theme of this chapter.

In the story of creation, Genesis chapter 1, we are told that God created light, and He "saw that it was *good*." He created land and seas, "and God saw that it was *good*." He created the plants on the third day, "and God saw that it was *good*." He made two lights, "and God saw that it was *good*." On the fifth day, life in the sea was created, "and God saw that it was *good*." On the sixth day, He created animals, "and God saw that it was *good*." Then God created man (Adam) and woman (Eve). He looked over everything that He had made, "and, behold, it was *very good*."[1]

The word *good* was used seven times in the story of creation. What did God mean by this expression *"good?"* *Webster's Collegiate Dictionary* lists one of the definitions as

> to be in harmony with the moral order of the universe.[2]

God was saying that he had created planet Earth and all its inhabitants,

---

[1] King James Bible, Genesis 1:31.
[2] Merriam-Webster G. & C., *Webster's New Collegiate Dictionary*, G. & C. Merriam Co. Springfield, Massachusetts (1977) p. 495.

and they were in perfect harmony with His laws for the universe. All of God's creations are under His fixed laws. His created intelligent beings are also under His moral law. The light shining forth from Calvary is a demonstration of the self-renouncing love of God and is the law of life for the universe. This love seeks not its own; its source is in the heart of God. Christ Jesus manifested at the cross the character of Him who dwells in the light which no man can approach.

Every part of creation was in balance and ministers to some other aspect of the creation. Only the selfish heart of man lives unto himself.

> "I do nothing of Myself," said Christ, "the living Father hath sent Me, and I live by the Father." "I seek not Mine own glory, but the glory of Him that sent Me."[3]

Here is set forth the great principle for life in God's universe. Christ the Son takes from the Father to give to the created beings; through the Son, life flows from the Father to all. From the created flows gratitude and love back through the Son to the Father, thus creating a great circuit of beneficence constituting the law of life.

LAW OF LOVE

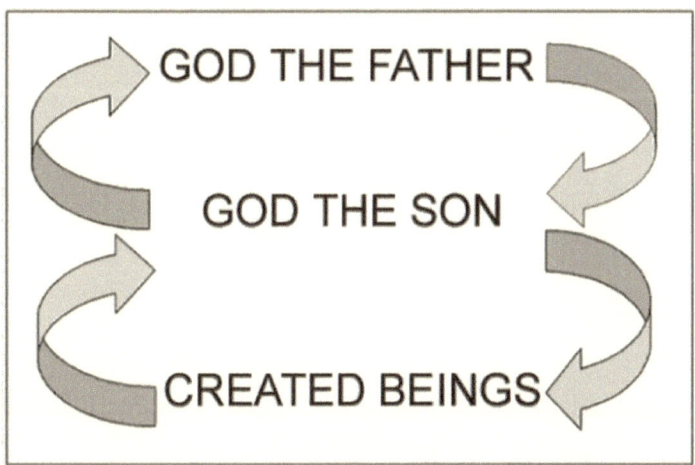

LAW OF THE UNIVERSE

Figure 1. Law of love.

---

[3] John 8:28; 6:57; 8:50; 7:18, (KJV)

Man was placed in a universe that is under the law of God. Government cannot exist without law. Immortality was promised them (Adam and Eve) on condition of obedience; by transgression they would forfeit eternal life.

God's law was first broken in heaven by Lucifer. Envious to be *first* was the driving force behind Lucifer's rebellion.[4] He desired that heavenly beings give him the homage due only to God and His Son. Through his own evil characteristics, Satan sought to invest the Son of God, deceiving angels and men. He led them to distrust and doubt the word of God.

The circle of love (law of universe) is broken when we give Satan the honor due God; his deceptions are designed to entice us to do just that.

LAW OF LOVE

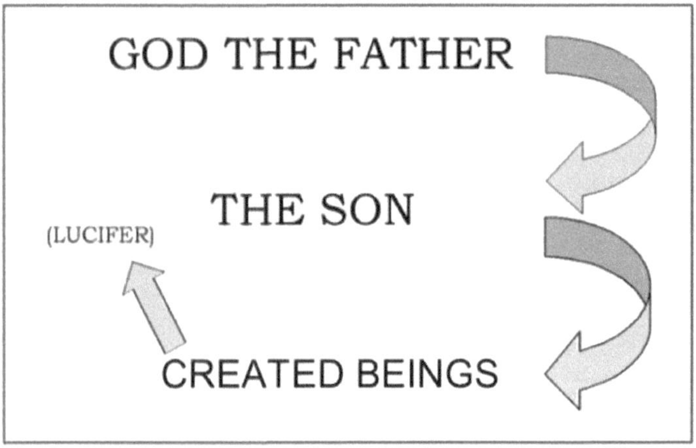

```
            GOD THE FATHER

                THE SON
   (LUCIFER)

            CREATED BEINGS
```

Figure 2. Law of love broken.

To deceive newly created man, Satan appeared to Eve in disguise. He chose the serpent as his *medium*. When Eve wandered from the side of Adam, she would undoubtedly feel some apprehension but felt she had sufficient wisdom and strength to discern evil and to withstand it. When she approached the tree of *knowledge of good and evil,* the serpent spoke to her; fascinated, she stayed to listen. She had stepped onto *Satan's ground*

---

[4] Isaiah 14: 9–14; Ezekiel 28: 13-18.

where he had access of influence. God had warned about that tree and its fruit.

She had no idea that the serpent was being used by Satan, about whom the angels had warned them. Satan, through the serpent, said that if she were to eat of the fruit of the tree, she would gain wisdom and know good and evil. She would become wise as God Himself, become a God. Eve did not design to rebel against God. However, in believing Satan's lie, she distrusted God and so came under the penalty of the law, which is death. We, in the judgment, will be held responsible for believing the truth and using opportunities to learn what is truth.

Satan's *great lie* is that disobedience to God does not result in death but rather will lead to a higher level of existence. He promised her that she would become wise like God, an insinuation that she would enter a wonderful field of knowledge.

So the first use of a *medium*, the serpent, to gain man's attention and then to draw him into rejecting God's instructions plunged the human race into sin and under the penalty of death. Satan has used the same pattern of deception since the fall of man. We are warned that the deception of the devil will be worldwide and greatly increased in power at the end of this world's history. Christ foretold this in Mark 13:22:

> For false Christs and false prophets shall rise, and shall show
> signs and wonders, to deceive, if possible, even the elect.

In Matthew chapters 24 and 25, we have an enlarged recording of the conversation referenced above in Mark 13. When asked by the disciples about signs of His coming and the end of the age, He spoke not only of certain physical signs but also of the real emphasis that was on the great deceptions that were to come so as to lead the saints astray. The parables in Matthew 24 are there to support the message of warning *to not be deceived*. He said that even the *elect* might be *deceived*. The entire passage is making the point that deception will be almost overwhelming and could cause us to reject salvation through Jesus Christ and instead follow the Prince of this world, Satan. Paul too warned of the great deception to come:

> Beware lest anyone cheat you through philosophy and empty deceit,
> according to the tradition of men, according to the basic principles
> of the world, and not according to Christ (Colossians 2:8).

The church in Colossus had been influenced by Hellenistic traditional teachings ("rudiments") which are similar to the neo-pagan teachings about us today. Paul, in his second letter to the Thessalonians, points to the special working of Satan in spiritualism as an event to take place immediately before the second advent of Christ. Speaking of Christ's second coming, he declares that it is:

> The coming of the lawless one is according to the working of Satan, with all power and signs and lying wonders (II Thessalonians 2:9). And no wonder! For Satan himself transforms himself into an angel of light. Therefore, it is no great thing if his ministers also transform themselves into ministers of righteousness, whose end will be according to their works (II Corinthians 11:14, 15).

Paul warned Timothy:

> Now the Spirit expressly says, that in latter times some will depart from the faith, giving heed to deceiving spirits, and doctrines of demons (I Timothy 4:1).

John, three times in the book of Revelation, wrote about this end-time deception:

> He performs great signs, so that he even makes fire come down from heaven on the earth in the sight of men. And he deceives those who dwell on the earth by those signs which he was granted to do in the sight of the beast; telling those who dwell on the earth, to make an image to the beast who was wounded by a sword, and did live (Revelation 13:13, 14).

> And I saw three unclean spirits like frogs come out of the mouth of the dragon, out of the mouth of the beast, and out of the mouth of the false prophet. For they are the spirits of demons, performing signs, which go forth unto the kings of the earth and of the whole world, to gather them to the battle of that great day of God Almighty (Revelation 16:13, 14).

> And the beast was captured and with him the false prophet who worked Signs in his presence, by which he deceived those that had received the mark of the beast, and those who worshipped his image. These two were cast alive into a lake of fire burning with brimstone (Revelation 19:20).

The last great delusion is soon to be upon us. Marvelous works by the Antichrist will be performed in our sight. The counterfeit will resemble the true so closely that it will be impossible to distinguish between them except by the Holy Scriptures.

Neo-paganism, often through the New Age Movement, has promulgated healing disciplines which have become nearly "Main Street," yet they have their origin out of the doctrine of ancient pagan religions. In the last thirty-five or so years, their acceptance and use has mushroomed to a place of common acceptance. Satan has laid his trap carefully and is preparing to join with the forces of religion in our time. He has been quietly at work to condition people's thinking until total control of their minds and the rejection of God and His law is accomplished. We have seen in recent years the amalgamation of Eastern religions and their spiritualism with occultism of the West. This neo-occultism and neo-paganism has been planting its seeds of doctrine through the healing disciplines.

For years, the West has been seeing changes in that which is taught in schools, even to an open attack on the Creator God. In the entertainment industry, we see efforts to change the views of people by devaluating Christian concepts and elevating atheistic and/or pagan ideas. This same shift is seen in music, games, comic books, movies, environmental movements, and in the special focus of this book, that of *health and healing*.

"...TENS OF THOUSANDS OF ENTRY POINTS TO THIS CONSPIRACY." --Marilyn Ferguson

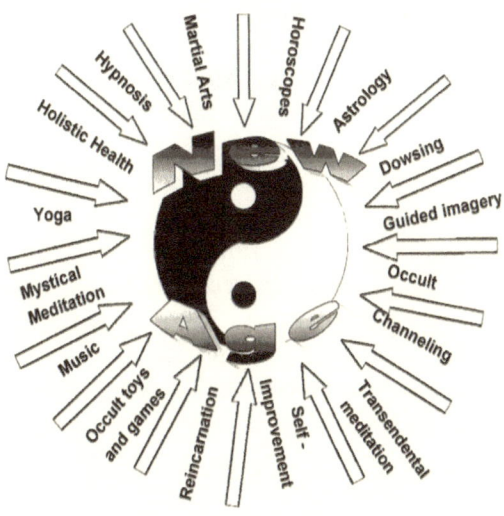

Figure 3. Points of entry.

Satan has developed his plan to deceive man until almost all external influences in our civilization are used as entry points to bring man's acceptance to his worldview. In his worldview, creation was not a six-day event and did not involve a sovereign God. God is nature and nature is god. We are gods, and we only need to learn how to bring this "god" within us to its full potential. One of the avenues that Satan uses to deceive man into paying homage to him is in the field of health and healing. He works to get the human race to accept his version of the *origin* of man and in turn, his false premise of the cause of disease. By accepting Satan's false concepts concerning the causes of disease and resorting to his unsound methods of treatment, man gives reverence to Satan.

> The pivotal book that officially launched the New Age Movement was Marilyn Ferguson's *The Aquarian Conspiracy* published in 1980. This book was "an important New Age manifesto that attempted to announce and popularize what the New Agers chose to publicly display in their Movement." The book set forth futuristic thinking that has become so commonplace in our culture that an entire generation has grown up believing its basic assumptions.[5]

> One of the key topics in this book was Ferguson's assertion that the radical overhaul of society could be based upon health-care "*reform*" —a "transformation" explained in the chapter "Healing Ourselves." Ferguson wrote, "The new paradigm of health and medicine enlarges the framework of the old, incorporating brilliant technological advances while restoring and validating intuitions about mind and relationships" (p. 247).[6]

Chapter 4 in *The Aquarian Conspiracy* titled "Crossover: People Changing" lists a number of medical disciplines that Ferguson refers to as *points of entry* and "psychotechnologies" to facilitate change in a person's worldview. They include biofeedback, autogenic training, music in combination with meditation and imagery, psychodrama, self-help programs such as "Twelve Step of Alcoholic Anonymous," all forms of meditation, yoga, ESP, Silva method of mind control, dream journals, Arica, Theosophy, *Science of Mind*, *A Course in Miracles*, all body disciplines and therapies, tai chi chuan, karate, Sufi stories, koans, whirling dervishes, etc.

---

[5] http://www.discernment-ministries.org, Feb 10, 2011
[6] *Ibid.*

In the chapter on *Changeover,* further explanation is made as to the steps involved in a change—transformation of an individual. *Step 1:* experimenting with an *entry point. Step 2: exploring* further the entry point and possible additional ones. This going deeper into the healing technique in search of something enticing, actually is a beginning of breaking the grip of one's deeply established core values and allows for changing to a new set of guide lines (pantheistic) for one's life. *Step 3: integration,* wherein the individual trusts an *inner guru,* a contact with an inner guide, an inner child, or as C. J. Jung says, "the divine child." This is a stage where contact is made with demons—fallen angels. *Step four, conspiracy* (defined as to breathe together) discovering additional sources of power and the ways to use it such as self-healing, healing others, and attempting to heal society, a conspiring for renewal. Is it any wonder that the New York Times referred to the book *The Aquarian Conspiracy* as the New Age Bible?

In 2 Kings 1, it is written that Ahaziah, king of Israel, fell and sustained serious injury. He sent a messenger to inquire of Baalzebub, god of Ekron, as to whether he would recover from his injuries. God sent Elijah the prophet to intercept the messenger of the king as he traveled toward Ekron. Elijah sent him back to the king with the question:

> Is it because there is no God in Israel that you go off to consult Baalzebub the god of Ekron? (2 Kings 1:3, NIV)

A captain and fifty soldiers were sent to arrest Elijah and to bring him to the king. When they attempted to arrest Elijah, fire from heaven consumed them. The king sent another fifty who suffered the same fate. The captain of a third group pleaded with Elijah not to allow fire to consume them, and God told Elijah to go with the captain to see the king.

As Elijah faced the king, he repeated the question:

> Is it because there is no God in Israel that you go off to consult Baalzebub the god of Ekron? (2 Kings 1:3, NIV)

Elijah told him that because of this inquiry of Baalzebub, he would not recover from his injuries but would die. We must be very careful not to be found "inquiring of the god of Ekron" regarding our physical status. Many sincere Christians are deceived by Satan and are indeed inquiring of the god of Ekron. If God's wrath was kindled by Ahaziah's act, then when mankind, who now has much greater understanding of physical disorder, turns from the source of truth and almighty power to inquire of the forces of darkness for healing, it must surely kindle God's wrath.

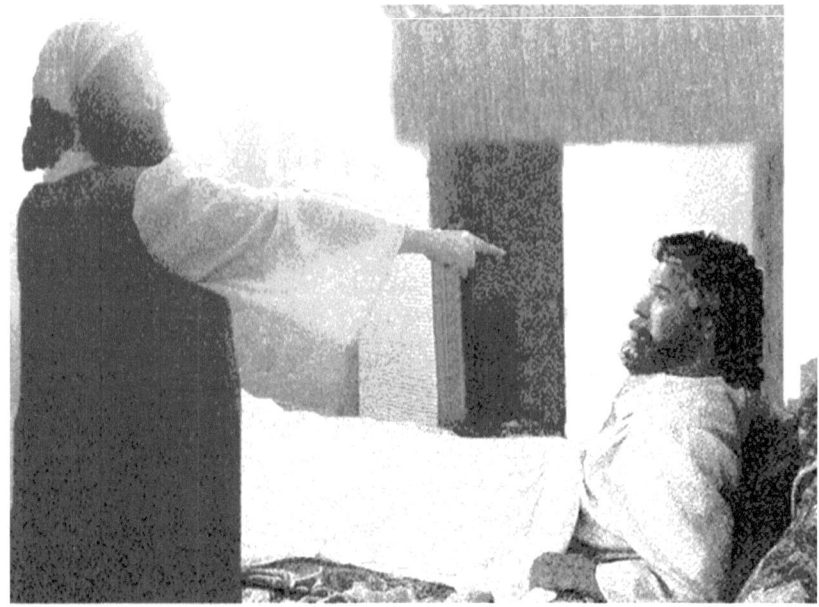

Figure 4. Elijah before the king.

Satan has long been preparing for his final effort to deceive the world. The foundation of his work was laid by the assurance given by the serpent to Eve in Eden:

> Then the serpent said to the woman, "You will not surely die . . . in the day ye eat of it, your eyes will be opened, and you will be like God, knowing good and evil" (Genesis 3:4, 5).

Little by little, he has prepared the way for his masterpiece of deception in the development of spiritualism. Spiritualism leads, by word and practice, to the belief in immortality (a spirit life after death), and it often involves communication with the spirit world. Satan has not yet reached the full accomplishment of his designs, but it will be reached in the last remnant of time. Let us again look at what the prophet John tells us will happen in the end of time.

> I saw three unclean spirits like frogs . . . they are the spirits of devils, working miracles, which go forth unto the kings of the earth and of the whole world, to gather them to the battle of that great day of God Almighty (Revelation 16:13, 14, KJV).

What is the fate of those who accept and partake of this end-time deception by the spirits of demons? In Revelation chapter 19, we find the answer. The scene depicted in this chapter is that final conflict, presented in symbolism, between good and evil, where the Son of God, King of kings, Lord of lords riding on a white horse leads the armies of heaven in the final battle between His armies and the kings of the earth. The losers, those deceived are cast into the lake of fire burning with brimstone.

Only as we trust by faith in power of His word will we be kept safe of the end-time deceptions. The whole world will be swept into the ranks of spiritistic delusions. The people are fast being lulled to a fatal security, to be awakened only by the outpouring of the wrath of God.

3

BABYLONIAN SPIRITUALISTIC MYSTERIES IN HEALTH AND HEALING FROM EDEN TO BABYLON

This chapter reveals how Satan created a counterfeit system of health and healing, which had its beginnings in the Garden of Eden, based on the lies that the serpent told Eve at the tree of the knowledge of good and evil:

> Then the serpent said to the woman, "You will not surely die." For God knows that in the day you eat of it your eyes will be opened, and you will be like God, knowing good and evil" (Genesis 3:4, 5).

In Colossians, Paul wrote:

> See to it that no one takes you captive through hollow and deceptive philosophy, which depends on human tradition and the basic principles of this world rather than on Christ (Colossians 2:8, NIV).

This verse points to the danger in man's philosophy and of blindly following the traditions of men. It especially points to the deceptions to come in earth's final events before the second coming of Jesus. The final delusions even now may be opening before us. The Antichrist is to perform marvelous works before our sight. The counterfeit will so closely resemble the truth we will only be able to differentiate between by the use of the scriptures. Every healing and every statement must be in harmony with scripture.

To be able to identify a counterfeit, we must know the truth. The foundation of the true system of health and healing can be found in the appropriate use of pure air, sunlight, abstemiousness (no use of harmful substances and temperate use of wholesome products), rest, exercise, proper diet, the use of water, and trusting in divine power. To trust in God means we not only acknowledge Him, but we also follow all his laws, both physical and spiritual. When we seek for our well-being through God's system, we will realize that God works through His laws, physical and spiritual, to impart health and healing.

When man is out of harmony with God's laws, changes occur that allow sickness and disease to manifest in our bodies. In Eden, following Eve's disobedience, a change began, which over time produced a condition that we call "disease." Disease is the body's response and change when the laws of health have been disregarded.

God has blessed us with considerable knowledge of nutrition and physiological principles that when applied often result in restoration of health. As we choose to be in harmony with God's physical laws of health, He imparts His healing power to us. God has given great knowledge of His laws through the sciences of chemistry and physics, and we are to use that part of science that is in harmony with His laws. Present-day medical science endeavors to learn more of the physical laws that govern our bodies.

However, there has been a movement among some clinical practitioners to accept types of treatment modalities that, I believe, are not in harmony with the physical laws of God. The objective of this book is to present information that will enable the reader to differentiate between therapy which follows the known physical and chemical laws (God's system) and the system of the great deceiver. Satan's counterfeit methods of treating disease have not been shown to be dependent upon these natural laws. The term *mystical medicine* is also used in reference to these treatment methods.

Those who believe in God are warned that at the end of time, God's people will face deception by "miracles." Revelation 13:14 and 16:14 identify the power behind those miracles as

>spirits of demons working signs (miracles).

The devil too, in his system of health, advocates the use of clear air, pure water, sunlight, exercise, rest, proper diet, and temperance; but instead of total trust in a Creator God's power to heal, he teaches that the power of healing is to be found within *self*. We are led to believe that by using certain varied treatment modalities, we can activate a *divine power* that is inherent in *self* to bring about not only restoration of health but also the elevation of one's consciousness to the level of godhood.

CREATION, TEMPTATION, FALL, DELUGE

When God called his creation "very good," He was saying it was not only perfect in design and beauty but also in total harmony with the laws of the universe.

Adam and Eve, as long as they remained in obedience to God's laws, were to enjoy immortality. To break from this harmony, they were told, would result in death. Eve's sin was that she did not believe God and accepted the lie told by the serpent that she would not die.

Satan charged God with withholding from man the knowledge that would make him wise like God. He said that God had withheld the knowledge of "evil" because it would balance with *good* and bring enlightenment and even *godhood* for themselves. There would be no death, as God had used the threat of death to scare them and keep them from this knowledge. He promised a new system which would bring harmony, equality, transformation, oneness, completeness, enlightenment, immortality, and finally *godhood* for man.

This promised utopia was already the experience of man, except he was created and never could become God. Lucifer (now Satan) had wanted to be God and was jealous of the Son of God. Eve was deceived into disbelieving God and believing Satan's lie to obtain what was already hers.

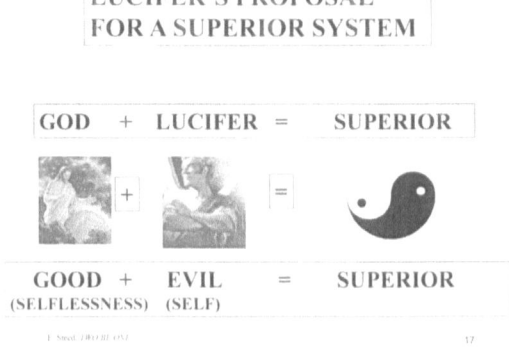

Figure 5. Christ and Satan.

The degree of influence this "pinch" of evil—self had become after more than fifteen hundred years is revealed in the following verse:

> Every imagination of the thoughts of his (man's) heart was only evil continually (Genesis 6:5, KJV).

God repented of making man, and He covered the earth with a flood.

POST DELUGE BABYLON, DISPERSION

Archeologists have discovered records and writings of past civilizations, which have been translated and studied. From these records, we get some knowledge of the concepts and beliefs of ancient times. Cush was the son of Ham and Ham the son of Noah. Of Cush, it is said that he developed numerics, astrology, geometry, and games of chance and hazard and devised alchemy.[1]

From the Bible, we learn that following the flood, Nimrod, a son of Cush, established the Mesopotamian civilization and that Babylon was one of its cities.[2]

The people of Babylon rejected God and attempted to build a tower that would reach to heaven, which they felt would protect them from another flood. God confounded the language of the people so they could not understand each other. From Babylon, the people spread out over the face of the earth, carrying with them the religion that had developed in Babylon, that is, paganism.[3]

ASTROLOGY, DUALISM, PAGANISM

The city of Babylon, "cradle of oriental civilization,"[4] located in the Mesopotamian Valley, was the origin of pagan religion—nature worship. The Babylonians believed that a great power maintained the universe. However, they did not credit this power to a living Being—God but rather

---

[1] Hislop, Alexander, *Two Babylons*, A.C. Black, Ltd., England (1916), p. 95; Steed, Earnest, *Two Be One*, Logos International, Plainfield, N.J., in Canada: G.R. Welch, Toronto, Ont., pp. 12–13.

[2] Genesis 10:8–12; Hislop, op. cit., pp. 19–25.

[3] Hislop, op. cit., p. 20; Garrison, Fielding H., *History of Medicine*, W.B. Saunders and Co., Philadelphia, Penn. (1929), p. 61.

[4] *Ibid.*

to a power called universal energy, universal intelligence, the creative principle, chi etc.

Universal energy was divided into *two parts* of supposedly opposing forces. These "opposing energies"—*dualism*—were given various designations, such as good and evil, male and female, positive and negative, dominant and recessive, dark and light, yang and yin, etc. Every entity was determined to be either one or the other. This concept was applied to minerals, plants, and animals.

> From the Mesopotamian Valley, the postdiluvians spread out east, west, south, and north, carrying with them the same basic idea for the unification of opposites —the one great philosophy to achieve life's secrets—obtain all wisdom and ultimate oneness. The ideas of Cush were carried into areas that are now Europe, China, and Asia. Except for those who worshiped the Creator God, their gods, few or many, were all allied to nature's opposites—the two most prominent being the *sun* and the *moon*. With the necessity for fire and fire allied to heat and heat to the sun, sun worship predominated. Sympathy, they believed, existed between all forces; consequently, identification of similarities resulted. Therefore, the sun symbolized the male and moon, the female.
>
> Looking back, we detect how astrology of the past, with its relationship by mankind to sun, moon, and stars, became paramount, built on the basis of correspondences and sympathy; thus, occultism soon guided the major activities of life.[5]

---

[5] Steed, Earnest, *Two Be One*, Logos International, Plainfield, N.J., in Canada: G.R. Welch, Toronto, Ont. (1976), pp. 12–13.

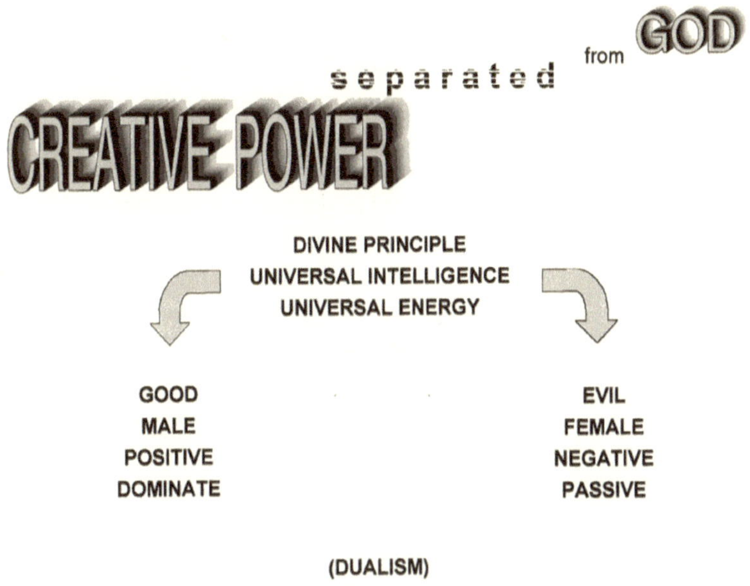

```
                                    from  GOD
                    separated
        CREATIVE POWER

                    DIVINE PRINCIPLE
                 UNIVERSAL INTELLIGENCE
                    UNIVERSAL ENERGY


        GOOD                              EVIL
        MALE                              FEMALE
        POSITIVE                          NEGATIVE
        DOMINATE                          PASSIVE


                       (DUALISM)
```

Figure 6. Creative power of God.

In the Garden of Eden, Satan proposed to Adam and Eve the blending of good and evil to improve God's government. Earnest Steed, in the book *Two Be One*, page 38, shares his perception of this principle used by Satan in his method of deception in the Garden of Eden, a pattern he has followed since. His mode of operation was not just introducing evil to counterbalance good. He "blended" *good* with *evil* so skillfully that evil was almost impossible to detect. It could be presented as follows:

            (selflessness)   (self)
            GOOD—versus—GOOD AND EVIL
    THE TREE OF LIFE—versus—THE TREE OF KNOWLEDGE OF
                        GOOD AND EVIL

It is this formula that has given Satan such power and success in his efforts.

After the flood, man's great goal was to achieve a proper *balance* among the cosmos, earth, and man, as it was believed that a perfect balance would result in utopia. Thus, the "knowledge of good and evil" involved not only a blending of good with evil but also the idea that harmony would only exist if this blending had universal application. This was and is the foundation of all nonbiblical belief systems.[6]

On the cover for the book *Two Be One* written by the publishers, the following comment appears:

> In his studies, Steed has uncovered a startling discrepancy: the teachings of Christ as recorded in the Scriptures comprise the only philosophy that does not fit into the world's basic pattern for unity. For throughout the ages, mankind has seen oneness, the conjunction of all opposites, as being the culmination of all their dreams and imaginations, the way to eternal happiness. Christianity looks for *separation* to provide the sought-after peace.

Utopia is not found by finding the proper blend with sin.

Having applied the concept of dualism to "universal energy," the great object then was to blend the divided energy back into *one*, covering every aspect of life. It became a supreme goal to blend opposites into proper balance to achieve life's secrets, obtain all wisdom and ultimate oneness.[7]

The creation of the universe (macrocosm) and man (microcosm) was thus explained as being derived from this blending of opposites.

> We have created our own body, within the framework of certain universal and immanent laws, says the Buddhist.[8]

Here, he refers to dualism. Actually, the doctrine of evolution is only a variant of dualism wherein the strong rises above the weak in the process of selection.

---

[6] Steed, op. cit., p. vii–ix.
[7] Steed, op. cit., p. 12–13.
[8] Govinda, Lama Anagarika, *Foundations of Tibetan Mysticism*, Samuel Weiser, now Red Wheel Weiser, Newberry Park, MA (1969), p. 159.

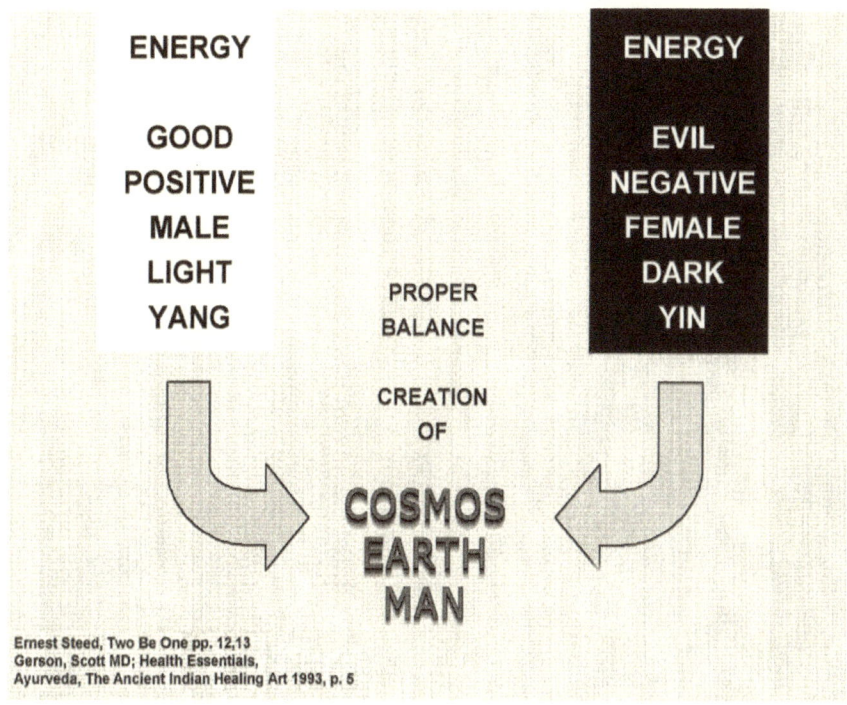

Figure 7. Blending together to create cosmos, earth.

CORRESPONDENCE, ASSOCIATION, SYMPATHY

In this explanation for the origin of the cosmos, earth, and man, the belief is that there is close correspondence, association, and sympathy between these entities. In Maurice Bessy's book, *Magic and the Supernatural*, a figure of two circles is shown, one outer circle and another inner circle, a man with outstretched arms, and legs is within the second circle. Surrounding the inner circle are the signs of the zodiac. Below this figure is the following explanation:

> A mirror of the world—"microcosm of the macrocosm." Man, as conceived in astrology, reflects the rhythms and structure of the universe in the same way as the universe mirrors the rhythms and the structure of Man himself. Everything is part of everything . . .[9]

---

[9] Bessy, Maurice, *Magic and the Supernatural*, Spring Books, NY (1970), pp. 73–74.

It was believed that changes in man or the cosmos influenced the other. The planting of seed, the choice of food, all acts of life—in short, every action, it was believed—should be guided by the position of the planets.

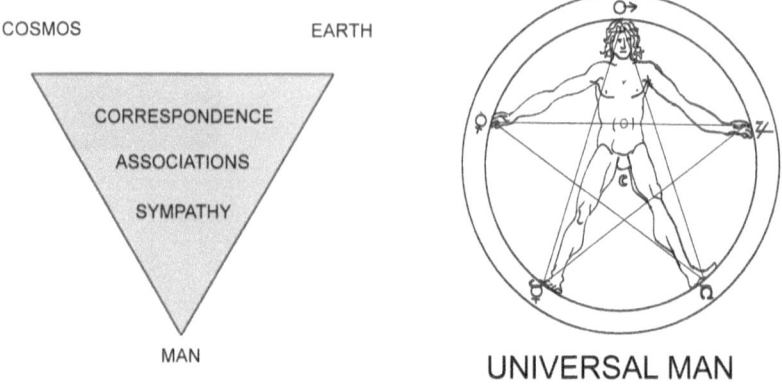

Figures 8. Triangle of correspondence and circle with man.

This symbol around man is known as a mandala, which in Sanskrit means circle. Although mandalas are of different designs, they all represent the same idea—revealing the relationship of the cosmos to man. The outer circle represents the cosmos; the inner circle represents the earth, with the figure of a man in the inner circle representing the "at-one-ment" of the universe, earth, and man. This is a counterfeit of the "at-one-ment" with God that Jesus obtained for us on the cross. This symbol is often seen in New Age health literature. The lines drawn from the arms to leg, hand and head form a five-pointed star (pentagram) which also represents the same belief.

J. E. Cirlot, in his book *Dictionary of Symbols* under the title of "Macrocosm-Microcosm," makes the following comment:

> This relationship is symbolic of the situation in the universe of man as the "measure of all things." The basis of this relationship—which has occupied the minds of thinkers and mystics of all kinds in all ages—is the symbolism of man himself, particularly as the "universal man" together with his "correspondences" with the zodiac, the planets, and the elements. As Origen observed: "Understand that you are

another world in miniature and that you are the sun, the moon, and also the stars.[10]

This implication is to be found in all symbolic traditions. Under the title "Man," the statement is made:

> Hence the pentagram (five-point star) is a sign of the microcosmos[11]

and is a sacred symbol in neo-paganism. The ancient Chaldeans promoted the idea of unity of all things and applied it to every aspect of life. The *zodiac* was formed as a tool to apply this concept to life on earth, and the practice of seeking guidance through the zodiac was referred to as reading ones *horoscope*.[12]

In time, the zodiac system was consulted when making most of life's decisions.

> For astrology itself was based on an understanding and interpretation of these symbols in terms of the complexities of life and its origin and meaning. The zodiac was likened to a wheel with the changing times and seasons but more so to the wheel of life. The Hindu sees it as the wheel of transmigration, the Buddhist as the wheel of completeness, and the Taoist of China, through the yang and yin and the circle of harmony; all visualize the correspondence or sympathy between opposites.[13]

The pagan religions originating in Babylon had their foundation in astrology, and the zodiac is based on the belief of the existence of sympathy between the planets, earth, and man. The sun was the preeminent planet in the zodiac. To participate in a belief system that has the zodiac as a part of its beliefs is paying homage to Satan.

---

[10] Cirlot, J.E., *A Dictionary of Symbols*, Philosophical Library, Inc., New York, NY (1962), p. 196.
[11] *Ibid.*, p. 197.
[12] Bessy, op. cit., pp. 67–74; Steed, op. cit., p. 15.
[13] Steed, op. cit., pp. 15–16.

PAGAN'S STORY OF CREATION

Out of chaos came pure light and collected to itself and then moved to form the sky. The darkness that remained traveled and out of itself formed the earth. Out of this activity arose the principles of yang and yin, darkness and light, earth and sky. This movement of "like to like" balanced the forces, and then there was growth and increase, resulting in the start of the ten thousand creation, all of which took sky and earth (yang and yin) as a mode. Contact between yang and yin produce water, fire, wood, metal, and earth.

> These five elements diffuse harmoniously and evolve into four seasons which proceed on their course. The two forces of maleness and femaleness reacting with and influencing each other bring myriad things into being. Generation follows generation, and there is no end to changes and transformations.

Insight Northwest "The Healing Transformation, Some Lesser God, Keep"[14]

The Hindu Creation Story:

> From this self, verily, space arose, from space, air, from air, fire, from fire, water, from water, earth, from earth, herbs, from herbs, food, from food, man.

Taittiriya Upanishad 2:1 reported in *Ayurveda*, Scott Gerson

The Buddhist says:

> We have created our own bodies.

Foundations of Tibetan Mysticism, Govinda, p. 159

These names of the proclaimed basic elements of creation (water, fire, air, earth, metal, and/or space) are not to be understood literally. They are words used in an attempt to describe creative spirit power believed to come from five planets (Mercury, Mars, Jupiter, Venus, Saturn) empowering the process of creation.

---

[14] Keep, Joan, Some Lesser God, *Insight Northwest* "The Healing Transformation," Dec-Jan 85/vol. 3 Number 6 p. 20.

Since the belief is that creation of all substance, animate and inanimate resulted from the balancing and proper mingling of the two aspects (good and evil, positive and negative, male and female, etc.) of so-called universal energy, it was felt that disease and illness were a result of an *imbalance* of these energies.[15] This energy, considered as "god," is pantheism. "All is one and one is all"—thus the belief that disease is a spiritual imbalance manifesting as physical disease.

It followed then that if an imbalance of energy caused health disorders, balancing would restore health. This led to a multitude of acts and practices designed to prevent and treat illness. As already noted, to treat an imbalance of energy, a myriad of methods were developed, which depended upon everything being categorized as good or evil, positive or negative, and yang or yin, etc. This approach to disease does not focus on following God's physical laws of health or recognizes disease as the body's response to violation of those laws.

Examples of substances used to restore balance are herbs, minerals, climate, temperature, spells, dances, animal matter of all types, stones, liquids, relics, spoken words, written words, colors, flowers, zodiac influences, charms of all types, psychotherapy, magnetism, acupuncture, moxibustion, meditation, divination, numerology, music, sound, spirits, pictures, aromas, talismans, crystals, alchemy, foods, etc. All were labeled as being either positive or negative in their influence. Medical historian Garrison tells us that medicine did not progress as long as it was founded in the supernatural.[16]

The Scriptures teach that *separation* from evil, *not blending* with evil, is God's way.

WORLDWIDE BELIEF IN ENERGY BALANCING

In the United States, many of the Native American Indians believe in dualism, and it is a principle they may apply in health and healing. Their therapeutic practices involve balancing animal spirits and/or energies. Navajo sand paintings are used to correct the believed imbalanced energies of those who are ill.[17]

Sand paintings are formed on the ground and may take an entire day to make. A variety of plants, seeds, and other natural substances are used in forming the painting. There are hundreds of varieties of sand paintings

---

[15] Steed, op. cit., p. 100; Garrison, op. cit., pp. 74, 88.
[16] Garrison, op. cit., p. 24.
[17] Bahti, Tom, *Southwestern Indian Ceremonials*, K.C. Publications, Las Vegas, NV (1987), p. 10.

and are said to be kept in the head of the shaman. A sick person sits on the painting for several hours. Then the painting is scooped up, taken, and buried as it is believed to have absorbed the excess spirit or energy of either the good or the evil influence causing illness.[18] The sand paintings are made with colors and patterns and represent dualism by containing contrasting objects, colors, or positions.

The shaman, or medicine man, may also use dances, "sings" (groups of people singing about the sick person), or a bag containing various objects, as well as certain sounds to influence the spirits and powers that cause sickness. These methods are used as sympathetic remedies.

In the past, Europeans associated particular organs of the body with the specific houses of the zodiac. The symbols of animals taken from the zodiac were assigned to specific organs. Aries the ram pertained to the head, while Pisces the fish was for the feet. When doctors determined an organ had an energy imbalance, they chose a treatment that supposedly would influence the correspondence between that organ and its zodiac house.[19]

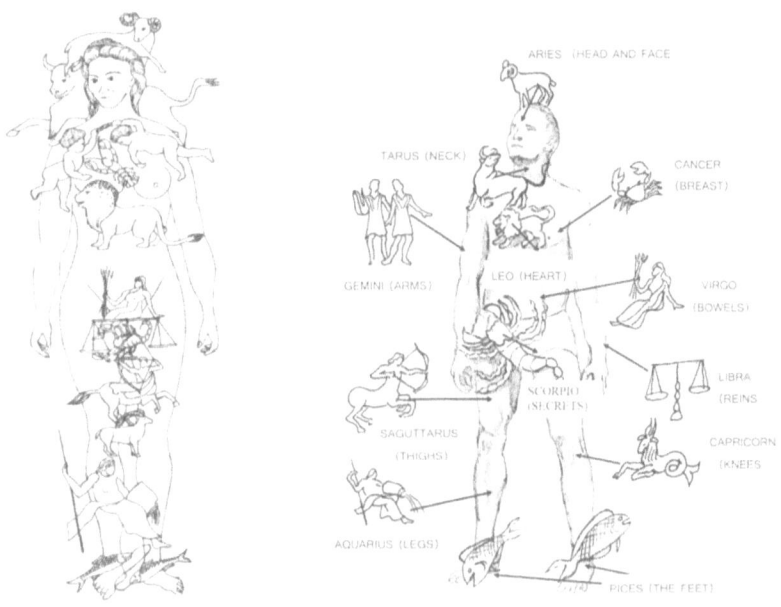

Figures 9. Man covered with animals representing association of man with zodiac.

---

[18] *Ibid.*, p. 10

[19] Bessy, op. cit. pp. 73–74; Garrison, op. cit., p. 37

Remember that the zodiac is based on the planets with the sun as chief, and sun worship is Luciferic (Satanic) worship. Satan's deceptions are received as from heaven, and faith in scripture diminishes in the minds of many until it is totally lost. Herein Satan receives the worship he desires. This core value change brings loss of virtue, and spiritualistic deceptions are accepted.

THREE WORLD CENTERS OF MEDICAL INFLUENCE

In the old world, there were three great centers of learning that influenced the concepts in medicine over the last thirty-five hundred years. The *first* was on the Island of Kos, where Hippocrates lived and practiced.[20] The *second* was the Indus River valley in India, from where came Ayurveda. It is also where the Hindu religion had its roots.[21] The *third* was in China, the place of origin of traditional Chinese medicine.[22]

The ancient Vedas, written in the Sanskrit language, contain the story of the origin of Hinduism and its health and healing concepts. These writings are thirty-five hundred years old and were written by "sages" (holy men) who retired into the foothills of the mountains and there

> produced India's original systems of meditation, yoga, and astrology.[23]

This healing system is called Ayurveda, the ancient Indian healing tradition. The Ayurvedic approach to health is not separate from Hinduism; *it is* Hinduism.

The *foundation* of all treatment for health and healing in Ayurveda is the *practice of meditation*. In fact, there is little help to be gained in other health and healing methods in Ayurveda without the use of meditation and yoga.[24] The practice of meditation is said to bring the inner self, the universal energy, the prana (air, breath), the *god* within us, to such a level

---

[20] Lyons, Albert S., MD, Petrucelli, R. Joseph, MD, *Medicine an Illustrated History*, Harry N. Abrams, Inc., Publishers, New York, NY (1978), p. 207.

[21] Gerson, Scott, *Ayurveda the Ancient Indian Healing Tradition*, Shaftesbury, Dorset (Element Books) Rockport, MA (1993), p. 3; Lyons, op. cit., p. 105.

[22] Lyons, op. cit., p. 121.

[23] Gerson, op. cit., p. 3.

[24] *Ibid.*, p. 78.

that it would allow us to interact with the spirit entities and eventually enter that same spirit state.[25]

The whole religious conquest of the Hindu is to escape this life and move into the spirit world. There is no separation between spiritual and physical in health and healing in Hinduism. It is said by an ex-guru, who is now a Christian, that:

> You cannot take Hinduism out of yoga and meditation, and you cannot have yoga and meditation without Hinduism.[26]

Turning our discussion now to Chinese traditional healing, a common symbol represents the summation of their Tao beliefs. The *Pa Kua*, or circle of harmony, also showing eight syndromes of disease (see chapter on "Acupuncture and Chinese Traditional Medicine"), represents constant transformation in order to achieve harmony and balance. It is a symbol of how another *universal energy* belief system, called chi by the Chinese, relates to our bodies.[27]

There seems to be no contention between the different groups—European, Indian, or Chinese—over the different explanations of the supposed manner of distribution of "universal energy" within the body.

Satan may use certain healing methods that may have some physiological basis, but it is wrapped up in his dogma. Those who believe in these concepts do not look to God as the restorer of health. The scriptures are our safeguard.

> Lest Satan should take advantage of us: for we are not ignorant of his devices. II Corinthians 2:11.

ENERGY BALANCING METHODS OF HEALING

The American Medical Association Committee for investigating alternative therapies has listed more than one hundred different methods of healing used and promoted today. The *Alternative Health Dictionary* lists more than four thousand names of various therapies of energy balancing. I list here some of the commonly used techniques. An alternative therapy would be defined as a therapy that does not have scientific evidence of effectiveness and usually has a history of use as a "folk medicine" therapy.

---

[25] Willis, Richard J.B., *Holistic Health Holistic Hoax,* Stanborough Press Ltd., Alma Park, Grantham, Lincolnshire, England (1997), Chapter 13.

[26] Video by Jeremiah Films Inc., Hemet, CA 1988.

[27] Lyons, op. cit., p. 125; Steed, op. cit., p. 46.

PSYCHIC THERAPY   AROMATHERAPY
ACUPUNCTURE   ESSENTIAL OILS
ACUPRESSURE   SONOPUNCTURE
MOXIBUSTION   LASERPUNCTURE
HOMEOPATHY   IRIDOLOGY
REFLEXOLOGY   POLARITY
MARTIAL ARTS   MARMA POINT MASSAGE
ROLFING   CHAKRA BALANCING
MAGNETIC HEALERS   REIKI
SOMA BODY WORK   COLOR THERAPY
RADIONICS   MERIDIAN THERAPY
MEDITATION   SOUND THERAPY
YOGA   GUIDED IMAGERY
TONING   VISUALIZATION
BIOFEEDBACK   ENERGY HEALING
TOUCH FOR HEALTH   VIBRATIONAL MEDICINE
THERAPEUTIC TOUCH   ABSENT HEALING
PENDULUM USE   MAGNETS
FLOWER ESSENCES   PAST LIFE REGRESSION
CRYSTALS   ORTHOMOLECULAR MED
TRANSCENDENTAL   CHANNELING
MEDITATION   TRANSCENDENTAL MEDITATION
SOUND THERAPY

In the following chapters, we will look carefully at several of these different healing methods. They all have the same basic foundation, that of moving and balancing a nonmeasurable, nondemonstrable vital force, energy, prana, chi, etc.

Why so many therapeutic approaches to balancing energy? Because none of them are based on true physics and science but on the paranormal or psychic. It really matters little as to the physical method of therapy. It has a lot more to do with the mental attitude and acceptance of the theory of *universal energy* or *intelligence*. It also strongly depends on the person administering the therapy and his connection to this unseen power. This *energy* has been given at least ninety different names, yet they all refer to the same thing. Of the men who gave so many names to this *energy*, it was found that the first fifty of them reviewed were spiritualistic channelers and psychics, and it may be that nearly all were.[28]

The rise and renewal of these ancient healing practices has been rapid, with no evidence of slowing. In the United States and other countries of the world, many of the medical teaching institutions have incorporated some of these practices in their curriculum. Physicians from around the world travel to China to take courses in traditional Chinese medicine. I have visited with medical students from Europe who were in China for a three-month rotation training in Chinese medical schools with the primary interest in learning traditional Chinese medicine. Probably 50 or more percent of hospitals in the United States have made available some type of *alternative therapy* because it is popular, and the hospitals are competing for business.

The interest in alternative therapies is strong among the people of the Western nations, partly because it is marketed as *natural* therapy (without the use of drugs). People do not know the history of these treatment methods, and many believe that new knowledge has led to their use. Others believe that old beneficial healing methods have been lost and are now being resurrected to our benefit.

A careful review of medical history will reveal that much of the philosophy behind alternative therapies comes from the ancient Indian healing methods called Ayurveda, from early European concepts of healing, and also from traditional Chinese medicine. Earnest Steed, in his book, *Two Be One*, chapter 4, traces the influence of astrology via the zodiac upon the above-mentioned ancient systems.

Historically, there is no evidence that the nations that depended on these therapies benefited from them. The following are quotes from some medical history books:

> It follows that, under different aspects of space and time, the essential traits of folk medicine and ancient medicine have been alike in tendency, differing only in unimportant details. In the light of anthropology, this proposition may be taken as proved. Cuneiform, hieroglyphic, runic, birch-bark, and palm-leaf inscriptions all indicate that the folkways of early medicine, whether Acadian or Scandinavian, Slavic or Celtic, Roman or Polynesian, have been the same—in each case an affair of charms and spells, plant-lore and psychotherapy, to stave off

---

[28] Wilson & Weldon, *Occult Shock and Psychic Forces*, Master Books division of CLP, San Diego, CA, (1980), p. 247.

the effects of supernatural agencies. Where this frame of mind persists, there is no possibility of advancement for medicine.[29]

Until recently, Chinese medicine has been what our own medicine might be had we been guided by medieval ideas down to the present time, that is, absolutely stationary.[30]

Where these therapies were used as the main method of medical treatment, there was no improvement either in the incidence of disease or in longevity. China had an average life span in 1949 of thirty-five years. The approach in China toward the cause of disease changed from an imbalance of energy, and a scientific approach was instituted, with the establishment of hygienic and basic disease prevention methods based on present-day science. The average life span increased to seventy by the year 2000 (World Health Organization). This is considered one of the great medical events of the past century.

We are warned in the Scriptures of the devil's attempt to deceive God's people, and at the close of earth's history, he will deceive all nations.[31] In health and healing, his power will be especially strong, and those who are not diligent Bible students will find it very difficult to tell the real from the counterfeit. The true power of healing will come from God, the author and sustainer of our lives.

The counterfeit teaches that the origin and power that sustains us is from within. Accessing this power from within is said to affect health and healing. The majority of alternative therapies today are ways of attempting to access power from within, to balance good and evil characteristics, and to bring about change and healing. Accepting these methods of treatment effectively means separation from God.

Revelation 22:14–15 shares with us those who will enter the gates of the new Jerusalem, "those who do His commandments" may enter the gates, "but outside are dogs and sorcerers."

This is the issue: Will we choose to follow God and have *eternal life*, or will we follow the devil (demons) and have *eternal death*? In the next chapter, we take a more in-depth look at this so-called universal energy that has been divided into two parts, resulting in the worldwide belief in dualism.

---

[29] Garrison, op, cit., p. 18.
[30] *Ibid.*, p. 73.
[31] Revelation 16:13, 14; Revelation 19:20.

4

Universal Energy

We live in an age of advanced knowledge of the sciences of physics, chemistry, and physiology. However, this does not seem to prevent a false science, the wisdom and arts of Satan from entering into this same field to deceive. We need to carefully and prayerfully consider healing methods not founded in solid science. Error often lies so close to truth that it is impossible to discern, unless the mind is enlightened by the Spirit of God.

Satan desired the worship of man, and to obtain such, he subverted the Biblical story of creation. He deceived man into worshiping the power and works of God but not God.[1] Shortly following the flood, nature worship appeared as the dominant form of worship. God is proclaimed as an *essence, an actuating energy* pervading all nature. Therefore, God would dwell in all men, and man needs only develop that essence power to attain holiness. There becomes no need for an atonement with God, and man becomes his own savior. This theory makes God's Holy Word of no value.

The essence, the *actuating energy* from which the universe, earth, and man are made, according to pantheistic theories, is called by many names. Different languages, cultures, religions, and leaders in pantheistic doctrine have created a large variety of terms which refer to the same theoretical power. Nearly one hundred of these different names have appeared in print. Listed below are some of the more commonly used terms referring to a "creative principle."

---

[1] *Romans 1:15–20.*

TITLE	ORIGIN
PRANA	HINDUISM
CHI (KI, QI)	TAOISM (TCM)
LOGOS*	GREEK
MANA	POLYNESIAN
ORENDA	AMERICAN INDIAN
ANIMAL MAGNETISM	FRANZ MESMER
THE INNATE	CHIROPRACTIC
ORGONE ENERGY	WILHELM REICH
VITAL ENERGY	HOMEOPATHY
ODIC FORCE	OUIJA BOARD
BIOPLASMA	RUSSIAN PARAPSYCOLOGY
THE FORCE	STAR WARS (GEORGE LUCAS)

Many English synonyms are used to refer to this supposed power. "Universal Intelligence" is a name commonly used, as is the term *energy*. I suspect each language likewise has many synonyms for this power. Listed below are several English synonyms:

    ONE
    SELF, HIGHER SELF, SUPREME SELF, DIVINE SELF, I AM
    PURER CONSCIOUSNESS, SUPREME CONCIOUSNESS, ETC.
    CREATIVE PRINCIPLE
    ESSENCE
    VITAL FORCE, VITALISM, LIFE FORCE

VIBRATIONAL FORCE, SOURCE
MONISM
ULTIMATE UNIFIED ENERGY FIELD
UNIVERSAL INTELLIGENCE, ENERGY
SUPREME ULTIMATE

In the world of pantheism, there are varying descriptions as to how the *energy* (of which they say man is made) exists within man. The system of Ayurveda (ancient Indian healing art) describes the energy as localized in seven centers within man. These are called chakras. Man is said to have an "aura" produced by the chakras, which is *life force, universal energy* (*electromagnetic force* to some New Age scientists) and extends *outside* the body. It is to this perceived energy force that many alternative healing modalities direct their focus.[2]

> Two key words, microcosm and macrocosm, are used to portray the primary opposites, heaven and earth, thought to be in correspondence or sympathy.[3]

Macrocosm stands for the sun, moon, and stars, while microcosm stands for the earth and man. In pantheism, these two opposites, macrocosm and microcosm, must harmonize. The use of the "zodiac" was established in Chaldea to guide in achieving this harmony.[4]

UNIVERSAL ENERGY'S SEVEN DIVISIONS

In the Oriental view of universal energy, there are *seven divisions* or levels of energy. This Eastern concept is accepted by neo-paganism (New Age Movement) of today. Understanding a little about this belief of divisions or levels of universal energy will be of value in comprehending the explanations of presumed power of various techniques applied in health and healing. At the same time, we will get a glimpse of some of the theology of the Eastern religions, making it increasingly clear that involvement in their

---

[2] Hill, Ann; *A Visual Encyclopedia of Unconventional Medicine*, Crown Pub. Inc. NY (1978), p. 46.

[3] Bessy, Maurice; *Magic and the Supernatural*, Spring Books, NY (1970), p. 74 Jaggi, O.P.; *Yogic and Tantric Medicine*, Atma Ram and Sons, Delhi, India (1973), p. 96

[4] Bessy, op. cit. p. 67.

techniques in health and healing might unsuspectingly lead to acceptance of their religious precepts.

Universal energy—life force energy—is said by the New Age healers to be of seven levels or planes in distribution and function. Of late, an occasional New Age scientist will call this perceived energy *electromagnetic energy*, which he believes to have specific vibrational frequencies at various levels. In this concept, the bottom level frequency of energy has *materialized* and formed the cosmos, earth, and man. Dr. Gerber, a medical doctor who is a very prominent New Age author, tells us in his text *Vibrational Medicine* that the other levels of universal energy have different and increasing frequencies above the speed of light.[5] The different levels of energy are believed to have specific progressive influences, first on the physical body and then on the spiritual path to godhood. The second and third levels are spoken of as having *subtle bodies*. In the days before the development of the science of physics, universal energy—life force energy—was explained by the term *spiritual power*, and different frequencies of light energy (not demonstrated by science) were not a part of their explanation.

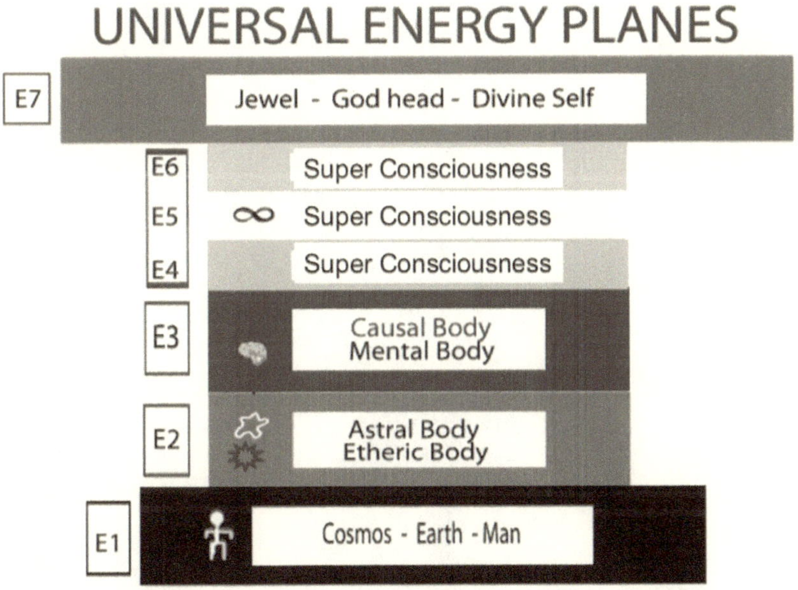

UNIVERSAL ENERGY PLANES

E7	Jewel - God head - Divine Self
E6	Super Consciousness
E5 ∞	Super Consciousness
E4	Super Consciousness
E3	Causal Body / Mental Body
E2	Astral Body / Etheric Body
E1	Cosmos - Earth - Man

Figure 10. Energy frequency levels.

---

[5] Gerber, Richard MD; *Exploring Vibrational Medicine*, Sounds True, Boulder, CO (2001), CD discs 1, 2.

The concept is that frequency level *one* contains the materialized cosmos, including man, and is believed to be composed of energy traveling at the speed of light. The *second* and *third* level of frequencies involves "*subtle bodies.*" These hypothesized bodies surround the physical body and are even supposed to be of different colors. The first body, *etheric body* or energy plane, is said to have the function of being an "electromagnetic" template of our physical body and is believed to be the controlling influence in the function of our physiology. When imbalance is present in the etheric body, eventually the physical body will present with malfunction or disease. Many healing techniques are aimed at correcting or balancing the status of the etheric body. The next higher body is called astral body, which functions in the "out of body," "light in tunnel," and "astral travel apart from body" experiences. The *third* level of frequency involves the *mental body* and is said to deal with higher thought processes: We then come to the *causal body*, which functions in reincarnation beliefs. It is said to store life experiences from *past and future lives.*

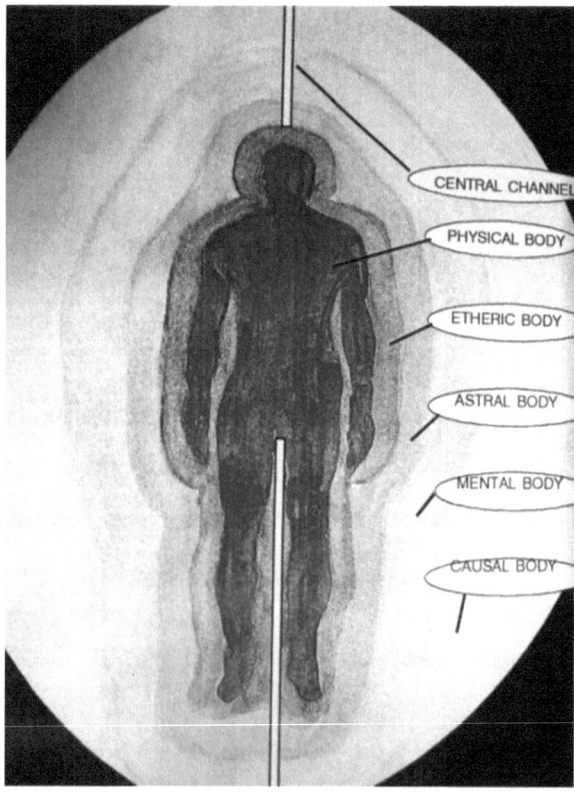

Figure 11. Multiple bodies.

Death involves the physical body, and it disappears, yet the "subtle" bodies continue on and receive the new reincarnated body in whatever form it presents, animal or human, possibly in a lower caste or, hopefully, at a higher status.

Levels 4 to 7 of universal energy frequencies deal with increasing levels of "consciousness," and at the top, level 7, symbolized by the *lotus flower* or the *jewel*, immortality—eternal life, is attained. This top level is said to interconnect with the energies of all the universe, and thus the expression *all is one and one is all* or *as above so below*. It is at this level that *godhood* is said to take place.[6]

A point of interest is the belief that plants contain high frequency levels of energy. Also by consuming plants as our diet, we can obtain from them higher levels of consciousness. This is one of the reasons vegetarianism is common within neo-paganism.

The goal of neo-paganism of the West and the religions of the East is to attain to the energy frequency level of the lotus and the jewel. All religious activities are directed to this concept. *Universal energy*, as described in this chapter, is the core foundational belief of Eastern religions and in Western occultism. The religious activities are for the purpose of raising energy frequency levels from the material, speed of light level, up through the higher frequency levels and eventually reach to the ultimate level. Illness is considered a burp, a blurb in the progress of ascending to higher frequency planes and to godhood. A multitude of acts and practices in these religions are designed with the idea that they will raise a person to the experience of Nirvana.[7, 8]

PANTHEIST'S EXPLANATION FOR CAUSE OF DISEASE

Illness and disease are explained in the pantheistic viewpoint as resulting from imbalance or blockage of the presence and flow through the body, of universal energy. Therapies are designed to balance, unblock,

---

[6] Green, Elmer and Alyce; *Beyond Biofeedback*, Knoll Pub. Co. Inc., Ft. Wayne, IN (1977), pp. 299–315.

[7] Gerber, op. cit., discs 1, 2.

[8] Prophet, Elizabeth Clare; *Djwal Kul Intermediate Studies of the Human Aura*, Dictated by Djwal Kul an ascended master also known as the Tibetan Master; Summit University Press, Colorado Springs, CO (1974), pp. 27–31.

restore, infuse, or otherwise manipulate invisible energies which allegedly exist or circulate within the human body.[9]

On the other hand, divine energy does not circulate within the body through psychic pathways whose imbalance causes disease. We cannot manipulate the power of God by putting needles in our skin, by massaging pressure points, by sitting in the yoga position, or by breathing exercises.

We have learned in the previous chapter of the foundational teaching of pantheism's explanation of our origin—that of blending two opposing parts of an imaginary universal energy. In this chapter, we have looked at the many different names and hypothesized different levels of speed given to this energy. The concept is that illness and disease result from the imbalance of the two parts (yin-yang) of energy in our system. Treatment of disease in Satan's system is an act of attempting to rebalance the energy. In the following chapters, we will look at various popular methods devised to affect balance and/or correct the vibration of universal energy in order to bring about health and healing.

That which takes our allegiance away from a Creator God and directs our allegiance to His counterfeit, will make void the grace of Christ toward us. It makes His word of no effect.

---

[9] Ankerberg, John; Weldon, John; *Can You Trust Your Doctor?* Wolgemuth and Hyatt, Brentwood, TN (1991), p. 67.

5

BABYLONIAN SPIRITUALISTIC MYSTERIES IN THE CHRISTIAN CIVILIZATION

An employee of a Christian publishing establishment in Russia missed work intermittently because of abdominal pain. Physicians could not discover the cause, and eventually, this person was unable to work. He then sought the services of an alternative medicine practitioner. By feeling the ear of this employee, the practitioner diagnosed an infestation of round worms in the stomach and intestines. Medicine was prescribed, which caused the worms to be eliminated. The pain ceased, and the employee returned to work.

A few months later, another employee developed abdominal pain. This individual heard an announcement on television about a certain healing technique and decided to try it. He sent to the TV healer a month's wages in rubles. He then taped a coin to the monitor of his television, and a healing current was supposed to be transferred to the coin. In turn, the coin was then taped to his abdomen. The coin was to transfer healing energy to cure his abdominal pain, even though no diagnosis had been established.

The above two incidents initiated my receiving an invitation in 1999 to organize a seminar on mystical medicine. The seminar was to be presented to Christian health educators in Russia and countries of the old Soviet Union. Many of the health educators were nurses, dentists, and physicians.

The use of similar healing methods in this part of the world is endemic. It was a sobering task for myself, as a foreign doctor who did not use such healing techniques, to attempt to convince the Eastern European doctors that these methods were wrong physically and spiritually. There was the need to demonstrate the intimate connection between those healing techniques and the core doctrines of paganism. The previous two chapters, combined with this chapter, is the foundational material presented. This information has proved to be a powerful influence in convincing individuals of the source of apparent healing power in most nonconventional healing techniques of which there are many methods.

To understand the rise, growth, as well as the coming out into the open of mystical medicine in our day, we have to understand its past and have a true understanding of its origins and author.

The pagan-nature worshiping civilizations continued in the philosophy of the zodiac with its mystical relational concepts, combined with the doctrine of "dualism," following their dispersion to the whole world from ancient Babylon. Satan, the great Counterfeiter, was able to influence the people of Israel through the Canaanites, who were idol worshipers and practiced the mysteries of Babylon. For over nine hundred years, Israel was harassed and intermittently succumbed to the influence of its pagan neighbors. Israel's captivity in Babylon in approximately 606–536 BC effectively ended Israel's involvement in idol worship.

Medical history texts present medical history by starting with ancient civilizations and progressing to modern times presenting the characteristics and advancements in treatment that each contributed to medical science. The Jewish civilization was the only one to promote prevention. It is interesting to note that information concerning the Jewish civilization is very brief, and no mention is made of any outstanding advancement in treatment methods. But there is one distinct difference. It was the only nation that practiced prevention and hygiene in dealing with disease. Careful study of the Bible will show that the health information God gave to Israel during the exodus focused on proper health habits and hygiene. No other civilization presented prevention as an approach to its health problems.

When the Jews returned to Israel from the Babylonian exile, Satan devised another plan of deception whereby he could usurp their loyalty to God. This he accomplished by the infiltration of the Babylonian mysteries into their religion by way of a secret society, the Kabbalah. Mystical healing methods were promoted by Kabbalah.

SECRET SOCIETIES

Sometime following the return of the Jews to their homeland after seventy years of captivity in Babylon (near 530 BC), a secret society began in Israel. No one knows for sure when this occurred, but it is believed by researchers that some of the Jewish priests, while in Babylon, began mixing their religion with Babylonian mysteries (the hidden knowledge based on astrology) and Zoroastrianism (religion of Persia). They carried back home with them this mixture in a society called the Cabala (Cabbala, Kabbalah, and/or Kabalah), which is based on the theoretical universal energy and dualism concept.

> But esotericism again presents a dual aspect. Here, as in every phase of earthly life, there is the "revers de la medaille" white and black, light and darkness, the Heaven and Hell of the human mind.[1]

Over time, the doctrine of the Cabala infiltrated and blended with Judaism to such an extent that one author described it as

> the heart and life of Judaism.[2]

> The modern Jewish Cabala presents a dual aspect, theoretical and practical; the former concerned with theosophical speculations, the latter with magical practices.[3]

The Cabala uses a mystical approach to illness and its treatment. One method uses numbers and letters on "talismans" applied near the bed of the sick.

In the hill country of Israel, north of Galilee, is a small Palestinian town with a Jewish section, located at the peak of a small mountain. The

---

[1] Webster, Nesta; *Secret Societies and Subversive Movements*, [Christian Book club of America, Hawthorne, CA (1924) p. 3 (Available through Emissary Publications), 0205 SE Clackamas Rd., No. 1776, Clackamas, OR 97015 (503-842-2050).

[2] Franke, Adolph; *La Kabbalah*, p. 288 (reported in *Secret Societies* by Nesta Webster p. 9); Stehelin, J.P.; *The Traditions of the Jews*, p. 145 (printed for G. Smith in London 1742–43) (Above reference reported in Webster (1922), op, cit., p. 9).

[3] Webster, op. cit., pp. 12–13.

Sea of Galilee can be seen in the distance. This city is Safed, considered one of the four "holy" cities in Israel today. As you enter the town, a sign will tell you that this is the location of the school of the Kabala.

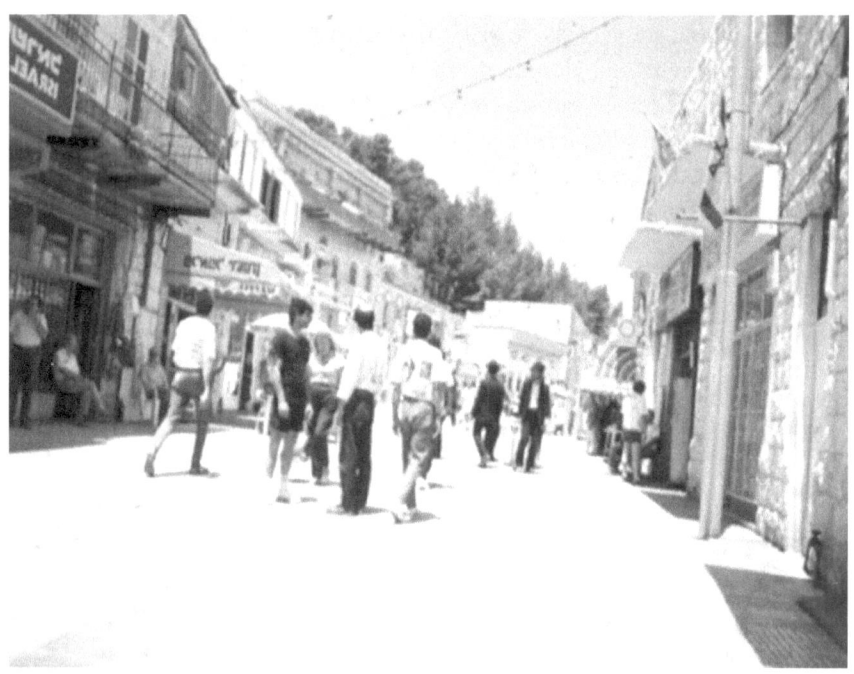

Figure 12. Main street in the city of Safed, Israel.

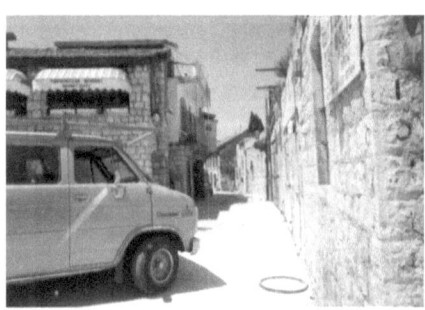 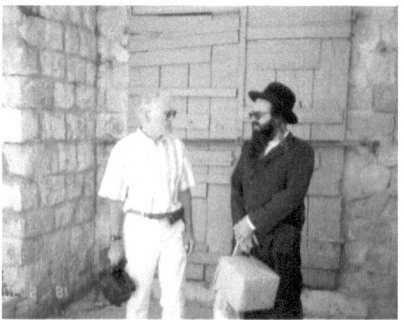

Figure 13. Jewish section of Sephat and Dr. Noyes talking to a Kabala teacher.

From the Kabala came the Gnostics, that sect which greatly opposed the Christian movement in the days of Paul and the Apostles.

> The Freemason, Ragon, gives the clue in these words: "The Cabala is the key of the occult sciences. The Gnostics were born of the Cabalists."[4]

Simon Magus, whom Peter rebuked because he tried to buy the power of the Holy Ghost for the laying on of hands (Acts 8), is known in secular writings as the founder of Gnosticism. He was also a magician and was involved with mystical medicine. Legend has it that he became sorcerer to Nero who had a statue made in his (Simon Magus) likeness and placed in Rome.

> In the *Dictionary of Christian Biography*, volume. 4, page 682, we read that "when Justin Martyr wrote his Apology (AD 152), the sect of the Simonians appears to have been formidable, for he speaks four times of their founder, Simon, and tells that he came to Rome in the day of Claudius Caesar (AD 45) and made such an impression by his magical powers, that he was honored as a god, a statue being erected to him on the Tiber, between the two bridges, bearing the inscription "Simoni deo Sancto" (i.e., the holy god Simon).[5]

The heart of the doctrine of these secret societies was *Divinity within—pantheism,* God in everything and everything God. The deification of humanity became a supreme doctrine of the secret societies. Nature worship too was a result.

A major reference book of the Masonic order, *Morals and Dogma of the Ancient and Accepted Scottish Rite of Freemasonry* by Albert Pike, has a forty-page discussion of Gnosticism and its connection to Freemasonry. Of Gnosticism, Pike wrote:

> The Gnostics derived their leading doctrines and ideas from Plato and Philo, the Zend-avesta and the Kabbalah, and the Sacred books of India and Egypt; and thus introduced into

---

[4] Ragon; *Maconnerie Occulte*, Emile Nourry, Paris (1853), p. 78; Reported in *Secret Societies* by Nesta Webster, p. 28.

[5] Griffin, Des; *Fourth Reich of the Rich*, Emissary Publications, Clackamas, OR (1989), (503-824-2050) p. 33.

the bosom of Christianity the cosmological and theosophical speculations, which had formed the larger portion of the ancient religions of the Orient, joined with those of the Egyptian, Greek, and Jewish doctrines, which the New-Platonists had equally adopted in the Occident.[6]

Pike, a past sovereign pontiff of Universal Freemasonry, traces the chronological growth and spread of the mysteries over the face of the earth from ancient Babylon to the present-day Masonic Order. In reference to the esoteric doctrines of the mysteries, he states:

> The communication of this knowledge and other secrets, some of which are perhaps lost, constituted, under other names, what we now call Masonry, or Free or Frank-Masonry. The present name of the Order, and its titles, and the names of the Degrees now in use, were not then known . . . But by whatever name it was known in this or any other country, Masonry existed as it now exists, the same in spirit and at heart . . . before even the first colonies emigrated into Southern India, Persia, and Egypt, from the cradle of the human race (ancient Babylon).[7]

These doctrines were preserved in the Christian civilization over the ages within the societies of the Kabalah, Gnosticism, Manichaeism, various secret orders of the Islamic countries, Sufis, Knights Templars, Rosicrucians, and Freemasonry. Notice the following conclusion by an author and researcher in this subject:

> Luciferian Occultism controls Freemasonry—Luciferian Occultism is therefore not a novelty, but it bore a different name in the early days of Christianity. It was called Gnosticism, and its founder was Simon the Magician.[8]

---

[6] Pike, Albert; *Morals and Dogma of the Ancient and Accepted Scottish Rite of Freemasonry*, Kessinger Publishing Co., Kila, MT (1925), p. 248 (original publication 1871 In Charleston, South Carolina).

[7] *Ibid.*, pp. 207–208.

[8] Miller, Edith Starr, *Occult Theocracy*, printed in France and no Publishing companies name given in the book (Originally Published in 1933, not printed for general sale, reprinted in 1980 Hawthorne, CA. By the Christian Book Club of America, p. 33.

Satan's goal is to pervert Christianity with these concepts, and *counterfeit healing* is the right arm of his message. So it continues to this day. From the time of the early church through the ages to our day, these spiritual and healing mysticisms have been kept alive in the Christian community via secret societies with the aim of promoting, in disguise, the worship of Lucifer. Healing modalities are used to attract people, progressing on to the philosophical and spiritual teachings of their theosophy—pagan theology (see glossary).

The Babylonian mysteries were the basis of paganism and nature worship of the people who dispersed from Babylon, which today we recognize as the old religions of Egypt, Persia, Greece, India, Oriental countries, Americas, etc. The common core philosophy is *the Divine within* (pantheism). Their cosmological beliefs and teachings through time are reflected in their approach to medical care.

From French Freemasonry (Grand Orient lodges), greatly influenced by Illuminism at the end of the eighteenth century, arose various American and European secret political societies, the international banking elite, Marxism, and eventually the World Council of Churches. Nesta Webster in her book, *Secret Societies*, reveals that the Freemasons of France gave support to the establishment in 1875 of the Theosophical Society in New York.[9]

NEW AGE MOVEMENT

In the 1970s, the influence of all of the above-mentioned and other pantheistic societies came together to bring about what is now known as the New Age Movement. The expression East-West refers to the joining of Western occultism with Eastern mysticism.

With reference to the teachings of these societies, Albert Pike made the following statement in July 14, 1889, to the twenty-three Supreme Councils of the World (his answer was recorded by A.C. De La Five in *La Femme et L'Enfant dans la Franc-Maconnerie Universelle*, p. 588):

> If Lucifer were not God, would Adonay (the God of the Christians) whose deeds prove his cruelty, perfidy, and hatred of man, barbarism, and repulsion for science? Would Adonay and his priests calumniate him? Yes, Lucifer is God, and unfortunately Adonay is also God. For the eternal law is that there is no light without shade, no beauty without ugliness,

---

[9] Webster, op. cit., pp. 297–310.

no white without black, for the absolute can only exist as two Gods: darkness being necessary to light to serve as its foil as the pedestal is necessary to the statue, and brake to the locomotive. Thus, the doctrine of Satanism is a heresy, and the true and pure philosophic religion is the belief in Lucifer, the equal of Adonay; but Lucifer, God of Light and Good, is struggling for humanity against Adonay, theGod of Darkness and Evil.[10]

Nesta Webster, in her book *Secret Societies and Subversive Movements*, credits the secret societies, more specifically the Masonic lodge of Paris called Grand Orient, controlled by the Illuminists, as the primary force behind the rise of anarchy, philosophy, encyclopedists, atheism and the French revolution.[11]

Napoleon's rise to power in France lessened control of the government by this spiritualistic power, but its influence continued "underground" and has grown worldwide in such movements as humanism, socialism, communism, etc. From the atheistic and spiritualistic movement of the French revolution sprang different organizations. Not all of them were atheistic. Some were deists; others were guided by ancient pagan doctrines somewhat similar to those taught by the modern Theosophical Society, which was started in New York in 1875. This society had great influence and ultimately helped usher in the New Age Movement, with all its mystical medical practices.

The doctrines found in spiritualism are that men are unfallen demigods; each mind will judge itself, that true knowledge places all men above the moral law; that all sins committed are innocent, for whatever is, is right, and God doth not condemn. These same teachings can be found in theosophy.

The Theosophical Society was founded in 1875 by Helen Blavatsky and Henry Olcott. Mrs. Blavatsky stated that she came from Tibet where she said she had been initiated into esoteric doctrines. Annie Besant, an English lady, was Blavatsky's successor in leadership of the Theosophical Society. She (Annie Besant) became vice president of Co-Masonry. In France, women had been allowed to enter the Masonic Order in this branch called Co-Masonry. Mrs. Besant led the movement for three decades.[12]

---

[10] Miller, op. cit., pp. 220, 221; Reported in Kah, Gary; *En Route to Global Occupation*, Huntington House Pub., Lafayette, LA (1992), p. 124.

[11] Webster, op. cit., p. 150.

[12] Kah, op. cit., pp. 89.

Alternative & Mystical Healing Therapies

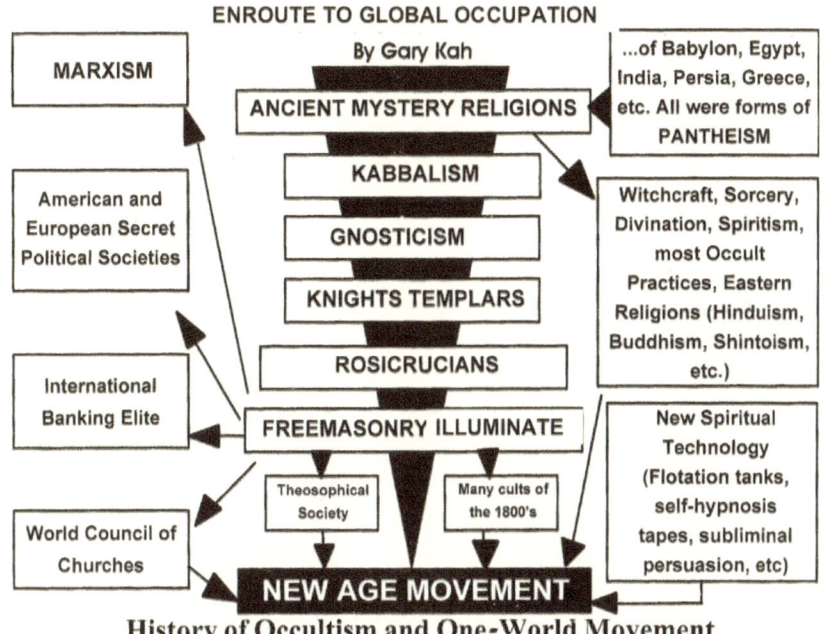

History of Occultism and One-World Movement

Figure 14. Graph of secret societies.

Cardinal Caro Y. Rodriguez, archbishop of Santiago, Chile, in exposing the Masonic Order, wrote:

> Madame Blavatsky, the promoter or founder of theosophy in Europe, was also a member of the Masonic Lodge; her successor, Annie Besant, president of the Theosophical Society in 1911 was vice president and great teacher of the Supreme Council of the International Order of Co-Masonry—and among us, in our city, the brother masons are the ones that contribute mostly to spread of the Theosophical Society.[13]

He summarized his comments on Co-Masonry as follows:

---

[13] Rodriguez, Cardinal Carl Y., *The Mystery of Free Masonry Unveiled*, Hawthorne, CA, Christian Book Club of America 1971, pp. 336, 238. Reported in Kah. op. cit., p. 90.

> It is understood: the theosophical doctrines on the nature of God and the soul are the same doctrines as taught in masonry; it is enough to read the books dealing with the history of theosophy to see that each theosophical center is founded, almost without a doubt by members of the Lodge.[14]

Nesta Webster, in *Secret Societies* and *Subversive Movements* (pp. 297–310), discusses the association of theosophy with the Grand Orient lodges of France.

The third leader in this movement was Alice Bailey who lived in the United States. Under the guidance of a spirit guide (Djwhal Khul, also known as the Tibetan Master), she wrote approximately twenty books from messages channeled from this spirit guide and which have been the foundation and guide for the New Age movement.[15] This movement is the major promoter of "mystical medicine" in the United States and around the world. It also has been very effective in drawing millions of people to the belief of theosophy.

Alice Bailey was closely connected to the Masonic Order. The following excerpt from her book, *The Externalization of the Hierarchy*, states:

> The Masonic Movement—It is the custodian of the law; it is the home of the mysteries and the seat of initiation. It holds in its symbolism the ritual of deity, and the way of salvation is pictorially preserved in its work.[16]

Constance Cumbey, in her book *The Hidden Dangers of the Rainbow*, on page 46, states that from her research, she learned that the Theosophical Society in 1875 received orders from "spirit messengers" that the organization was to remain secret for one hundred years. They worked quietly but were still able to spread their dogma to the world. In 1975, they went public with their presence and programs.[17]

EAST-WEST

---

[14] *Ibid.*

[15] Cumbey, Constance; *The Hidden Dangers of the Rainbow*, Huntington House Inc., Shreveport, LA (1983), pp. 49–50.

[16] Bailey, Alice; *Externalization of the Hierarchy*, Lucis Publishing Co., New York, NY (1983), p. 511. Reported in Kah, op. cit. p. 89.

[17] Cumbey, op. cit., p. 46.

In 1989, I began receiving at my medical office a journal called *New Age*. It contained only holistic-type medical articles. All of its advertisements were for products relevant to holistic health practices (techniques based on pantheistic concepts). I had no idea who sent it to me. (It was an expensive magazine.) In 1992, I read in a book, *En Route to Global Occupation,* by Gary Kah, that someone had been able to make contact with the publishers of this journal (*New Age*) and inquired about advertising. They received a letter in return, and on the letterhead, these words identified the source of this journal: *"Ancient and Accepted Scottish Rite of Free Masonry."* Finally, I had the answer as to who was sending the journal to my office. The magazine soon thereafter changed its name to *East-West.*

Michael Howard (who is not a critic but a sympathizer of this pantheistic theology) writes the following:

> A very important work of the *secret societies* has always been the *ultimate unification of the world religions.* This aim was based on the restoration of the pre-Christian Mystery Tradition, which had been persecuted by the early Church and forced to go underground in medieval Europe, and the recognition that all religions had originated in a universal spirituality referred to as the *Ancient Wisdom.*
>
> It forms the basis for the ancient Egyptian mysteries, Gnosticism, esoteric Christianity, the Cabbala, the Hermetic Tradition, Alchemy, and societies such as the Templars, Freemasons, and Rosicrucian's, the occult doctrines of geomancy, alchemy, astrology, and sexual magic taught by these secret societies were used as symbolic metaphors illustrating the progression of the individual from material darkness to the spiritual light of understanding[18] (emphasis added).

These organizations are some of the powers behind the New Age Movement and its pagan system of health and healing which has been the right arm of their missionary endeavors. The following chapter will deal in more detail and specific healing practices.

---

[18] Howard, Michael; *The Occult Conspiracy: Secret Societies: Their Influence and Power in World History*; Destiny Books, Rochester, VT, p.170, 171.

6

MEDITATION: AYURVEDA THE ANCIENT HEALING TRADITION OF INDIA

Part I

THE GREAT WISDOM OF THE EAST?

While attending a mini seminar on alternative medicine, I was impressed by the enthusiasm of those putting on the demonstration. When asked how these treatments work, the answer was "we do not know, but it works." There was comment about the "great wisdom from the East." It was insinuated that great knowledge of healing from the past had been abandoned, but it was being resurrected, and we were being recipients of it.

This comment brought to memory that which I had learned of the healing methods of the past, from the West and East, but I could not recall any knowledge in the history of medicine that we were neglecting. In fact, I could only give thanks that we had left most of the old knowledge to the past. This was especially true of the basic concepts of anatomy, physiology, and disease including the old concept of its cause. The old worldview explaining man's existence, his purpose in life, and his future is definitely not in harmony with the biblical worldview.

Therefore, I determined to prepare a presentation about the ancient healing methods of the East. The West has its own history in occult healing modalities, and today we see a blending of the two, hence the expression "East-West." Outside of God's original plan for health and healing, the oldest continuous system of medicine is called Ayurveda. It had its beginning in the Indus River Valley in Northern India sometime before 1700 BC.

> It was established by the same ancient sages (holy men) who produced India's original system of meditation, yoga, and astrology. Ayurveda has both a spiritual and practical basis.[1]

The word *Ayurveda* is derived from two words of the Sanskrit language. *Ayus* and *vid,* meaning life and knowledge, respectively. Ayus, or life, represents a combination of the body, the sense organs, the mind, and the soul. The Ayurveda healing tradition is an integral part of the Hindu religion. *Vedas* are ancient Hindu books of knowledge said to have been "divinely revealed" to ancient sages (holy men). The Vedas, written in Sanskrit, were started more than three thousand five hundred years ago.[2] The Vedas are believed to embody the rhythm, knowledge, and arrangement of the universe, the secrets to sickness, health, and healing. As the living sage of astrology in India, Dr. B.V. Raman has written:

> The influences of planets on human diseases appear with such persistence that it is impossible to ignore their effect. The sun and the moon provide the strongest influence on human healing, and their movements indicate changes not only in the seasons but also in human health and behavior.[3]

> According to Ayurveda, everything in the material creation is composed of combinations of the five elements: space, air, fire, water, and earth. These five elements derive from, and are the manifestations of, an unmanifest and undifferentiated *Creative Principle*, which is One (universal energy).[4]

The Creative Principle is believed to manifest throughout the universe as *two great antagonistic forces* which continually create, sustain, and destroy all that exists in the universe. These forces (in Sanskrit) are called rajas

---

[1] Gerson, Scott, MD, Ayurveda, *The Ancient Indian Healing Art,* Element Inc., Rockport, Mass., (1993), p. 3.

[2] Lyons, Albert S., MD, Petrucelli, II, R. Joseph, MD, *Medicine: An Illustrated History;* Harry N. Abrams, Inc., Publishers, New York (1978), p. 105.

[3] Warrier, Gopi; Deepika Gunawan, MD, *The Complete Illustrated Guide to Ayurveda,* Barnes and Noble Books (1997), p. 170.

[4] Gerson, op. cit., p. 3.

and tamas, to the Chinese, yin and yang (dualism). In Ayurveda, there is a belief that three psychic forces govern the mental and spiritual health. This system and its explanation are derived from astrology. The Chinese zodiac utilizes the movement of 108 planetary bodies through our galaxy for use in divination. These heavenly bodies are, in the occult world, symbolic of deities, false gods of paganism. The spirits of *five of these planets* are believed to be *elemental energies/creative spirits* involved in creation and its continuation. Synonyms for these astrological elemental energies/spirits are shown here: Jupiter/Zeus/Wood; Mars/Ares/Fire; Saturn/Cronos/Earth; Venus/Aphrodite/Metal; Mercury/Hermes/Water. Everything in Hinduism, Buddhism, and pagan religions' cosmologies are based on these astrological roots.

> The basis of all treatments in the Ayurvedic system is the balancing of the life energies within us.[5] Meditation is a primary and fundamental tool in this balancing therapy which uses diets, herbs, mineral substances, and aromas as well.[6]
>
> Ayurveda teaches that the "mind-body" has the intelligence and ability to heal itself. This intelligence is believed to operate in the macrocosm (cosmos)—which also directs the yearly migration of birds, the seasons and their changes, the movement of tides, the positioning and movement of the planets and stars in the universe, and also the human physiology referred to as the microcosm. It is the sole function of Ayurveda to promote the flow of this great intelligence (universal energy) through each and every human being.[7]

In the Hindu thought and in Ayurveda healing tradition, the Creative Principle, as an indescribable force, might be referred to as the unified energy field which underlies all of creation. Ayurvedic physicians see man simultaneously as energy and matter and view diseases in the same way.

The previous paragraphs have given very briefly the basic astrological—cosmological foundation from which Ayurvedic medicine is derived. We will now look at how it is applied. The dominant healing practice of India was Ayurveda. It is interesting that there was also conventional medical care. India was known for its advanced surgical skills during the dark ages, while Europe

---

[5] *Ibid.*, p. 5.

[6] *Ibid.*

[7] *Ibid.*, p. 6.

Alternative & Mystical Healing Therapies

lost its skills and knowledge. So we had alongside each other, without apparent conflict, astrological-based practice of healing, as well as medical practice that was not based on the Hindu religion and cosmology. The basic therapeutics developed in Ayurvedic medicine gradually spread to the world, first to Tibet and then on to China, Japan, and to the rest of the East. It also spread to Persia and the Arabian Empire in the eleventh century. In the Middle Ages, it showed up in Europe.[8] And it is evident that in the United States, its influence was present in methods of treatment in the 1700s and early 1800s.

In Ayurvedic medicine, two forces make up these supposed divisions of energy, together called life force. A third division of energy is added and is made up of parts of the other two. Man is said to have had his *origin* from the mingling of these forces in a proper balance. In Ayurvedic teachings, health depends upon the perfect balance among the three forces.

When imbalance is present in these energy divisions called doshas, dysfunction or disease supposedly occurs. It is believed that balancing the doshas will restore health. Ayurvedic medicine has, as *its goal—the balancing of doshas*, these divisions of energy.

> The doshas are identified with the three supposed universal forces: sun, moon, and wind.[9]

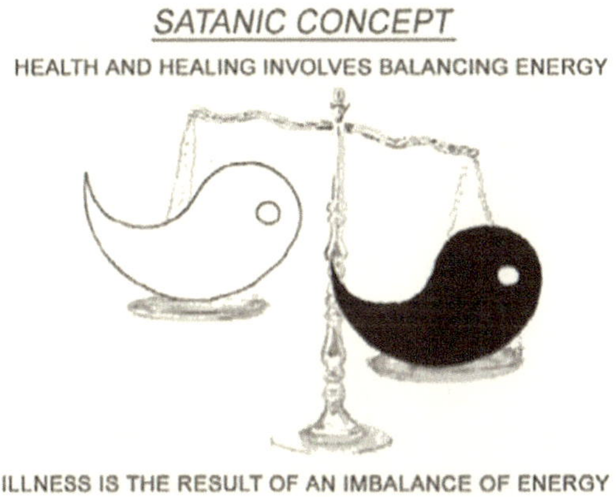

SATANIC CONCEPT
HEALTH AND HEALING INVOLVES BALANCING ENERGY

ILLNESS IS THE RESULT OF AN IMBALANCE OF ENERGY

Figure 15. Scales with yin and yang.

---

[8] Lyons, op. cit., p.105.
[9] Raso, MD, RD, *Mystical Diets*, Promethius Books, Buffalo, NY (1993), p. 87.

CHAKRAS–AURA

Ayurveda teaches that there are *seven* centers of concentrated, focused universal energy in the body, which collectively form an *aura*, an invisible light to the "nonsensitive," which surrounds a person. There are *sensitives* who say they can see the colored light of the aura. These energy centers start at the coccyx area and then are said to be located in the sacral, mid-abdomen, heart, throat, behind the eyes, and on the top of the head, all having connection to or close association with the spinal cord. A center is called chakra, meaning "wheel," which can be considered a "whirling vortex" of energy. Think of a cyclone as a vortex of swirling cone-shaped energy powered by hot air beneath and cold above, representing dualism. Dualism is incorporated in the explanation of the swirling energy of the chakra as being powered by doshas (rajas and tamas) to bring energy balance. Dualism is a foundational concept in Ayurveda and oriental religions.

Chakras are supposed to promote and regulate the spread of universal energy to the organs of the body, each center focusing on distributing energy to certain organs in its anatomical area. The energy is distributed from the chakras via *nadis*, which are invisible nonanatomical channels proceeding out from the chakras to carry energy. There is said to be seventy-two thousand *nadis*.

Ayurveda is founded upon the belief in the universal energy theory and postulate that all living objects have an energy field outside of and surrounding the body, which is said to influence other energy fields. Seven rays of colored light constitute this energy field, believed to represent seven endocrine glands. The harmony and energy balance of the individual is believed to be ascertained by observing this aura. Ayurveda also teaches that:

> Every animate and inanimate substance, provided its function is not impaired, has an "aura," which exists because of the life forces inherent in the natural constituents of its form. This life force, whether from mineral, vegetable, animal, or human sources, creates a common auric realm or plane, which is a storehouse of pure, untapped energy. On this plane, the mineral and vegetable kingdoms are constantly engaged, through their own channels of communication, in transferring their particular life force to the more subtle natures of animals and humans.

Thus, the aura depicts the sum total of all these qualities and presents a complete and whole picture of the subject.[10]

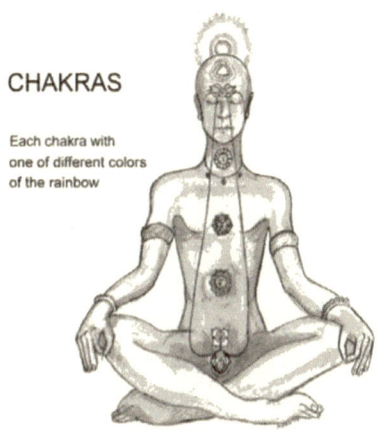

Figure 16. Chakras.

Ann Hill, in her book *A Visual Encyclopedia of Unconventional Medicine*, describes the *aura* as seven rays of the *presumed* human unified energy field, forming seven colors. Each individual is said to have different frequencies of these rays. She tells us that the aura can be drawn by a trained *sensitive*, viewing the aura or by observing some object an individual has handled. A *sensitive* of special skills is said to be able to determine a person's mental and spiritual state, as well as to diagnose illness if present, by inspection of the aura. The nature of the color, bright or dull, reveals and determines the physical condition and/or health and also a person's spiritual status.

This *aura* or *magnetic energy field* cannot be demonstrated by science. It can be perceived only by persons who are *sensitive* or *mediumistic*.

In the chapter on universal energy, we learned about the hypothesized concept of the division of universal energy into seven electromagnetic frequency levels. The lowest frequency level is at the speed of light, and all other levels are at a greatly increased frequency speed. This concept is not in harmony with known laws of physics that are understood today. The subject of the seven chakras is not the same as seven frequency levels. The lower chakras in the anatomical positions are said to handle and process

---

[10] Hill, Ann, *A Visual Encyclopedia of Unconventional Medicine*, Crown Publishing Inc. NY (1978), p. 46.

energy at low levels of frequency and that higher chakras handle high frequency levels. Chakras are supposed to be able to act as transformers and convert low frequency levels of energy to higher levels, passing the energy up the chain of chakras and vice versa with the top chakras transforming high frequency energy into lower levels, passing it downward to the lowest chakra which is able to pass this energy into the physical body.

The higher frequency levels of energy are believed to come from the cosmos through the top chakra at the top of the head to be passed down the other chakras and eventually throughout the body. As a person is able to raise, by meditation and yoga, his *subtle energies* to the level of the top chakra, those energies are interchanged with the energies of the cosmos. Also, plant food is believed to possess midlevel frequencies of energy; this, in turn, influences the middle-level chakras. Universal energy also comes to the body via the air (prana) we breathe, which is believed to be a major source of subtle energy. The *aura*, which is supposedly produced from the sum total energies of the seven chakras and emanates light outside of the body, can be felt, seen, and influenced by an *aura* of another, by coming into close proximity, by application of hands, and with special procedures of sending energy over a distance to another.

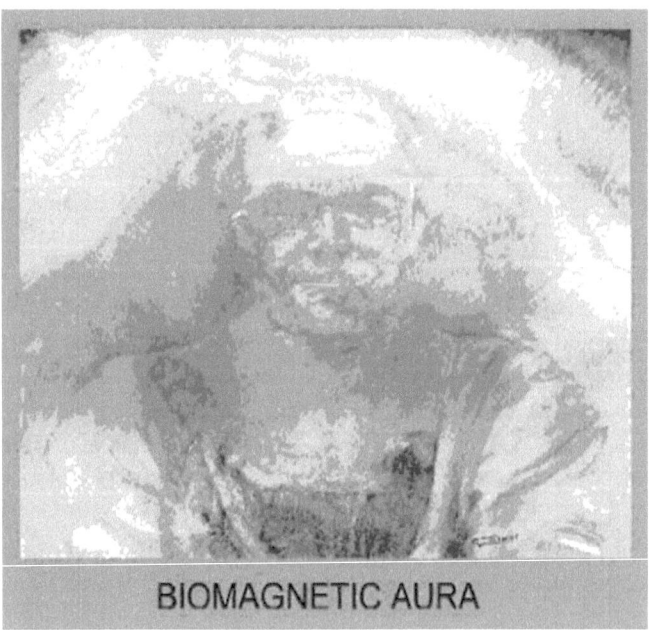

Figure 17. Picture of biomagnetic aura.

The root chakra (chakra no. 1 at the coccyx) is also regarded as the seat of *kundalini*. The *kundalini* is symbolized as a coiled serpent within the sacral/coccygeal region. The coiled serpent represents a powerful subtle force that is poised and waiting to spring into action. Only when the proper meditative and attitudinal changes have occurred does this force become directed upwards through the appropriate spinal pathway and activate each of the major chakras during its ascent to the crown. The *kundalini* is the creative force of manifestation which assists in the alignment of the chakras, the release of stored stress from the bodily centers, and the lifting of consciousness into higher spiritual levels.[11]

The chakras are said to be in the colors of the rainbow, with each chakra having a specific color. Each aura has a frequency of resonance or vibration and emits a fine electrical current and in turn can receive vital energies from external influences. This is the source of belief in *"vibrational medicine."* The human body is said to be a symphony of color, including the skeleton. The various colors we apply to the body with

> (a) clothing, walls, illumination, or (b) by mental image-making, counseling, and guided meditation, (c) through projection, on the spiritual level, to any person anywhere, is believed to build the forces and strength of the chakras and the aura to effect healing.[12]

When "magenta," an eighth color is added, an octave is produced, and then music is also able to influence the chakras. Gems are known to refract light, dividing it into different colors. Sunlight consists of seven colors of the rainbow, so it is believed these refracted sunrays from gems can increase the energy (vibrations) of the chakra specific to each hue of sunlight.

> The seven natural colors, with the added eighth (magenta), are used in therapy when there is an energy imbalance. The colors are red, orange, yellow, green, turquoise, blue, violet, and the added eighth color, magenta. It is believed that these colors correspond with three musical octaves and with twenty-four

---

[11] Gerber, Richard, MD, *Vibrational Medicine, The No. 1 Handbook of Subtle Energy Therapies*, Bear and Co., Rochester, Vermont (2001), p. 389.

[12] Hill, op. cit., p. 219.

vertebrae of the spinal column. Two additional octaves have been added so that infrared can be applied to the sacrum and ultraviolet to the skull. Employed by the music therapist and astrologer *to dowse* (use the pendulum) out the problem areas of a patient and thus determine which color is to be used in treatment.[13]

Color therapy is also performed by placing water in a colored glass vessel and letting the sun shine through it. The water is then ingested, thereby applying color therapy to correct imbalances in the aura. This type of treatment is still practiced. It is not necessary to visualize color, as therapy can be administered even to blind people with equal benefit, it is believed, by having them drink the sunlight-exposed water.

Nutrition and dietetics figure importantly in many of these healing systems. For example, in the yoga-oriented *Spiritual Nutrition and the Rainbow Diet* (1986), Gabriel Cousens, MD, states,

> By putting foods of various colors over each chakra (spiritual center of the human body), I was able to determine which colors were most enhancing for each chakra.[14]

The aura (composite energy) of a person is also believed to be influenced by sound and/or music. Music therapy is another method of restoring an imbalanced aura.

Each animate and inanimate object is also believed to have a specific energy frequency or vibration. (Not all believers in the aura accept that inanimate objects have an aura.) These vibrations are altered when disorder is present in the body. It is claimed that detection of altered vibrational forces can be done by the hands, Kirlian photography, or by radiesthesia using electronic instruments. Energy therapies and vibrational therapies, of which there are many varieties, seek to understand this continuous energetic aura and to interact with it in order to facilitate health and healing.

The above-described beliefs and teachings of Ayurvedic medicine form the foundation of many ideas that are widespread in the field of alternative therapies today. I wish to make it clear to the reader that the above-described beliefs are not accepted in the sciences of medicine,

---

[13] *Ibid.*, p. 218.

[14] Raso, op. cit., p. 13.

physics, and physiology. The detection of the basic energy, which is the center core belief of alternative therapy, cannot be found or measured by even the most sensitive instruments, a discrepancy that cannot be explained by its adherents.

I recommend an article found on the Internet, "Human Auras and Energy Fields" by Don Lindsay,[15] which discusses the subject of auras and whether or not science can demonstrate such. The following is his summary:

> Humans do not have auras. There is no kind of "energy field" consistently found around humans. I say this for a bunch of reasons:
>
> * It is the consensus of the scientific and medical communities.
> * Proponents have had a lot of years to produce positive evidence.
> * Negative evidence from equipment.
> * Negative evidence from photography.
> * Negative evidence from those who see auras.
> * Negative evidence from those who feel auras.

For those readers who might wish to further investigate the argument that there is proof of auras, I suggest the following specific article that claims there is scientific proof:

> Spring Wolf's Spiritual Education Network
> Chakras and Magic
> The Aura
> The Colors of Life[16]

It is important not to confuse the claimed energy of the chakra and aura of Ayurveda, with the bioelectrical activity of living matter. There is certainly electrical activity within our bodies as is demonstrated by electrocardiographs, electroencephalographs, electromyography, etc. To do any of these tests, it is necessary to either place needle probes into and under the skin or to prepare the skin by sanding the outer layer of

---

[15] *http://www.don-lindsay-archive.org/skeptic/* HYPERLINK *"http://www.don-lindsay-archive.org/skeptic/auras.html""* HYPERLINK "http://www.don-lindsay-archive.org/skeptic/auras.html"" HYPERLINK "http://www.don-lindsay-archive.org/skeptic/auras.html" auras.html

[16] http://sacredwicca.jigsy.com/chakras.jigsy

cells free to make good electrical contact on the skin. With the proper contact, electrical activity is then demonstrated in muscles and nerves. No electrical machines have shown electrical activity of a chakra or of an aura inside or outside of the body. There is instrumentation that is one million times more sensitive than the living tissue of our bodies. However, these electrical measuring instruments do not show evidence of chakras—inside the body or auras—outside the body.

Not all practitioners of Eastern mysticism accept the explanation that universal energy can be explained by conventional physics and object to the term *electromagnetic* in describing such. They believe that universal energy is a spiritual entity and that it cannot be described by common scientific terminology. Many modern scientists who are believers of Eastern mysticism do, however, attempt to explain their beliefs by scientific terms. Some psychics claim to be able to see the aura in color around individuals. When put to the test on these claims, they failed. If light from the believed *aura* did surround our bodies, we might see rainbows about us when we are in the rain and the sun shines through the clouds. It would be very easy to demonstrate the colors of the rainbow by an optical prism held near the body if light was flowing from us, but this does not happen. The colors of the rainbow are light wave frequencies that are detected by the eyes of all of us, not just psychics or sensitives.

Dr. Elmer Green, who has his doctorate in physics and is a lifetime believer in Eastern mysticism, explains this concept: This universal energy, which is in question with science, exists in seven levels or degrees. The first level is the materialization of the energy, and that is the material world around us. The other six levels are not measurable by instruments because those levels are beyond instrumentation detection. Only the human body is capable of detecting such (see chapter 19 on biofeedback). It is taught that these different levels of energy can exist simultaneously within the human body.

Oriental religions have, as their purpose and goal in life, to escape the cycle of reincarnation in which they believe they are caught up and to join the spirit world. They do this by a lifelong pursuit of raising the energy levels in the body up through the chakras to bring it to its peak performance at the seventh chakra on top of the head. The religious activities of the Hindu and other oriental religions are all for the purpose of maintaining an unhindered flow of universal energy so as to raise the energy level to its zenith at the top chakra. Meditation and yoga are believed to raise kundalini and clear the chakras to allow the rising of universal energy, and their existence is solely for this purpose. When the universal energy comes in full power to the top chakra, a person's energy level has meshed with the energy of the universe, and one experiences enlightenment, the supreme self, lotus, jewel, *godhood* status. The reincarnation cycle is then broken, and at death of the physical body, the soul will assume its position with the spirit world of nirvana.

During the pursuit of immortality status described above, disorder or illness of the physical body may occur. This is understood simply as an interruption of flow of universal energy through the body, and corrective measures have been invented to correct and bring about the continued free flow of energy. It is those therapeutic methods that constitute many of present-day alternative medical therapies. It is vital to have understanding of the foundational doctrine of the oriental religions so as to recognize their counterfeit of God's healing system and the false science proclaimed.

Meditation and yoga are simple yet powerful techniques believed to open, activate, and cleanse congested or blocked flow of energy in chakras. Their most common use in America is for "relaxation"; however, meditation is far more than that. It opens the mind to connect to the cosmic energies, the universal mind, the *higher self (the pantheistic god)*. We are told that the higher self holds the solutions to many of our problems.[17]

Understanding the tenets of Ayurveda and Hindu's basic dogmas is critical to understand therapeutic methods to be exposed later in this book. A vast amount of New Age doctrines and therapies are based upon the principles of what has been presented.

MEDITATION

Ayurveda uses meditation as a primary and fundamental tool for healing. It also promotes yoga, diet, herbs, mineral substances, cleansing practices, and aromas for maintenance or restoration of energy balance. Meditation and yoga are fundamental *tools* of Hinduism for progression to a higher spiritual plane, with the goal of leaving this life on earth and moving on into the spirit world. In Ayurvedic medicine, meditation is fundamental to accessing the powers of the cosmos in order to bring increase and balance of the energies within a person. It is also a process, physically and mentally, of trying to elevate the believed *divine* attributes within oneself and connect with the god of the cosmos (Brahman), the ultimate deity of Hinduism. Meditation, whether for health or spiritual reasons, is a way of *connecting with the spirit world*. It is through meditation that blending of the sun and moon energies are said to occur. When a perfect blend is achieved, immortality is said to be the result. Immortality is believed to bring perfect harmony with Brahman, the ultimate Hindu deity.

---

[17] Gerber, op. Cit., p. 391.

The above is the Hindu plan of salvation (counterfeit of God's plan), the journey to nirvana, their heaven. It is centered in the dogma of *self—divine within*. By physical and mental acts, it is believed that the divine within can be manipulated, resulting in progression to immortality, nirvana, and godhood. Physical disorders are considered simply a spiritual malady. Therapeutics are anticipated not only to relieve physical and mental distress but also to restore the individual to the path of progression to godhood.

Ayurveda declares the *essence* of the human being to be the *One*, the *Creative Principle*, the *Eternal Essence*. A Hindu physicist might describe this essence as the *ultimate unified energy field*, which Ayurveda says underlies all of creation. Humans are seen as energy converted to matter and disease as deranged energy. This life energy, also called prana, is believed to be enhanced through meditation, yoga, deep breathing, herbs, cleansing, and foods. Life energy (prana) is proclaimed to increase with deep breathing of air *through the nose*.

> Of all the many forms of treatment described in the Ayurvedic texts, there is one which holds a pre-eminent position—*the practice of meditation*. This is the fertile soil upon which all other forms of therapy take root. Strictly speaking, without meditation, the true healing potential of Ayurvedic medicine cannot be realized.[18]

The English word *meditation* has two definitions:

1. Study, contemplation, pondering on or about a subject by an active thought process
2. Putting the mind into a passive, neutral—no thought mode, stilling the mind, ridding our mind of all thoughts, *the silence*, and so develop an altered state of consciousness

In our discussion of *meditation* in the Ayurveda system, we refer to this second definition. To enlarge upon the above definitions, think of it in this way: study, contemplation, and pondering can be thought of as looking outward and upward, while the passive mode puts our thoughts inward and downward.

How does one bring about the nonthinking state? We find an answer in *Meditation as Medicine* (page 25) by Dharma Singh Khalsa, MD. It is achieved by the powerful effects of:

---

[18] Gerson, op. cit., p. p. 78, 79.

1. the breath
2. a mantra (repetition of word or phrase)
3. focusing the mind
4. posture and movement including finger positions[19]

Of the four acts given above in performing meditation, the *two* most common and important are attention to *breath* and repetition of a *mantra*. As the mind focuses on the breathing pattern and at the same time on the repetitions of a word or phrase, a thoughtless state of the mind is triggered. The word *mantra* is from the Sanskrit language with the syllable *man*, meaning "to think," and *tra*, referring to "liberation of thinking." By an act and process that stops the mind from thinking, the mind is *stilled*. The subject of movement will be explored further in the discussion of yoga. Meditation and yoga go together like a hand in a glove. Yoga will be presented later in the next chapter.

Meditation is practiced in many forms and by many names; some we probably have not recognized as being meditation. In his book *Meditation as Medicine*, Dr. Khalsa lists the following practices as being considered meditation using a common element—relaxation.

- Prayer—contemplative prayer, breath prayer, silence; (uses breath and mantra)
- Visualization—an *act of creation* by imagination, using god—power from within
- Sufi meditation—found in Islam, "whirling dervishes," feverish dancing
- Guided Imagery—similar to visualization, minimizes thinking in words
- Mindfulness—Buddha-type meditation, mind wanders as it focuses on breath
- The Relaxation Response—meditation, named so as to disguise, by H. Benson, MD
- Transcendental Meditation—with secret mantra, brought to USA by Maharishi Mahesh Yogi and popularized by the Beatles
- Zen Buddhist Meditation—way to enlightenment, worldview—one is all, all is one
- Native American Meditation—drums, psychedelic herbs, crystals
- Movement Meditation—tai chi, qigong, martial arts, *yoga exercises* (added by author)

---

[19] Khalsa, Dharma Singh, MD, Stauth, Cameron, *Meditation as Medicine*, fireside Rockefeller Center, New York, NY (2001), p. 25.

- Medical Meditation—meditation combined with yoga and specific postures of body, limbs, and fingers. Khalsa says, it is the most powerful type of meditation.[20]

Continued practice of meditation over time causes gradual changes in the mystical subtle energy flow through the chakras. They are slowly activated and cleared of any obstruction of flow, such as past traumatic emotional events, that of frustration or anger, etc. Overtime meditation will initiate a rise of *kundalini*—serpent power which is believed to be in the bottom chakra, forcing its climb up the subtle energy pathways (chakras) and within the spinal cord on its journey to the crown chakra and *enlightenment—godhood*.

Meditation and yoga are fundamental *tools* of Hinduism for progressing to a higher spiritual plane, with the goal of leaving this life on earth and moving into the spirit world. In Ayurvedic medicine, meditation is fundamental to accessing the powers of the cosmos in order to bring increase and balance of the energies within a person. It is also a process, physically and mentally, of trying to elevate the believed divine attributes within oneself and connect with the god of the cosmos (Brahman), the ultimate deity of Hinduism. Meditation, whether for health or spiritual reasons, is a way of connecting with the spirit world. It is through meditation that blending of the sun and moon energies are said to occur. When a perfect blend is achieved, immortality is the result of being in harmony with Brahman, the Hindu deity.

Transcendental meditation was brought to the USA by Maharishi Mahesh Yogi in 1957 and popularized by the Beatles music group and is a slight variant style of meditation. A secret mantra word is given to each initiate. Unbeknownst to the initiate, the word is a title or name of a Hindu god. Hunt and Weldon comment on this secret mantra in *America: The Sorcerer's New Apprentice* (page 31) stating that from authoritative texts, not only is the mantra the name of a Hindu god, but also by reciting it over and over, one is calling on that god to possess them. TM (Transcendental Meditation) worked its way into the New Jersey Public School system, and parents sued saying that it was a religion, but TM lawyers argued that it was a science. The New Jersey Federal Court decided it was a religion and banned its presence in the schools (Malnak v. Yogi, 440 F. Supp. 1284–1977). The decision was appealed, and on February 2, 1979, the first court decision was upheld. TM thereafter took out every word in their written material that would indicate that it was religious, and it has since

---

[20] *Ibid.*, p. 40

spread across the United States as *science*. Below is the pledge to Maharishi that every teacher of TM has to sign:

> "Serve the Holy Tradition and spread the light of God to all those who need it." Yet every TM teacher claims in his public lecture, "TM is not a religion."[21]

Dave Hunt in *Yoga and the Body of Christ* (pages 12–16) exposes the planned and designed missionary movement of Hinduism that has spread to the world. He shares with the reader that the largest missionary organization in the world is Hindu—India's *Vishva Hindu Parishad* (VHP). Also, in January 1979, this organization sponsored a second "World Congress on Hinduism" in Allahabad, India, and with sixty thousand delegates attending. This organization had first attempted their mission activities by promoting religion, but that was not successful. So they made a change by presenting it as science. A speaker at the 1979 congress made the following comment:

> Our mission in the West has been crowned with fantastic success. Hinduism is becoming the dominant world religion, and the end of Christianity has come near.[22]

The VHP organization has centers all over the world, with a branch in the USA called Vishwa Hindu Parashad of America, Inc.

A writer with exceptional discernment and perception warned long ago concerning that mind therapies and spiritualism would deceive many by coming in as a science. The comment was made that in later days when skepticism and unbelief so often appear in a scientific garb, we need to be cautious. Through this means, the great adversary is deceiving thousands and leading them captive. The advantage the devil takes by use of the sciences, *sciences which pertain to the human mind*, is tremendous. Here, serpentlike, he imperceptibly creeps in to counteract the work of God.

The practices of yoga and meditation are not without their dangers. Suicide is high among the instructors: demon possession, psychopathology, psychosis, epileptic seizures, hallucination, blackouts for hours, eyesight problems, extreme stomach cramps, mental confusion, sexual licentiousness,

---

[21] Weldon, John, *The Transcendental Explosion*, Irvine harvest House (1976), pp. 23–24; reported in Wilson and Weldon, *Occult Shock and Psychic Forces*, Master Books, a Division of CLP, p. 35.

[22] Hunt, Dave, *Yoga and the Body of Christ*, The Berean call (2006), OR, p. 13.

severe nightmares, antisocial behavior, recurrence of psychosomatic symptoms, and depression requiring psychiatric care. *America, the Sorcerer's Apprentice* (page 51) states so severe and so common are abnormal reactions to meditation and yoga that in 1980 Johns Hopkins University School of Medicine professor Stanislave Grof (expert in LSD) and his wife Christina (instructor in hatha yoga) organized the "Spiritual Emergency Network" (SEN), now headquartered at the California Institute of Transpersonal Psychology in Menlo Park, California. By 1988, the organization (SEN) was coordinating thirty-five regional centers and utilizing one thousand five hundred professionals in attempting to handle psychological emergencies resulting from the mind-altering practices of meditation and yoga.

Dr. Khalsa tells us in his book that the *Relaxation Response*, which Khalsa identifies as a *form of meditation*, was made popular by Harvard's Herbert Benson, MD.

> He [Benson] made meditation palatable to the medical community.[23]

The Office of Alternative Medicine, or OAM, which is a part of the National Institutes of Health, has funded many studies on meditation. A 1994 report stated that:

> "Over a period of 25 years, Benson and colleagues have developed a large body of research. "Meditation in general and the relaxation response in specific have slowly moved from alternative to mainstream medicine, although they are still overlooked by many conventional doctors."[24]

The techniques used in Benson's *The Relaxation Response* are identical to those used in all other forms of meditation, namely concentration on breathing, posture or position of comfort, passive attitude, and use of a mantra. Unfortunately, there have been people who have not recognized the relaxation response for what it is and using a biblical term or verse as a mantra have felt it was just what its name speaks of, a simple measure to bring relaxation. Unfortunately, it is much more than that. It, too, is a technique to still the mind, to bring in passivity to the thinking, and to allow an altered state of consciousness. There are physiologic changes in our autonomic nervous system when the relaxation response is used such

---

[23] Khalsa, op. cit., p. 7.

[24] *Ibid.*, p. 41.

as in the amount of oxygen consumed, and apparently, many healthful changes can occur without use of drugs. Yet in that state, we open our mind up to the possibility of contact with and control by powers of darkness.

These meditation or relaxation techniques have demonstrated decrease in oxygen consumption by the body, lower hydrocortisone blood levels, increase in immune factors (including increased leukocytes), and it calms brain wave activity. These benefits remain for several hours following meditation. Yes, these methods do have an effect on our physiology; however, we must determine the source of this power and influence upon our systems.

Has there been a comparison of this apparently harmless technique with other forms of meditation? Yes, it was compared to transcendental meditation, the results of which are summarized in the following statement:

> Tests at the Thorndike Memorial Laboratory of Harvard have shown that a similar technique used with any sound or phrase or prayer or mantra brings forth the same physiologic changes noted during transcendental meditation: decreased oxygen consumption; decreased carbon dioxide elimination; decreased rate of breathing. In other words, using the basic necessary components, any one of the *age-old* or the *newly derived* techniques produce the same physiologic results regardless *of* the mental device used.[25]

Are these changes from simple relaxation of our nerves, or is there another power apart from our Creator God at work? If another power, then from where? That is the question. Have I made accusation against innocent techniques? A question I have asked multiple times of myself. Well, I find that those involved in leading out and teaching in the field of meditation and yoga have included the relaxation response technique as one of their own but simply changed to an acceptable name.

How an individual becomes interested in or starts practicing yoga and/or meditation has much to do with whether they continue. When a doctor recommends this practice to deal with certain medical problems, the tendency to stay with it greatly increases. Frequent articles appear in medical literature proclaiming the medical benefits of yoga and meditation, so we see an ever increasing acceptance by the medical profession.

---

[25] Benson, Herbert, MD, *Relaxation Response*, Wings Books, distributed by Outlet Books Company, Inc., Avenel, New Jersey (1990), pp. 162–163.

Herbert Benson, MD, a Harvard University Medical School professor and president of the Mind/Body/Medical Institute in Chestnut Hill, Massachusetts, tells in his book *The Relaxation Response* that his research group has studied all the forms of meditation used down through millennia by various religions. His research found certain essential acts paramount to reaching the altered state of consciousness and/or autonomic nervous system influences sought by the act of meditation. These are: comfortable position; muscular relaxation; deep rhythmic breathing; use of a mantra—all to bring the mind to a state of *passivity*. The mantra can be a word, a phrase, a sentence, or even a Bible verse.

You may have been surprised to see "prayer" listed as one of the forms of meditation. How can that be? Is not prayer a dialogue with God? The Bible has recorded many prayers, and Christ prayed and taught his disciples to pray. Daniel chapter 9 reveals Daniel pleading with God to forgive Israel and fulfill His pledge to return them to Canaan; John 17 contains a prayer that Christ prayed to His Father in heaven the night of his arrest. Are we to look at those prayers in the Bible as falling under the definition of "meditation" as we have previously defined it? The King James Version of the Bible has fourteen places where the word *meditate* is used and six times *meditation*. King David utilized that word the most, with Psalms 119 as the focus of it use:

> O how I love your law! It is my meditation all the day (Psalms 119:97).
> But his delight is in the law of the LORD; and in His law he meditates day and night (Psalm 1:2).

What is the real difference in the use of the words *meditate* and *meditation* as they are used in the Bible, in contrast to their meaning in the preceding paragraphs? Prayer, as found in the Bible, reveals man seeking God and opening his heart to him, inviting Him to be Lord of his life. The definition, as understood in the use of meditation in previous paragraphs, is the same definition as for a "mystic" that is:

> Someone who uses rote methods to tap into their inner divinity.[26]

Biblical-style prayer:

---

[26] Yungen, Ray, *A Time of Departing*, Lighthouse Trails Publishing Company, Silverton, Oregon, (2006), p. 34.

Alternative & Mystical Healing Therapies

> And when you pray, do not use vain repetitions as the heathen do, for they think that they shall be heard for their many words. Therefore do not be like them. For your Father knows the things you have need of before you ask Him (Matthew. 6:7, 8).

Few Christians would choose to be involved in the standard meditation and yoga practice, but is it possible that they might choose to do so when it has been given a new name and are told it is a way to come closer to God? Is that happening? Yes, it is sweeping through the Christian world community. The words of Paul ring out:

> Now the spirit expressly says that in later times some will depart from the faith, giving heed to deceiving spirits and doctrine of demons (I Timothy 4:1).

An early book to reach millions of people by promoting an apparently benign form of meditation was *Creative Visualization* in 1978 by Shakti Gawain. Ray Yungen tells us that this book could well be called the mystics bible. This book promoted improved creativity, career achievements, relationships, health, relaxation, and peace. It caught on with the public as few books do and gained the attention of people that were not of the New Age community. Below is a quote from the book:

> Almost any form of meditation will eventually take you to an experience of yourself as source, or your higher self . . . Eventually you will start experiencing certain moments during your meditation when there is a sort of "click" in your consciousness, and you feel like things are really working; you may even experience a lot of energy flowing through you or a warm radiant glow in your body. These are signs that you are beginning to channel the energy of yourself[27] (emphasis authors).

Ray Yungen, an Evangelical minister, has researched and followed for thirty years the movement that is promoting a special type of prayer referred to as contemplative prayer, centering prayer, sacred space, silence, etc. The methods used in these prayers fit the criteria for mystic meditation. Yungen has written a book *A Time of Departing* which identifies and traces

---

[27] Gawain, Shakti, *Creative Visualization*, Novato, California, National Publishing (2002), back cover, reported in Yungen, op. cit., p. 19.

the origin, ancient history, recent history, and present influence and use of these mystical prayer techniques. He lists in his book authors who have written books promoting these prayer practices. These books have sold beyond belief. One set of authors sold fifty million copies, another author twenty million and a third seven million. Since then, there have been scores of books on the same topic by as many different authors.

What makes the practice of these special prayers so popular is that mediators using the prayer methods do get the *"click"* that Shakti Gawain spoke of. People are convinced they have been touched by the Holy Spirit and have experienced God. Eastern doctrine of *pantheism*—god *is* everything—has been altered a bit and made more deceptive to the Christian by teaching that God *is in* everything—*panentheism*. This becomes the worldview of those using the mystical prayer practices. The Bible does not support these views.

> For in Him dwells all the fullness of the Godhead bodily: and you are complete in Him who is the head of all principality and power (Colossians 2:9, 10).

> I am the Lord, that is my name; And My glory I will not give to another. Nor my praise to carved images (Isaiah 42:8).

Contemplative prayer (and synonym names) uses the basic principles of regular meditation, that is, position of comfort, deep rhythmic breathing, and use of mantra. This mantra may be some Bible name or verse but used in repetition. Then there is the emphasis on bringing the mind to a passive state, emptying of the mind by concentration on the breath and mantra. This alters consciousness, which is the key to all occult training, and can bring the individual to the "click" spoken of before, and now the individual is certain he has experienced the Holy Spirit and God.

Yungen traces the ancient history of the contemplative (meditation) movement to medieval monks known as the Desert Fathers living in the wilderness of the Middle East, who, in turn, most likely had borrowed the practice from the Far East. The Catholic mystics (*especially Ignatius Loyola*) over centuries kept the practice of meditation through prayer alive. It was picked up again in our age by Thomas Merton (1915–1968), a Catholic scholar who was to the contemplative prayer movement as was Martin Luther King to the Civil Rights Movement. So too Catholic scholar Henri Nouwen (1932–1996) had a strong part to play in promoting contemplation prayer to Catholics and mainline Protestants as well. The movement continued to pick up momentum as two monks joined in the fray, Thomas Keating and Basil Pennington. Yungen tells us that these monks blended their Catholic Christianity with Eastern mysticism and produced *centering prayer.*

The movement is also referred to as Spiritual Formation. One of its centers for spreading the contemplative prayer in this country is the Shalem Institute located near Washington DC and founded by Episcopalian priest Tilden Edwards. Its purpose is to spread the practice of mystical prayer to Christianity. Thousands have taken training at this center, trained to be spiritual directors propagating mystical prayer. Another Episcopal priest, Matthew Fox, has influenced not only Catholics but also mainline Protestants in promoting "God in everything." In his book, *The Coming of the Cosmic Christ,* Fox makes the following comments:

> Divinity is found in all creatures . . . The cosmic Christ is the "I Am" in every creature.[28]

> Without mysticism there will be no "deep ecumenism," no unleashing of the power of wisdom from all the world's religious traditions. Without this (mysticism), I am convinced there will never be global peace or justice since the human race needs spiritual depths and disciplines, celebrations, and rituals to awaken its better selves.[29]

Mysticism is leading many Christians into what is termed interspirituality (a merging together of all faiths). It has as its basic tenet that divinity (God) is in all things, and the presence of God is in all religions, and through mysticism, this state is recognized. Once again, let us consider the words of Ray Yungen:

> Former New Age medium, Brian Flynn, in his fascinating book, *Running Against the Wind,* explains it as a uniting of the world's religions through the common thread of mysticism. Flynn quotes the late Wane Teasdale (a lay monk who coined the term interspirituality) as saying that interspirituality is "the spiritual common ground which exists among the world's religions."[30]

---

[28] Fox, Matthew, *The Coming of the Cosmic Christ,* New York, NY, HarperCollins Publishers, 1980), p. 154: reported in Yungen, op. cit., p. 68.

[29] *Ibid.,* p. 68.

[30] Yungen, op. cit., p. 50.

In time, evangelical Protestants were infected with this movement. Richard Foster wrote a book, *Celebration of Discipline,* and is a prominent leader. He brought in "breath prayer"— that is, picking a single word or phrase and repeating it in conjunction with the breath. There have been scores of other ministers leading the charge and writing books, continuing its spread like a tsunami. The movement of mystical prayer has powered the formation of the Emerging Church, which is an ecumenical movement, including pagan, animist, Hindu, Catholic, Protestant, Islam, and all religions. The goal of the Emerging Church is to gather all religions under one banner. *Feelings,* not *thus saith the Word,* seem to be the measuring criteria in this movement.

If you consider carefully the above history of the development of the mystical prayer movement, you will recognize that spiritual formation, contemplative prayer, centering prayer, silence, mysticism, and interspirituality have been introduced and promoted by clergy, not coming from the laity. The watchman on the wall will need to keep their eyes on fellow watchmen and sound the alarm when mysticism is recognized in the church. I have only touched on this subject, but that is enough to put out an *alert*. I suggest you obtain the book by Ray Yungen, *A Time of Departing,* and read it carefully. You will be shocked, I am sure, but will gain a deeper understanding as to where we are in time.

I will close this section with the following quote from Ray Yungen:

> Mysticism *neutralizes* doctrinal differences by sacrificing the truth of Scripture for a mystical experience. Mysticism offers a common ground, and supposedly, that commonality is *divinity in all*. But we know from Scripture there is one God, and there is no other but He.[31]

---

[31] Yungen, op. cit., pp. 196, 197.

7

MINDFULNESS MEDITATION

Mindfulness meditation has captured the interest of the world in the field of psychology and stress management the past few years. Interest in it has swept across America like a tidal wave, and there seems to be no end in sight. We have been exposed and grown accustomed to Hindu-type meditation and yoga over the past fifty or more years. But what is this *mindfulness* you speak about? You say it has grown and spread everywhere, yet I have not heard of it, and what's more, I do not understand the word *mindfulness*.

Courses of mindfulness meditation are offered in many businesses, universities, government agencies, counseling centers, schools, hospital, religious groups, law firms, prisons, military, and other organizations. The business world has taken a strong interest in the technique evidenced by articles in the business press, in books on leadership, and on the Internet. A book with the title *Resonant Leadership: Renewing Yourself and Connecting with Others through Mindfulness, Hope, and Compassion* by Boyatzis and Mckee,[1] along with many other books, have added force to this popular subject.

The University of Massachusetts Medical School Center for Mindfulness in Medicine, Health Care, and Society, as well as Carroll's book, *The Mindful Leader*,[2] published in 2007, amplifies the widespread

---

[1] Boyatzis, R.E., McKee, a., *Resonant Leadership: Renewing Yourself and Connecting with Others through Mindfulness, Hope, and Compassion*, Boston: Harvard Business School Press (2005).

[2] Carroll, M. *The Mindful Leader: Ten Principles for Bringing Out the Best in Ourselves and Others*, (First Edition) Boston (2007): Trumpeter.

utilization of this style of meditation. Many fortune five hundred companies utilize "mindfulness" for training programs as well as the CEOs of some companies practice such.[3] This university center has promoted the integration of mindfulness meditation in mainstream medicine and health care through patient care, research, academic medical, and professional education. These activities have been directed by Saki F. Santorelli, EdD, MA, and with the founding of the center by Jon Kabat-Zinn, PhD. Eighteen thousand people have completed an eight-week mindfulness-based stress reduction program offered by this center.[4] Mindfulness meditation has and is making itself felt throughout the discipline of psychology.

What is mindfulness? How does it differ from other meditative techniques? What is the advantage? What is its origin? Is it spiritually safe? The term *mindfulness* is a translation of *Sati* of the Pali language into the Sanskrit word *smrti*, meaning "that which is remembered." David explains:

> Sati is literally "memory" but is used with reference to the constantly repeated phrase "mindful and thoughtful"; and means that activity of mind and constant presence of mind which is one of the duties most frequently inculcated on the good Buddhist.[5]

Shambhala Publications Presents *A Guide to Buddhism* and lists the basics of Buddhism:

> Four Noble Truths; The Eightfold Path: (1) Karma; (2) Attachment; (3) The Three Marks of existence; (4) Koans: *Mindfulness;* (5) Bardo; (6) Heart Sutra; (7). Loving-Kindness; (8) Pure Perception[6] (numbers added by author).

This article on the Internet on Buddhism continues in attempting to define *mindfulness*. The Pali word *Sati* in English translation is *mindfulness*. Sati is an activity, but what is that? There is no exact answer in words. *Words* are formulated by symbols in the mind and attempt to describe

---

[3] *Ibid.*
[4] http://www.unassmed.edu/content.aspx?id=41252.
[5] Rhys Davids, tr. T.W., *Buddhist Suttas*, Clarendon Press (1881), p. 107; Reported in http://en.wikipedia.org/wiki/Mindfulness_(Buddhism).
[6] http://www.shambhala.com

reality from such. Mindfulness is presymbolic and not fixed to logic yet can be experienced with ease and can be described but with limitations.

> They are not the thing itself. The actual experience lies beyond the words and above the symbols. Mindfulness could be described in completely different terms than will be used here, and each description could still be correct.[7]

This meditation technique referred to as *mindfulness* was introduced by the Buddha about twenty-five centuries ago and is a set of mental activities aimed at experiencing a state of *uninterrupted mindfulness.* The article elaborates further with a comment that when this mindfulness meditation is prolonged, using proper techniques, the experience is profound, and *it changes one's entire view of the universe,* from a Judeo-Christian worldview toward Eastern pantheism. This article is spread over three pages with additional paragraphs attempting to describe what mindfulness is. I will share the first sentence in several different paragraphs describing mindfulness to illustrate the difficulty in understanding *mindfulness meditation.*

Definitions presented by this article are as follows: it is a nonrecognized process presently being used, mirror-thought, nonjudgmental, fair watchfulness, nonconceptual awareness, awareness of the right now, and nonegotistical alertness.[8]

I finally found a paragraph that had a sentence that made sense to me. *"Mindfulness is not thinking."* Just reading this article and others like it in the attempt to explain this technique brings about feelings of mental confusion. Are you with me? Are you beginning to sense what "mindfulness" is? It is simply the Buddhist's word for bringing the mind into the silence, passive mode, an altered state of consciousness—Eastern-style meditation? Then this altered state of consciousness opens to the possibility for the mind to be influenced and/or controlled by occult forces.

This two-thousand-five-hundred-year old Buddhist-style meditation has been "secularized" for use in coping with stress, chronic pain control, immune disorders, anger, fear, greed, thoughts, feelings, attention, emotions, skills, addictions, performance, creativity, and changing the structure of our brains. It is proclaimed to change our relationship to life. It involves "inward investigation" to promote well-being. It is partaking

---

[7] http://www.shamhala.com/
[8] *Ibid.*, p. 2.

of an ancient Eastern practice to inform, affect, and compliment life. It now is said to be based in science but was once in the realm of mystics and philosophers.[9]

"Contrast the above with the counsel of the prophet Isaiah for dealing with stress.

> You will keep him in perfect peace, whose mind is stayed on You: because he trusts in You" (Isaiah 26:3).

Ron Kurtz is a psychologist, a Buddhist for more than thirty-five years, and the author of the online text *Hakomi Method of Mindfulness-Based Body Psychotherapy*. Hakomi is a name he gives to his psychotherapy which, in turn, utilizes mindfulness as a principle component of therapy. We connect to Ron Kurtz's online book *Hakomi Method of Mindfulness-Based Body Psychotherapy*.

- Mindfulness is undefended consciousness. It has been defined as "the clear and single-minded awareness of what actually happens to us and in us at the successive moments of perception."
- It is a skill; it improves with practice. *It is a traditional form of meditation*, especially for beginners. It is a traditional method of self-study.
- In mindfulness, there is no intention to control what happens next. It is a deliberate *relinquishing of control*. That is why the first focus in traditional practice is often on the breathing. To pay attention to the breathing and not control; it is more difficult than one might imagine, especially when we think about how little attention we ordinarily pay to breathing and how well it works outside of our conscious control. Mindfulness is a way of *surrendering*.
- In mindfulness, one attempts to calm the mind, to *silence thoughts*.
- One focuses inward on the flow of one's experience.
- In Hakomi, we use it in small doses (thirty seconds to a minute)[10] (emphasis added).

In literature, espousing Hakomi-style psychotherapy, there is claim made by its practitioners that unconscious *core beliefs* of an individual can be made conscious through use of the *mindfulness* technique, and that, in turn,

---

[9] Smalley, Suan, Winston, Diana, *Fully Present: The Science, Art, and Practice of Mindfullness*, DaCapo Lifelong, Cambridge, MA (2010), pp. xvii, xviii.

[10] *http://www.shambhala.com*

offers the opportunity to alter and change those fundamental core beliefs. A person's worldview—"where did we come from," "why are we here," and "where are we going" are as a result of being placed in "mindfulness" subject to change.[11] "Mindfulness practice is a spiritual discipline."[12]

Ron Kurtz, in his book, tells us that when a person has attained a state of mindfulness, the person becomes very still and the *eyelids flutter up and down over closed eyes*. This movement of the eyelids is almost always an accurate sign that the client is in mindfulness. Kurtz states that he uses this sign "all of the time."[13]

Psychologist Kurtz elaborates further in his use of mindfulness in his practice. He tells when a person makes a change in their state of consciousness, their voice may become childlike, and vocabulary and speech are as a child. Past emotions and emotional memories from childhood may present; the face may express past childhood emotions. When this happens, Ron Kurtz says the psychologist needs to contact that *inner child* by directly speaking to it, such as "you are feeling your youth again," etc. He further comments:

> When the child appears, you want to contact it . . . . This childlike state is a very fruitful state to work with. The client is, in a sense, innocent and open, ready to be helped by an adult. I like to engage a client's adult self in the process of working with the child. I want the adult to help me understand what's going on with the child. I want to help the client self-engage with her child in a nourishing way, more nourishing than the child experienced in her formative relationships.[14]

This is a dialogue wherein the patient communes with *another voice*, her or his *own youthful voice*. Is this a disguised spirit-demon contact?

There are varying stages of entering into hypnosis. The first stage is entered by focusing on something, anything such as a light, sound, flame, or breathing. This is done until fatigue occurs and the awareness of outside activities wanes. Relaxation follows next, etc. The Bynum Scale

---

[11] Kurtz, Ron, *Hakomi Method of Mindfulness-Based Body Psychotherapy*, http://www.scribd.com/doc/6673762/HAKOMI-Methode p.4 (on line book by Ron Kurtz now deleted from scibd.com)

[12] *Ibid.*, 36

[13] *Ibid.*, p. 124

[14] *Ibid.*, p. 23.

of Hypnotic Susceptibility lists the following first five of thirty levels of hypnotism:

- No Objective Change
- Relaxation
- *Fluttering of Eyelids* (emphasis added)
- Closed Eyes
- Complete physical relazation.

To summarize the issue of *mindfulness,* it is ancient *Buddhist meditation* with the possibility of progressing to higher levels of hypnotism and at times channeling of spirit entities—demons. We are advised that the religious association is discarded in the present-day practice of mindfulness meditation. How does one remove the spiritual influence from a practice solely designed and practiced to connect one with the spirit world by an Eastern religious discipline for two thousand five hundred years? It does not separate; it is Satan's ground. Do not be seduced.

Certain definitions of a more pleasing form of spiritualism comes to mind, helping in this struggle to clear the confusion created in my mind in attempting to understand and describe the great variety of explanations for this word *mindfulness.* Spiritualism teaches that man is progressive; his destiny is to progress toward godhood. The throne is within one; this type of reasoning supports progression for sure. Progression not upward but downward.

The Apostle Paul counsels us to:

> And be not conformed to this world: but be ye transformed by the renewing of your mind, that ye may prove what is that good and acceptable, and perfect renewing will of God (Romans 12:2).

8

YOGA-YOGA EXERCISES AND CLEANSING: AYURVEDA: THE ANCIENT HEALING TRADITION OF INDIA

PART II

Forty years in the past, yoga was an activity that most Americans considered as Hinduism and associated with pagan idol worship. The Christian community tended to consider its practice as a denial of faith. In the intervening years, many Americans have been conditioned to accept it as a healthy part of Christianity. The term *Christian yoga* is often heard or read. Its practice has spread through clubs, sports, schools, television, businesses, churches, youth groups, medicine, entertainment industry, and for many individuals simply a practice at home. It has even been especially prepared and presented to the very young and promoted as a "family activity." Yoga has moved into wellness programs primarily through yoga exercises which have become popular in many churches, especially with young women.

Has the Christian community carefully analyzed yoga and found it to be an appropriate adjunct to the Judeo-Christian doctrines? Has there been any concern that it might be a "wolf in sheep's clothing?" Some pastors give warnings about its practice, while some others are encouraging its practice. We need to look carefully at the origin of yoga and its place and purpose in the Hindu worship for the past three thousand five hundred years. Then we need to answer the question, is its use spiritually safe for the Christian? Read carefully this chapter and learn more about this controversial subject.

YOGA

Yoga is an intrinsic part of Hinduism. Laurette Willis, who was led into New Age occultism through yoga and then delivered through faith in Christ and obedience to God's Word, explains:

> The goal of all yoga is to obtain oneness with the universe. That's also known as the process of enlightenment or union with Brahman (Hinduism's highest god). The word *yoga* means *union* or *to yoke* . . . Yoga wants to get students to the point of complete numbness in their minds (to open them to this force). God, on the other hand, wants you to be transformed by the renewing of your mind through his Word.[1]

We read an opposing viewpoint:

> Yoga is a science as well as a method of achieving spiritual harmony through the control of mind and body. The *asanas* (yogic postures) and *pranayama* (breath control) are practices that not only help us to acquire perfect health, but also develop the inner force that enables a believer to withstand stressful situations with a calm and serene mind.[2]

B. K. S. Iyengar, the founder of hatha yoga (style used in the United States), makes the following statement regarding the goal of yoga:

> The means by which the human soul may be completely united with the Supreme Spirit pervading the universe and thus attain liberation (escape reincarnation) . . . *Yoga Journal,* May/June 1993, p. 69.

Yoga is an ancient physical practice of postures and movements established to *join* the mind, body, and spirit. Yoga means to hook up, to join, to unite. The primary purpose of posture and movement of yoga is to facilitate the

---

[1] Hunt, *Yoga and the Body of Christ*, The Berean Call, page 35
[2] Warrier, Gopi; Deepika Gunawan, MD; *The Complete Illustrated Guide to Ayurveda*, Barnes and Noble Books (1997), p. 166.

flow of energy through the body and chakras, especially kundalini energy. As stated previously, yoga is associated with meditation like a glove is with the hand. Dr. Khalsa tells us in *Meditation as Medicine* that he combines yoga with meditation to obtain a more powerful response in healing.

Swiss psychiatrist C. G. Jung, a spiritist and anti-Christian, brought yoga to the West ninety plus years past and was a devotee of it. He strongly emphasized that the spiritual cannot be taken out it (see quote below).

> The numerous, purely physical procedures of yoga (unite), the parts of the body ... with the whole of the mind and spirit, as in the pranayama exercises, where prana is both the breath and the universal dynamics of the cosmos ... the elation of the body becomes one with the elation of the spirit.... Yoga practice is unthinkable and would also be ineffectual, without the ideas on which it is based. It works the physical and the spiritual into one another in an extraordinarily complete way.[3]

Later, Yogi Paramahansa Yogananda popularized yoga in this country in the later part of the twentieth century by introducing it as science in the guise of health enhancement. Yoga was presented as a purely physical practice nonrelated to religion. Hatha yoga, often considered only as physical yoga, has for its center of instruction the "Temple of Kriya Yoga" in Chicago. Yogananda initiated approximately one hundred thousand people into Kriya yoga (or hatha yoga) for the purpose of "self-realization" (to realize one's oneness with God). The leaders in this movement have been "yogis" or holy men.

> These techniques were all precisely developed over centuries to induce subtle changes in states of consciousness leading to "self realization." They were not developed for physical benefits.[4]

Medical newspapers and journals frequently print articles reporting yet another medical condition that improves with the use of yoga and/or meditation. A government survey of thirty-one thousand adults revealed that 8 percent of Americans use yoga as an alternative medical therapy. As of 2004, Wal-Mart Web site listed 990 and Target 4,235 yoga products

---

[3] Jung, C. G. trans. R.F.C. Hull, *Psychology and the East*, Princeton University Press (1978), pp. 80, 81: reported in Hunt, Dave, *Yoga and the body of Christ*, The Berean Call, Bend, Oregon, p. 9.

[4] Hunt, Dave, *Yoga and the Body of Christ*, The Berean Call, Bend, OR, p. 18.

for sale.⁵⁵ Richard Hittleman, a leader in the "physical yoga" movement in the USA, makes the following comment:

> As yoga students practiced the physical positions, they would eventually be ready to investigate the spiritual component which is "the entire essence of the subject."⁶

Yoga is sweeping the West. Multiple millions practice yoga not intending to embrace Hinduism yet using the fundamental tools of Hinduism and placing their minds under its influence. They do not contemplate on God while in yoga meditation. Instead, they try to empty their minds of all thought or concentrate on a single thought so as to achieve mental rest or "passivity of mind." The end result, however, allows opportunity for Satan to control one's mind. We are to contemplate on God through prayer and study scriptures of the Bible while inviting the Holy Spirit to direct our thoughts.

Yoga is also a commercial business. Consider the financial impact of this movement:

> Nationally, Yoga is a 22.5 billion-dollar industry. Advertisements for yoga books, videos, clothes, wellness retreats, and even yoga business training classes can be found in the back of magazines such as *Yoga Journal,* and the phenomenon in now reaching into the mainstream . . . 35 million Americans who will try yoga for the first time this year. Once confined to New Agers with an interest in Eastern spirituality, yoga is catching on among young men, fitness fanatics, aging baby boomers, and other unlikely enthusiasts who claim the mind-body practice does everything from healing illness to tighten abs.⁷

Contrast yoga meditation with Christian meditation which really is best called *study* or *concentration*. The Christian attitude is that of allowing God to direct his thoughts and life. He does not look inward in an attempt to raise his divinity to godhood but outward and upward to the Creator God as the source of power and redemption. This is directly opposite to Ayurvedic principles. Can one take a fundamental act and practice, physical and mental, from a pagan religion (Satan's ground) and make it Christian? The *Christian yoga* term is an oxymoron. As the Hindu

---

⁵ httn://www.letusreason.org/NAM1.htm.

⁶ *Yoga Journal,* May/June, (1993), p. 68.

⁷ http://www.letusreason.org/NAM1.htm.

holy men tell us, we cannot take yoga out of Hinduism, nor can you take Hinduism out of yoga.

Reflecting upon the subject of meditation and yoga in the 1950s, I cannot remember that the subject was ever thought of or considered Christian compatible by people with whom I associated. In the 1960s, a change was observed occurring on college campuses, such as style of dress, long hair on men, etc. Standards were changing, and to a person not involved in the culture change of the youth, it was not well understood. Many influences were creating the outward changes we were seeing, and most of us did not understand what was happening. One of the greatest influences for change came from the influence of psychedelic drugs and the popular music of the period. Timothy Leary is a name that comes to mind when this subject of psychedelic drug use is mentioned. He championed the use of LSD; other substances such as peyote, marijuana, amphetamine were easily available. The mind trips experienced with these substances blew away old norms and created a desire for ever expanding "consciousness." Drug using musicians, Presley, the Beatles, Rolling Stones, and many other music groups came on the scene captivating the youth and opening up the drug use as nothing else could do. This was a stepping stone to even more exhilarating practice of yoga and the "trips" that could be taken in this manner without purchasing drugs.[8]

The Beatles spent time in an *ashram* in India learning meditation and yoga and then returned to the music performance circuit, promoting yoga. They had learned that mind trips, equal and beyond what drugs give, could be experienced by yoga without drugs. Yoga was now on a roll. Meditation and yoga is not a novelty any longer; it has gone "main-street" even in many of our leading hospitals. An altered state of consciousness is a prerequisite to experience mind trips and obtaining a "spirit guide."

> In view of the nonphysical nature of consciousness, it is intriguing that those who practice divination techniques for initiating contact with "spirit" dimension all agree that the secret is in achieving the requisite *state of consciousness* through drugs, yoga (other forms of Eastern meditation), hypnosis, and mediumistic trance. It is not surprising then that this "altered state of consciousness" and the contact it brings with "spirit guides" has always been the traditional shamanistic method of achieving paranormal or

---

[8] Hunt, Dave, McMahon, T.A., *America, the Sorcerer's New Apprentice*, Harvest House Publishers, Eugene, Oregon (1988), pp. 233–252.

psychic powers. It has also often opened the door to what has become known as possession[9](emphasis by author).

YOGA EXERCISES

Yoga is an act whereby a person assumes a physical posture in Sanskrit called asana. There are more than fifty different postures in yoga. The purpose of yoga is to facilitate liberation from reincarnation (rebirth) as taught in pagan religions and yoke (yoga) together the individual soul with a pagan deity. By the practice of yoga, the agitated mind is said to be brought under control. In the meditation-yoga system, the mind is controlled by focusing on obtaining to samadhi, lotus, supreme self, godhood. At this level of attainment in meditation and yoga, the individual knows that he is a real entity having a life that will go on in spite of the destruction of the body. Meditation is an integral part of yoga practices, and all that has been said about meditation is equally applicable to yoga. Szurko, an ex–yogic master, explains:

> The importance of asanas (physical postures), pranayama (breath control) . . . to the yogi pursuing liberation lies partly in the belief that the body is the microcosm of the universe; that is to say, whatever exists in the universe may be found in the body, which is a "universe in miniature." Thus, the yogi finds within himself all bodies; all truth; heaven and hell; all the expanses of space and the whole of time as well as of eternity; spirit, the gods, and deity.[10]

The knowledge of the universe is said to be found in self; all healing is to be found in self. Yoga is less of a treatment for illness and more for preventative measures. The Hindu believes that yoga exercises decreases congestion and blockage of energy and facilitates its flow. Sitting straight during meditation or even without meditation, it is believed, will allow for release of the congestion and blockage of the universal energy, making it flow smoothly through various organs. The yoga exercises are supposedly to stimulate the *chakras*, which in turn allows the energy to flow freely and maintain health.

---

[9] *Ibid.*, p. 155.
[10] Davies, Gaius, *Stress*, Kingsway Publication, Eastbourne, England, 1988, p. 241; reported in Willis, Richard J.B., *Holistic Health Holistic Hoax?* Pensive Publications, 10 Holland Gardens, Watford, Hertfordshire, WD2 6JW (1997), p. 231.

The above concept has been accepted by western mysticism and magic in whole and forms the philosophical basis of most alternative medical therapies yet to be discussed.

The positions of the yoga postures are important in its concept because each position is proclaimed to direct prana or universal energy to specific parts of the body. In hatha yoga, the spine is to be kept straight so that the latent kundalini, or serpent force, supposedly coiled up at the base of the spine from birth, will be able to ascend through the chakras (energy centers of Hinduism) toward the top chakra. All these acts are directed at "stilling the mind." Hatha yoga is the most popular in the United States. *Ha* means sun, and *tha* is moon. Breathing through the nose in the left nostril will bring in the moon energy and, in the right nostril, the sun energy. Both sun and moon energy then travel downward through special (nonexistent) passages, one on each side of the body, and go to the bottom chakra at the coccyx area. This energy will then ascend up through the body by the help of yoga postures and exercises until the energy comes into full force at the top chakra, signifying that eternal life has been attained.

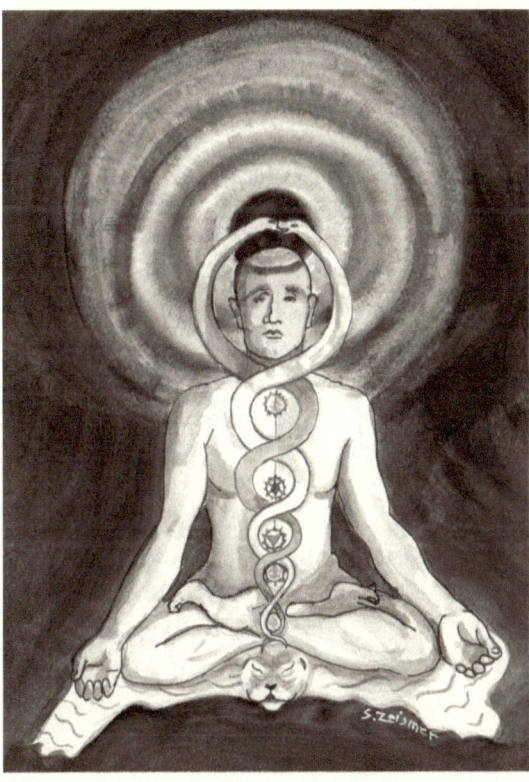

Figure 18. Kundalini—serpent power.

Let Us Reason Ministries placed an article about yoga on the Internet titled "Yoga: Today's Lifestyle for Health." The author of the article, once a practitioner of yoga, tells of becoming involved in yoga meditation as a result of practicing the yoga exercise positions. He cautions us that the physical yoga is not separate from the whole of Eastern metaphysics.

How popular are yoga exercises? Let Us Reason Ministries' article on this gives just a glimpse of the interest.

The YMCA teaches hatha yoga in their physical education programs as physical exercise in health spas and on TV programs. Most of the clubs offer yoga classes. Churches have bought into this movement as well, calling such Christian yoga with the idea that they are simply physical exercise and condition of the body and the mind. Stress reduction is the explanation for its use as well. "Touted as scientifically proven is more an assumption that is really at worst, a presumption."[11]

The response that so often comes from participants of yoga exercise is that they are only doing "stretching exercises." What could be wrong or dangerous with that? The answer is given by the author of the article submitted by Let Us Reason Ministries:

> The poses that they so diligently practice in their stretching are named after Hindu gods, and what one is actually doing is calling on them. In that worshipful pose, they are bowing and, for all intents and purposes, worshipping that god. Our God says: "You shall not bow down to them or worship them; for I, the Lord your God, am a jealous God" (Exodus 20:5).[12]

Another yogic or Hindu mystic, Sri Aurobindo, taught that all yoga, including hatha yoga, "has the same goal—unity with the supreme." Many people think they are just taking a physical fitness activity when they join a yoga exercise group. The master mystics and the yogis tell us you cannot separate the physical from the spiritual. Szurko, an ex-mystic, says:

> When I taught yoga, it became apparent that for many people, the spiritual dimension of the discipline was self-manifesting—it could be ignored at first but not for long.[13]

---

[11] http://www.letusreason.org/NAM1.htm p. 1.

[12] http://www. letusreason.org/NAM1.htm p. 6.

[13] Szurko, Christtian, *Can Yoga be Reconciled with Christianity?* The Church Medicine and the New Age (1995) p. 107; reported in Willis, op. cit., p. 232.

I quote Yogi Ramacharaka:

> The beginner will also do well to study "hatha yoga" in order to render his physical body healthy and sound and thus give the spirit a worthy temple in which to manifest.[14]

Theos Bernard states:

> Great masters, through the potency of hatha yoga, breaking the scepter of death, are roaming in the universe.[15]

Combined with yoga exercise is the emphasis placed on breathing. In Eastern medicine this is paramount. Air (*prana*) is believed to carry the universal energy (life force) into an individual, and breathing in a certain manner (through the nose) increases the amount of this universal energy, intelligence, consciousness, or creative principle in a person. Ramacharaka also tells us:

> The yogi practices exercises by which he attains control of his body and is enabled to send to any organ or part an increased flow of vital force "prana," thereby strengthening and invigoration the part or organ ... He knows that by rhythmical breathing, one may bring in the unfoldment of his latent powers. He knows that by controlled breathing he may not only cure disease in himself and others, but also practically do away with fear and worry and the baser emotions.[16]

The Complete Illustrated Encyclopedia of Alternative Healing Therapies tells us:

> The exercises of yoga are all designed to direct the flow of "prana" and to release the body's internal energy to create spiritual awareness. Yoga is thus a form of preparation of the mind, body, and spirit, which must be unified through conduct,

---

[14] Ramacharaka, Yogi (1960), *The Hindu-Yogi: The Science of Breath*, London: L.N. Foweler and Co. Ltd. p. 78; reported in Willis, op. cit., p. 233.

[15] Bernard, Theos, *Hatha Yoga*, Arrow Books, London (1950), p. 19; reported in Willis, op. cit. (1997) p. 233.

[16] Ramacharaka, Yogi (nd), Raja Yoga, Ondon: L.N. Fowler & Co. Ltd. (1960), p. 10; reported in Willis, op. cit., p. 233.

right thinking, and meditation before the ultimate merging of the self with the universe or the totality of all that is—the equivalent of God or the Hindu goal of "nirvana." In this wider context, the postural and breathing exercises of hatha yoga are simply a means of promoting meditation and internal balance, through which the final goal of "oneness" can be achieved. Hatha yoga is a yogic system in its own right, although in the West emphasis is generally placed on its exercises.[17]

Taking air in through the right nostril is said to be breathing in the *sun* energy. Breathing through the left nostril is said to be breathing in the *moon* energy. In the nostrils are believed to be two channels for carrying universal energy. These channels are called *ida* (left) and *pingala* (right) and are believed to start at the nostrils and go down to the lower end of the spinal column. They are said to be related to the activities of the lunar and solar forces in the body. The mystic moon of the body (microcosm) is said to be located in the head, pouring with its milky rays the elixir (amrita), which serves the channel *ida* on the left side of the body, etc. The antagonistic principle of devouring solar heat is supposed to be situated at the lower pelvis area of the body.[18]

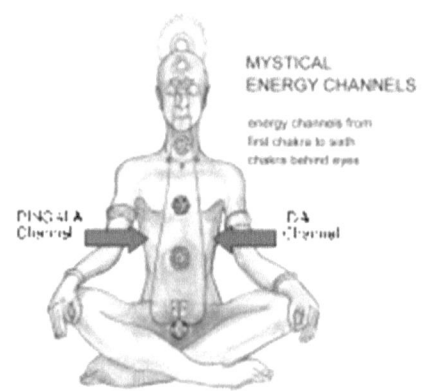

Figure 19. Man in yoga position with IDA AND PINGALA.

---

[17] Shealy, Norman, MD, PhD, *The Complete Illustrated Encyclopedia of Alternative Healing Therapies*, Element Books Inc., Boston, MA (1999), p. 52.

[18] Jaggi, O.P., MD, PhD, *Yogic and Tantric Medicine*, Atma Ram and Sons, Delhi, India (1973), p. 62.

Hatha yoga, by definition, means *union of sun* (ha) *and moon* (tha). At a little higher level of yoga called pranayama, the two channels in the nostrils become stimulated, and union of the two breaths takes place at the "agya," the important chakra between the two eyes. One set of yoga exercises called *surya namatura* (salutation to the sun) is a set of easy movements and postures not held as long as most exercise postures. These exercises present a

>spiritual salutation to the rising Sun, the source of all energy for life, and are found in many religious and pagan societies.[19]

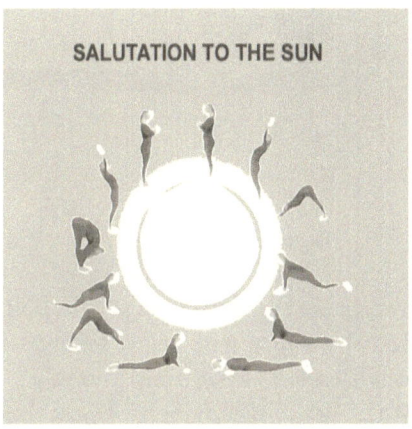

Figure 20. An artist's depiction of yoga Surya Namatura exercises.

Hinduism teaches that there is a great "latent" power within each person. Said to be located at the base of the spine, it is called kundalini, also referred to as the serpent power, as this is the definition of this Sanskrit word. To attain godhood, this *serpent power* must be awakened and moved up the body through the Hindu chakras to the highest one at the top of the head. The movement of this kundalini is believed to be accomplished by practicing meditation and yoga. Yoga asanas (postures) and exercises were designed to force flow of this serpent power up through the chakras and the body to the crown chakra on top of the head. The exercise positions are specifically designed to be snakelike in motion and are named after Hindu gods. One such position is called the cobra. Along with the positions of the exercises, great emphasis is placed on breathing. Remember *prana*, the *universal energy* of Hinduism, is believed to be in the air we breathe.

---

[19] Shealy, op. cit., p. 55.

In so-called Christian yoga (an oxymoron), there may be practiced what is called the breath prayer, a pagan practice given a Christian name, not unlike the centuries wherein paganism entered the church by simply giving Christian names to pagan customs.

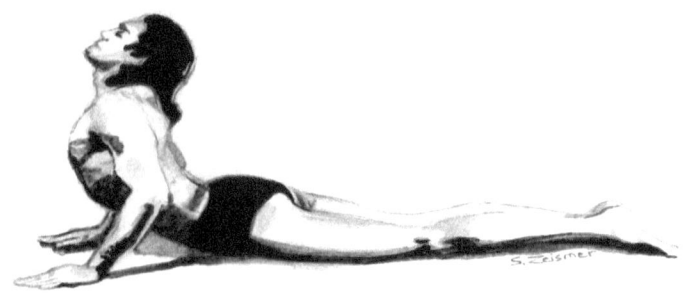

Figure 21. Cobra position.

When the universal energy delivered to the body by breathing has traveled to the lower chakra, it will begin to ascend in an undulating manner, going through the chakras until it reaches the seventh crown chakra at the top of the head, whereupon one receives *immortality*. This may take many lifetimes to accomplish.[20] Yoga is a counterfeit of being yoked to Christ.

> Come unto me, all ye that labour and are heavy laden, and I will give you rest. Take my yoke upon you, and learn of me; for I am meek and lowly in heart: and ye shall find rest unto your souls. For my yoke is easy, and my burden is light (Matthew 11:28–30).

Spreading across the world like a forest fire is the popular activity of yoga exercise and the breathing exercises that go with them. There may or may not be meditation involved, but most formal yoga sessions end with a few moments of meditation. This can easily lead to spiritualism experiences. Because the spiritual philosophy that is a part of Hinduism is not presented in a verbal manner with yoga exercises or with meditation, people totally disassociate the Hindu religion and its "worldview" of man's

---

[20] Jaggi, op. cit., p. 123.

Alternative & Mystical Healing Therapies

origin from doing the yoga exercises. Yoga exercises are alleged to be purely physical with no mysticism involved. Yoga is yoga, and those various movements and stretching are designed to raise *kundalini* up through the chakras to join with the universal god of Hinduism. Partaking of these exercises places oneself on *Satan's ground*. He has used such activities for more than three thousand years and for his purposes only. Will we move his counterfeit system into our lives and into the church as paganism moved in during the fourth to fifth centuries and call it *Christian?* An ex-Hindu guru, now a Christian, has stated a very clear truth about the influences of participating in yoga. He said:

> There cannot be Hinduism without yoga, and there can be no yoga without Hinduism.[21]

A most dangerous concept is that we can separate yoga and yoga exercises from their roots, practice them, and be free of their spiritual influence. Connie J. Fait is a former Tibetan nun, yogi, and head of a Tibetan Buddhist temple who practiced, studied, and taught yoga and its traditions for forty years prior to converting to Christianity. She warns of the spiritual association of the practice of yoga exercises and postures even devoid of meditation. She makes the following comments (see http://womenofgrace.com/blog/?p=29077 posted April 7, 2014):

> The knowledge of the yogic tradition is deeply hidden in mystery, and only understood by accomplished yogis who have passed on those secrets orally to one another for five thousand years. *Yoga asanas are recognized as the main tool* to realizing these secrets and is accomplished only through a process of experience. Anyone who is doing yoga asanas is in that same process—*whether or not they are aware of it or intend it* (emphasis added).

She further explains that yoga asanas are the basis for the theology of Hinduism. From the start of Hinduism, recluse yogis sat, yearning for union with their believed creator "Brahman." As they sat in the mystical mind's altered states, spontaneous physical movements occurred, referred to as kriyas now called asanas. In the practice of these postures, they would experience high meditative states and experience contact with deities who appeared to them. Specific poses were named for those gods.

---

[21] *Gods of the New Age*: Video Tape 1988, Jeremiah Films Inc., Hemet, CA.

Remember the goal of yoga—to escape reincarnation by becoming one with Brahman and entering the spirit world. Lyengar Yogacharia believes that only two forms of the eight limbs of yoga are necessary to accomplish this goal, that of the asanas and pranayama (the controlled breathing). He further shares that the breathing aspect need not be taught as it will occur spontaneously as the asanas are perfected. Likewise for meditation, as it too will be experienced, and eventually ultimate union with Brahman, other gods, and various deities (demons) occurs. Connie tells us that eventually physical distress of various natures often will afflict individuals that have advanced in yoga, but they will have no clue as to its origin.

The highest goal of the Eastern religion is to *realize one's own believed divinity, to make contact with the spirit gods*, and *to escape the cycle of reincarnation* and joining them. These religions teach that this goal can be accomplished by our own works, not necessarily by good deeds but by practicing meditation and yoga and its exercises. These practices were designed for these religions (by Satan's directions) to facilitate an alteration in one's state of consciousness wherein Satan can exert his power over them and lead the person to believe he has attained godhood and will at death join the spirit world.

To participate in these practices is to accept the foundation pillars of Hinduism. It is akin to dancing around the tree of knowledge of good and evil, and since it seems safe, eventually the urge to reach out and touch and eat of its fruit is too strong a temptation to resist.

MASSAGE

Ayurveda teaches that the body has special channels which not only carry nutrients throughout the body but also additionally conduct subtle energies which link mankind with the cosmos. Disease in Ayurveda medicine is said to be determined by knowing which of these channels is affected. Massage and yoga exercises are used to open these channels when they are blocked or are not flowing freely. The congestion of these channels is considered a source of disease.

In Ayurveda, it is taught that there are 107 points on the body called trigger points (or *marma points*) and that by massaging these points, we are able to facilitate the flow of energy that may be stagnant, blocked, or in some way congested. By massaging specific *marma points* with *essential oils*, then there is free flow of energy (prana). Different types of *essential oil*s are used for different types of illnesses, and in turn, these oils will be chosen for application to particular trigger points. The various trigger points are said to be associated with particular areas or organs of the body. None of the above comments is substantiated by science.

It is very important to understand that the "trigger points" in Ayurvedic medicine should not be confused with the expression "trigger point" as is used in today's conventional practice of medicine. A very frequent complaint encountered in family practice is a localized point of pain on a specific muscle. Examination will reveal a firm, tender nodule in the muscle. A "twitch" of the muscle group will occur when the tender nodule is touched or pressed on. The cause of the nodule is most likely a section of muscle fibers in constant contraction. It can be very painful and can last days, weeks, or even months. There are various methods of treatment. Firm pressure held on the tender nodule for ten minutes may alleviate it. Injecting the nodule with a local anesthetic may also bring relief, and use of ultrasound over the nodule works well. I have personally treated hundreds of these tender nodules. They have no relationship to the "marma points" of Ayurvedic medicine.

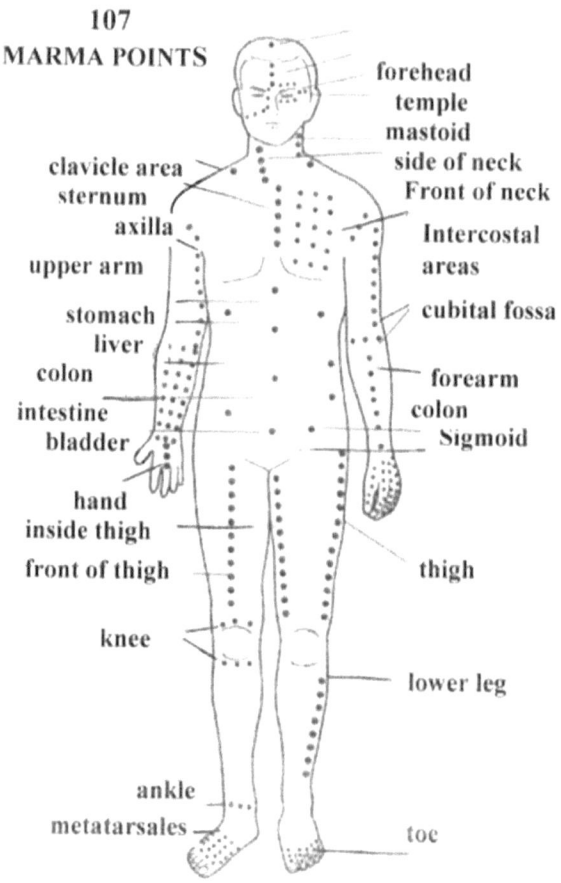

Figure 22. Marma points.

Through memory of past emotional experiences, the Hindu believes we sometimes adopt postures and physical behaviors which create congestion of prana. Massage, above all else, involves the movement of energies, relieving congestion, thereby supposedly rejuvenating the mind and body.

Essential oils (oil of a plant) are extracted from plants having specific aromas and are placed on specific marma points and massaged into the skin. Different marma points may require specific oils applied when massaged. These oils are used because they are believed to contain "spirit"—universal energy of high frequency.

In Ayurveda, food also imparts universal energy (prana) to the body. The diet philosophy is complex. There is a strong bent toward vegetarianism. Another Eastern religion diet is the Zen Buddhist macrobiotic diet; it consists of seven steps with progressive restriction of diet choices. It is believed that food brings a type of energy (universal energy) apart from the energy obtained from the metabolism of food. It is also believed that foods of animal origin are stronger in rajas-tamas, yin-yang, and fruits and vegetables are more neutral in yin-yang and do not upset the energy balance, thus an additional reason for the choice of vegetarianism.

One may hear of *live enzymes*, which can refer to the enzymes of plants unaltered by heat or to the universal energy believed to be carried by the enzymes and not a biochemical condition of the enzymes. A normal body will produce all the appropriate enzymes we need, and it is not necessary to assimilate *live enzymes* from plants for proper metabolism. (However, there are a number of genetic diseases wherein the body does not produce specific enzymes.) The enzymes in plants are for facilitating the biochemical actions in the plant and do not function in our biochemical reactions. Previously stated in chapter five was mentioned the choice of vegetarian diets because of the belief that eating plant food facilitated receiving energy from higher levels, or planes, which are then transferred to an individual's higher chakras.

HERBS AND MINERALS

The use of herbs has been a fundamental practice in all ancient health and healing systems. Herbs are considered helpful in "bridging" the cosmic energies which are said to be internal and external to the body. In Ayurvedic practice, herbs are always to be used in conjunction with meditation, diet, and other Ayurvedic approaches to health. According to these theories, benefit from herbal therapy will depend upon it being added to other therapies; also, we must acknowledge the *consciousness* of the plant, or it will be of no value or effect on us. Little to no benefit is to be expected when it is used alone.[22] A later chapter, "Mystical Herbology," will expound on the use of herbs in Ayurveda medicine.

Aromatherapy and the use of *essential oils* are very popular as a method of influencing universal energy within a person. The aroma is obtained by using oil concentrates of flowers and plant substances. It can be applied as oil or placed in vaporizers and diffused through the air. Many times, plants are placed in water and then placed in the sunshine for several hours. Sunlight is supposed to increase the "essence" of the plants. They are then

---

[22] Gerson, op. cit., p. 90.

processed by steam distillation of other methods of extraction into oils which are usually rubbed into the skin. This is one more way in which it is believed that the universal energy (prana) is absorbed by the body. This subject will be dealt with in detail in a later chapter.

PANCHAKARMA: CLEANSING, PURIFICATION

Disease, by Ayurveda understanding, is the result of an abnormal accumulation of dosha (yin-yang) energies in the tissues of the body. One very interesting part of the Ayurvedic healing system belief is *panchakarma* or purification treatment. It is believed that cells in the body contain residual impurities deposited in them as a result of improper digestion. The goal of purification is to rid the body of *ama* or impurities which imbalance doshas.

Ayurveda teaches that there is a "fire" in the body (called agni), which we call metabolism, that drives all of the vital chemical processes. It directs and supports digestion. If digestion is impaired by too little agni or for any other reason, then impurities (ama) are produced. The ama is supposedly a *white sticky substance* (not recognized by scientific medicine) that is absorbed by channels (nondemonstrable by the anatomist), spreads to the tissue of the body, and if not cleaned out, often develops disease by causing imbalances of the dosha energies. The diseases might be called gallstones, cancer, heart disease, etc. Ayurveda recognizes two types of disease—outside disease and inside disease. Ama is said to be the root of all inside diseases.[23] The purification procedures are used as both preventative and restorative therapy.

The five cleansing therapies of Ayurveda are:

- Nasal administration of substances that are believed to clear out the imbalanced doshas, or energies, from the head and neck area.
- Emetics to induce vomiting, which clears the energies from the lungs and abdominal area.
- Laxatives and strong purgatives to cleanse the blood, liver, spleen, small intestine, and sweat glands.
- Medicated enemas to cleanse the colon, rectum, lumbar-sacral region, and bones of excess energies. "Ayurveda regards medicated enemas (Ayurveda lists over one hundred different ones) as the most important purification method of all because of the importance of the large intestine in health and disease." The loosened doshas (yin-yang, rojas-tamas) are believed to be washed out through the intestinal tract.

---

[23] *Ibid.*, p. 49.

Alternative & Mystical Healing Therapies

- Bloodletting had long been a practice in Ayurveda until a change (140–150 years ago) when using herbs was substituted for taking blood. The concept behind drawing blood was that it eliminated toxins and excess energies from the blood, lymph, and deep tissues. The purpose for bloodletting was to treat skin disorders, enlarged liver and spleen, gout, fevers, abdominal tumors, jaundice, etc. There are other cleansing practices such as the topical application of plasters and herbal pastes, etc. Bloodletting has nearly ceased, and herbal use has been substituted in its place.

Ayurveda medicine is strongly connected to astrology: for this reason, the zodiac was used in determining which area of the patient's body should be bled.

> The sun and moon have the strongest influence on health and healing, and their movements indicate changes not only in the seasons but in human health and behavior.[24]

Another believed-in (supposed) cleanser is urine, applied topically, by drinking, by enema, and even by injection into the body.

> In traditional Ayurveda, alcoholism, poor appetite, nausea, indigestion, ascites (free fluid in abdominal cavity), and edema are treated with goat feces washed with urine; constipation is treated with a mixture of milk and urine; impotence is treated with 216 kinds of enemas (some including the testicles of peacocks, swans, and turtles), and epilepsy and insanity are treated with ass urine.[25]

These remedial substances were administered in enemas. Urine is the body's process of elimination of a multitude of waste chemicals. To drink or use urine waste in any way is simply putting back into the system a concentration of impurities. I have systematically presented the fundamental principles in Ayurvedic medicine because even today, these practices are commonly promoted. It is common to hear of coffee or medicated enemas or an electrical machine, repeated enemas, herbs, etc., to remove toxins caught in body tissues. Various cleansing practices of Ayurveda are accepted and used by many who have no idea of its origin.

---

[24] Warrier, op., cit., pp. 170, 172.
[25] Raso, op. cit., p. 89.

In the practice of panchakarma (purification) in Ayurveda, the organs selected for stimulation to supposedly facilitate the removal of toxins from the system are not all organs science recognizes as designed to eliminate impurities and toxic substances from the body. Ayurveda sometimes may apply irritating and/or toxic substances to the sinuses, stomach, lungs, and intestines, which in turn causes them to secrete mucus and fluids, to vomit, or to have bowel movements. This is not a process of ridding the system of impurities; it is a method of adding impurities, which in turn causes the body to react.

The sciences of anatomy and physiology recognize the function of the lungs, kidneys, liver, and skin as the prime organs for processing and eliminating toxins from the body. The intestinal tract is not a prime detoxifying organ. However, it does carry out of the body the detoxified impurities discharged from the liver. Our bodies also need fresh air, water, and exercise to facilitate the elimination of toxins.

A simple approach to bodily cleansing follows: eat a nonrefined plant food diet; drink at least five to six glasses of water per day; breathe clean, fresh air; exercise an hour per day, and bathe daily. Abstain from coffee, tea, alcohol, and tobacco. In addition, it is prudent to be regular in habits of sleep, rest, and eating. Allow for five or more hours between meals, with nothing at all, except water between meals. The fiber in a nonrefined diet of plant foods will absorb many chemical by-products from the bowel and will promote elimination. There are several thousand types of phytochemicals in plants and some counteract various types of toxins. With this approach, the skin, lungs, kidneys, bowels, and liver are able to function at their best so as to eliminate impurities.

A fast for a day or even up to three days will allow the eliminating organs to neutralize and rid the body of substances we do not want in our systems. In the case of heavy metal poisoning such as lead, medical care is indicated.

I will share with you a clinical "gem" for promoting bowel function and avoiding constipation that I shared with patients in my medical practice. When first arising in the morning, drink two or three large glasses of quite warm to near hot water. It must be drunk as a bolus and not in sips. Do not eat any food for at least fifteen minutes. This is most effective with a high-fiber diet for bowel regularity. Do this daily for the rest of your life. I have had patients tell me that this solved their lifelong problem with constipation.

COMPARISON OF HINDUISM AND THE BIBLE'S PLAN OF SALVATION

The path for the Hindu to reach nirvana (spirit heaven) is by meditation—yoga, visualization (see next chapter), and with clearing the chakras by cleansing techniques such as nasal irrigation, cathartics, purgatives, and repeated colon irrigations. This is a self-work method, a counterfeit of the Bible's plan. The holy scriptures guide us to seek God through prayer and a mental process that is active and guided by the Holy Spirit, facilitated by the imagery of the Bible to point our minds to the great saving truths found in the scriptures. The Hindu looks to his various "cleansing" techniques to clear the spiritual impurities so as to better move energy through his chakras, which he believes will then carry him into the spirit world of nirvana. In sharp contrast, the Christian by faith trusts in the *merits of the shed blood of Jesus Christ* to cover (cleanse) his sin and be accepted into heavenly paradise by God the Father.

> Then one of the elders answered, saying to me, "Who are these which are arrayed in white robes? And where did they come from? And I said to him, "Sir, you know." So he said to me, "These are the ones who come out of great tribulation and washed their robes and *made them white in the blood of the Lamb.* Therefore, they are before the throne of God, and serve Him day and night in His temple: and He who sits on the throne shall dwell among them" (Revelation 7:13–15).

> Then I heard a loud voice saying in heaven, "Now salvation, and strength, and the kingdom of our God, and the power of His Christ have come, for the accuser of our Brethren, who accused them before our God day and night, hast been cast down. And they *overcame him by the blood of the Lamb*, and by the word of their testimony; and they loved not their lives to the death. Therefore rejoice, O heavens, and you who dwell in them (Revelation 12:10–12) (emphasis added).

CONVENTIONAL SCIENCE VERSUS VIBRATIONAL MEDICINE

For the past three centuries, the discipline of *science* was developed by experimenting, measuring, analyzing, and reproducibility. Conflict in beliefs occurred between the proponents of universal energy, vitalism, life force, etc., and modern science. The characteristics of the universal energy could not be measured, demonstrated, or explained by the known laws of physics. When electricity was discovered and its laws of action understood, the proponents of universal energy felt that life force energy would now be demonstrated and explained to the nonbelieving skeptic scientists. It did not work out that way, and there is still a gap in belief between the two.

In recent years, instruments for testing electricity and electromagnetic energy fields have been greatly expanded and have become more sophisticated. Still, scientists cannot find common ground with those believing in and teaching the universal energy hypothesis.

The scientist who believes in Eastern mysticism and energy hypothesis presents his work as proof. Points of "proof" proclaimed by universal energy adherents are:

A. Auras

> All living things (people, plants, animals, etc.) are made up of a complex combination of atoms, molecules, and energy cells. As these ingredients coexist, they generate a large magnetic energy field that can be sensed, felt, and even seen around the physical body. This (hypothesized) energy field is called an aura. [26]

Are there energy fields around the human body? Yes, sort of, but there are energy fields almost everywhere. The body's energy fields are commonly measured by medical devices such as electrocardiograph, electroencephalograph, or electromyography. To obtain a measurement with these devices, it is necessary to either insert needles into the skin to make electrical contact or sandpaper the skin to prepare it for the application of an electrode that can pick up an impulse that reveals the electrical field. If either of these methods is not used, the machines will not be able to detect an electromagnetic field.

The scientific world of physics has very delicate instruments for measuring an electrical flux; for instance, one quantum of electromagnetic force can be detected. This is more than a million times more sensitive than living tissue. These instruments do not have the limitations of tissue which is warm and wet. Cooling something to hundreds of degrees below zero will make them superconductive.

> Even if the human nervous system turns out to be a thousand times better than I think, devices would still be hugely better at measuring energy fields.[27]

---

[26] http://paganspath.com/   Q—aura.

[27] http://www.don-lindsayarchive.org/skeptic.

The human body has been measured with powerful machines that would detect an aura if such existed. The MRI machine is composed of extremely powerful magnets. When they are turned on the hydrogen atoms in a person's body shift in position and when the magnets are turned off the hydrogen atoms return to prior position. The movement of the hydrogen atom creates an electrical force that is measured by the instrument and the computer converts the information into a picture of the body's anatomy. No auras have been detected by MRI machines.

B. Kirlian photography

In 1939 in Russia, Semyon Kirlian discovered by accident that if an object placed on a photographic plate was subjected to a high-voltage electric field, an image would be created on the plate. The image, though somewhat nondiscreet and fuzzy, was accepted by believers in auras as proof.

This phenomenon has been shown to be the result of moisture or gases around the test object reacting with the generated electrical field and therefore reacting on the photographic plate. When Kirlian photography is done in a vacuum where no moisture or gases can exist, the "aura" vanishes from the photographic plate (Hines 2003). In spite of the scientific explanation, Kirlian photography is still referred to as *proof* that auras surround living and nonliving objects.

C. Radiating energy fields are said to be projected from the hands

James L. Oschman, in his book *Energy Medicine: The Scientific Basis*, makes the comment that energy fields can be detected around the hands of "suitable trained therapists." Another author states that these same phenomena can be measured on "sensitives" but not on nonsensitives. (As an illustration of energy radiating from hands, Oschman uses the story of Mesmer and his power of healing as done by magnets and then as he changed to using only his hands for healing. See chapter on hypnosis.)

D. Claims that energy fields or auras can be felt

Therapeutic touch healing method is based upon this claim.

> The spring issue of *Scientific Review of Alternative Medicine* reports a rare test of therapeutic touch designed by James Randi. The practitioner (of TT) was unable to detect the presence or

absence of a human arm in a "sleeve." The test involved a patient flipping a coin.[28]

After each flip, they either did or didn't insert their arm into a sleeve. For the first twenty flips, the patient was in plain view, and the TT practitioner was 100 percent successful (twenty out of twenty) in determining if the arm was or wasn't in the sleeve. The patient was then screened from the TT practitioner's view, and another twenty flips were done. The practitioner did no better than random (guessing) at telling if the arm was in the sleeve. They were asked if they would like to go on, and they refused.

Emily Rosa, a nine-year-old girl, did a test of a similar type with the same results for a science project in school. Her project was written and appeared in three medical journals—*Lancet*, *The British Medical Journal*, and *The Journal of the American Medical Association*. Her experiment was also reported on nationwide television.

E. Psychics and sensitives can see *auras*

Ten thousand dollars was offered to any psychic who could accurately identify auras. A test was set up with twenty partitions on a large stage. The psychic, Berkeley Psychic Institute's best, was to identify which partitions had a person behind it. This was a live test on the *Bill Bixby* television show. The psychic agreed that the test was fair. Prior to placing the people behind the partitions, the psychic was asked if she could see the auras of the people. She said yes and that they were from one to two feet above their heads. Six people were placed behind partitions, but fourteen did not go behind partitions and stayed out of sight. The psychic saw auras behind all twenty partitions. There is now a one-million-dollar offer for the psychic that can pass this same test.[29]

F. Magnetic therapy is used in conventional medicine

Pulsating electromagnetic waves are used to facilitate bone healing, with ongoing research exploring its use in soft tissue injury. It is now recognized that with an injury to tissue, there is an electromagnetic field *inside* the body surrounding the wound, but none on the outside. Pulsating electromagnetic forces can affect this energy field, stimulating healing by attracting repair cells. Powerful magnetic pulses can be used in severe cases

---

[28] http://www.don-lindsay-archive.com/skeptic   Q—aura.

[29] http//skeptic.com   Q—aura.

of depression; however, there may be significant memory loss. There is no evidence from double-blind studies that any benefit occurs from using stagnant magnets. It may be asked: why use terms such as electromagnetic frequencies, radio frequencies, etc., throughout this book relating to supposedly emanating energies from our bodies? The reason is that there are no proper terms to use for an energy that does not really exist. I have used the terms that appear in writings of those supporting, believing in, and teaching the universal energy hypothesis. For example, from the book *The Way of Energy* by Lam Kan Chuen, we find this:

> *You are a miniature field of the electromagnetic energy of the universe.*[30]

I must use the terms appearing in the literature so readers can relate the information in this text to that which they may read. A more accurate term might be *Satan's electric currents*. There are many highly trained scientists who are believers in Eastern mysticism. Several are superb authors. They are able to convincingly present the subject of the aura and hypothetical electromagnetic energy as radiating from our bodies and hands, which is said to be able to influence and correct the energy fields of others. I present two paragraphs from a book review which appeared in the *British Homoeopathic Journal* (volume 87, July 1998) about one such author.

Dr. Richard Gerber, a physician practicing in Livonia, Michigan, USA, is by many considered the authority on what is called energetic medicine. His book titled *Vibrational Medicine: The No. 1 Handbook of Subtle-Energy Therapies* brings together a large variety of alternative and complementary therapies such as acupuncture, homeopathy, magnet therapy, body or soma therapy, flower essences, etc., linking their perceived properties with a common denominator, that of electromagnetic vibrations and/or *vibrational medicine*. A synonym would be *energy medicine*. He contrasts style of medical practices; one method (orthodox) he says is based in Newton's mechanical physics, while another approach (energy medicine) is explained by quantum physics. Gerber is an excellent writer, and the reader has to stop at times and consider very carefully what his book is saying to avoid being persuaded in some of the esoteric concepts he makes simple.

> Gerber describes nonchemical information exchange between cells, which ultimately forms the basis of his theories on how

---

[30] Chuen, Lam Kam, *The Way of Energy*, Simon &and Schuster Inc., p. 12.

these therapies may work. He creates a working hypothesis that embraces the ideas of chakras, meridians, and energetic force fields. He expands on traditional Eastern philosophies of chi and prana, blending them together with fascinating results; there is a blending of scientific fact and esoteric philosophy that captures the imagination.[31]

Dr. Gerber presents in his book, *Vibrational Medicine* (and on DVDs), that universal energy frequencies above the first level or plane are faster than light frequencies. He refers to a William Tiller, a previous physicist of Stanford University for his authority on this subject. *This hypothesis is not entertained in conventional physics.*

I have listened to Dr. Gerber's explanation of vibrational energy medicine. He is highly trained in conventional science and medicine. He is so smooth and convincing that I began to wonder about my own beliefs. I have repeatedly experienced this same *self-questioning* after reading other well-trained scientists and skilled authors who are oriented in Eastern religion and metaphysics. I found that I had to back away from the immediate discourse and evaluate the overall picture that each of these doctors present. Where are they heading with this concept and their explanations of the physical workings of the universe?

As I continued to listen to Dr. Gerber, the subjects of astral travel, astrology, numerology, reincarnation, clairvoyance, channeling, psychic abilities, spiritual evolution, and divine self were presented as wholesome objectives and realities. He teaches that we have a divine nature and are divine lights. There is the idea of chakras being the processors of energy which moves us onward in the spiritual climb toward the supreme self or godhood. Attaining perfection is a process of self-works which is obtained by the development of a higher energy level. Dr. Gerber is not the only scientist holding such beliefs.

I asked myself how it is possible that highly trained scientists, such as Drs. Gerber, Green, and Oschman arrive at conclusions so far from the accepted laws of conventional physics and chemistry. They at times speak of *intuition* as the source of their information. What is intuition? As I understand it, they are speaking of receiving intelligence from the universe that they are able to tap into. This is analogous to receiving *divine revelation*. The information received or arrived at by intuition and then is accepted as superseding conventional science.

---

[31] http://www.minimum.com/reviews/vibrational-medicine.htm.

Elizabeth Clare Prophet claims to have received seven dictated messages from Djwal Kul, an "ascended master" (demonic spirit) which she placed in a book. These messages are a:

> discussion of the chakras within the body as transmitters of light energy which is essential to the understanding of spiritual evolution.[32]

He, Djwal Kul (Djwhal Khul in some other writings), presents numerous meditations and techniques for "clearing the chakras" to facilitate their expansion and projection into the "macrocosmic-microcosmic interchange." These messages by Djwal Kul are a guide for the Pagan's pilgrimage and pathway to immortality and godhood.

In Kul's messages the *aura* is an extension of god "himself" in us and that the size of the aura is directly related to the mastery of god's energies within our chakras. The "god" spoken of in this book is not the God you and I think of. In reality, it is Satan. However, the description given in this esoteric book is that it is the highest plane (plane 7) of universal energy. It is believed to be the level of energy which imparts *immortality* and *your divine self.*

Why write about such blasphemy? What does it have to do with spiritualistic practices in health and healing? The alternative and complementary methods of treatment are about balancing body energy. They are not based on being in harmony with God's laws of health. If we choose to use these "energy" methods, we are accepting that they indeed may work in providing health and healing. At the same time, we have accepted (perhaps not consciously) the energy hypothesis, which is the foundation and core of Hinduism and pagan religions.

DEEPAK CHOPRA, MD

Deepak Chopra, MD is a name you may have heard as a lecturer or in interviews on a TV show. He has authored nineteen books promoting Ayurvedic medicine, produced many CDs teaching his style of Ayurveda, and established the American Association of Ayurvedic Medicine in 1991. In 1995, he opened the Chopra Center for Well-Being in La Jolla, California, where he is educational director. His books are in twelve languages and sold around the world. The books have sold more than

---

[32] Prophet, Elizabeth Clare, *Intermediate Studies of the Human Aura*, Summit University Press, Colorado Springs, CO, p. 6.

ten million English copies. He has produced TV and radio programs promoting his Ayurvedic teachings.

Chopra is a graduate of All India Institute of Medical Sciences; he took several years training in the United States at Lehey Clinic and University of Virginia Hospital, becoming certified in internal medicine and endocrinology. He taught at Tufts and Boston University Schools of Medicine and was elected chief of staff at New England Memorial Hospital. He also established a private practice. Then his interests changed to Ayurvedic medicine. He no longer practices medicine but applies his skills to the teaching and promotion of Ayurveda.

What does Chopra teach that catches so many people's interest? Central to his philosophy is that the human mind has latent potential and self-knowledge. To bring this potential to fruition, he supports meditation, nutrition, yoga and exercise, herbal medicine, massage, sound, movement, and aromatherapy. He teaches detoxification and purification by fasting and enemas. His influence in this country and other nations has been vast. There are other medical doctors who also have taken up Ayurveda teachings and have great influence in this country—Drs. Weil and Coussens. They promote the association of Western scientific medicine with Eastern mysticisms which is called integrative medicine. See chapter "Those Who Do Magic Arts."

Dr. Oz

A physician of more recent public interest is a Mehmet Oz, MD, a faculty member of Columbia University. Dr. Oz was introduced to public several years past by Oprah Winfrey on her TV show. He has gone to have his own show and his name is seen in print on a regular basis. He is a surgeon but has been promoting dietary advice that nutrition experts have serious questions of. Recently, a panel of ten physicians asked Columbia University to rescind Dr. Oz's faculty position because of what they called egregious lack of integrity and promoting quack treatments.

Lighthousetrails.com had a recent article commenting on his connection to Rick Warren's "Daniel Plan." Dr. Oz. In January 2011 Rick Warren initiated "The Daniel Plan," a fifty-two-week wellness program sponsored by Rick Warren and the Saddleback Church and directed by Dr. Mehmet Oz, Dr. Daniel Amen, and Dr. Mark Hyman. Although these three physicians are all involved with New Age teachings, they describe themselves respectively as a Muslim, a Christian, and a Jew. Eastern style meditation is a strong component of their health plan.

Amidst this media blitz focusing on some of Dr. Oz's questionable medical practices, there is another side of this story that has affected mainstream Christianity. Rick Warren and the church seem to be totally unfazed by Dr. Oz's New Age occult spiritual practices. Author Warren B. Smith states that for Rick Warren to invite Dr. Oz into the church (through the Daniel Plan) is "the inconceivable equivalent of the first century church inviting Simon the sorcerer into the church to help it become more healthy."[33]

Dr. Oz has involved himself with a number of occultic practices, one being his association with psychic John Edwards who supposedly helps people to talk to their dead loved ones. Oz and Edwards did one TV show together titled "Psychic Mediums: Are They the New Therapists?[34] Find out if talking to the dead is a new form of therapy in which the answer to this question from both men was *yes*. Oz has also written the forewords to a number of New Age and occultic books including *Transcendence: Healing and Transformation through Transcendental Meditation* and *Quantum Wellness: A Practical and Spiritual Guide to Health and Happiness.*[35]

Warren Smith states:

> One can only wonder if the prophet Daniel's vision of the end days included a look at Rick Warren's Daniel Plan—a compromised pastor and three New Age doctors with their psychics, spirit guides, tantric sex, necromancy, yoga, Reiki, transcendental and Kundalini "sa ta na ma" meditations, and more—all in Daniel's name. If so, it is no wonder the Bible records that he (Daniel) "fainted" and became "sick" for a number of days (Daniel 8:27).[36]

Just Exercise?

---

[33] http://www.lighthousetrailsresearch.com/blog/wp-admin/post.php?post=17243&action=edit&message=1#py
[34] *Ibid.*
[35] Smith, warren, Lighthousetrils.com, *Dr. Oz*, April 23.2015.
[36] *Ibid.*

Former Yogi Says Spiritual Effects of Yoga Occur Spontaneously

I frequently hear a comment like this: "I know yoga, and yoga exercises have an ancient origin in paganism, but I do not think about the spiritual aspect and reject such interest when I participate in the practice." For many Christians, there seems to be no concern of a spiritual influence in participating in yoga or its stretches and exercises because of the belief that it is possible to separate the physical from the spiritual, but is this really possible?

Connie Fait, a Tibetan nun, yogi, and director of a Tibetan Buddhist temple spent forty years in the practice and study of yoga and its traditions. She has placed a short blog on the Internet sharing her experience and wisdom in regard to the concept that it can be practiced separate from any of its spiritual trappings. She has had a Christian conversion after her long life in the Buddhist religion and wishes to make clear to the unsuspecting public that there is a spiritual influence in the practice of yoga and/or its asanas (postures/stretches) whether one desires it or not. She refers to practicing yoga and/or the asanas without a person applying any attention to spiritual thoughts, actions, or meditation.

Fait explains that yogic tradition is deeply hidden in mystery, and those who do understand it are accomplished yogis. The asanas (postures/stretches) are "tools" by which the secrets of the tradition are to be understood. Note her following words: "Anyone who is doing yoga asanas is in that same process—whether or not they are aware of it or intend it." (http://womenofgrace.com/blog/?p=29077)

Her article continues in explanation. Yoga asanas are the foundation of Hindu theology. The initiators of Hindu religion sat in mystical altered mental states yearning to have union with their believed-in *creative force* of the universe, Brahman, chief of the gods to the Hindu. In this mystical state, they experienced visitation of deities (demons) who moved their bodies into movements (kriyas), which today are the postures (asanas) that are practiced in yoga exercises. While performing these exercises/asanas, they experienced high meditative states wherein they encountered directly "gods and deities" whose names are given to the poses. To assume that pose, one is inviting that deity to possess.

Lyengar Yogacharia, a leader in yoga, teaches that the goal of yoga (to yoke with the chief deity Brahman) can be accomplished by two actions.

First, practicing the asanas which will in time bring in "pranayama" (controlled breathing), the second action, and which will occur naturally with perfection of the asanas. Meditation will also follow spontaneously without ever being desired or being taught.

In this article, Connie Fait summarizes as follows: "The well-known Yogacharia, who has taught people of the West, has made clear that if performed well, asanas will bring about a spontaneous pranayama response in the body. In other words, the breathing aspect of yoga need not be taught in a class because it occurs naturally with perfection of the asanas. Meditation is never taught as it is also a result of the perfection of the asanas and alleged prana moving in the body, which leads to experiencing the meditative state and eventually ultimate union with Brahman, gods and deities, or demons" (reference from the above Web site address).

SUMMARY

Presented in this chapter are the basic principles of the Ayurveda system of health and healing. It is based on belief in astrology and the idea that man originated from the cosmic energy called the creative principle or universal energy. This is the "wisdom from the East" that so many consider superior to the knowledge gained through present-day science. It can be seen that many of the old practices of the West in past centuries were primarily the practice of Ayurveda without the spiritual names. There is a carryover of many of the old practices that have been slow to disappear.

In the Bible, we are told that God gave Solomon *wisdom*:

> Solomon's wisdom was greater than the wisdom of all the men of the East, and greater than all the wisdom of Egypt." "Men of all nations, came to listen to Solomon's wisdom, sent by all the kings of the world, who had heard of his wisdom (I Kings 4:29–34, NIV).

God had blessed His people Israel, through the prophet Moses, with instructions for healthful living. Remember, Israel is the only nation in the history of the world to have a primary system of disease prevention. Today, we can give praise to God for the instructions in health and healing as given through the Bible and science, providing us with the most advanced knowledge in the world for healthful living. The end results have shown this to be true. Why would we even consider looking back to the wisdom of the East and of Egypt (paganism and sun worship) and reject God's directions for health and healing?

At this time of great advances in science, when this knowledge has been applied with great benefit, we see widespread belief in and the following after these ancient methods that have no history of being effective for improving the health of man. There is no evidence that shows these practices have extended the life of man by even one day. The medical history in the areas of the world that practiced these methods has shown that health was dismal and never improved until the science that follows the physical laws of God, chemistry, physics, and hygiene were followed. How can we accept and use these pagan methods if we believe in a God who spoke and created by His power? We are sustained by His power and not by some power in us that can be turned off and on or stimulated by the practices presented in this book.

Why put so much effort into exposing the Ayurvedic system of health and healing? Because this system has had great influence on health and healing as practiced over the world for millennia. This system is being used as the right arm of the religious message of Hinduism and spiritualism. Ayurveda cannot be separated from Hinduism, and Hinduism cannot be separated from Ayurveda. Ayurveda has its basis in astrology. The sun is the all-powerful tenet of astrology, and to give homage to the sun is equivalent to Luciferic worship. To participate in these so-called healing methods is to partake of the *tree of the knowledge of good and evil.*

9

ACUPUNCTURE AND CHINESE TRADITIONAL MEDICINE

Chinese traditional medicine practices were little heard of in the West until the early 1970s. I became involved in medical education in 1954, and not until the 1970s did I hear of acupuncture or other traditional Chinese healing methods. The march toward scientific medicine in the first fifty years of the twentieth century had been almost complete. The medical disciplines of eclectic medicine, homeopathy, osteopathy, and naturopathy had either converted toward scientific medicine or had slowly faded and/or ceased to exist. Medical students were told about some past medical treatments, such as the use of heavy metals, emetics, blistering compounds, purgatives, and bloodletting, but I heard no mention of Ayurvedic or traditional Chinese medicine, such as acupuncture or moxibustion.

Since the late 1970s, there has been widespread acceptance of the oriental healing methods. Most of the older physicians rejected them, but a large number of younger doctors did not, and amazingly, some of the alternative therapies have gone "main street." For some practitioners, it has been mainly a financial interest; but for others, it has been a belief in these alternative methods. Now we see in many medical training institutions and at the National Institutes of Health research being done on alternative treatment methods, acupuncture being one of the more common.

Segments of the Ayurvedic system have been used more widely than has Chinese traditional medicine. However, the Chinese methods are often used along with Ayurveda. Let us examine the roots of the traditional Chinese system of healing. You are probably very familiar with the symbol of two fish swimming in a circle with eight trigrams of all possible combinations of the two, which in Chinese is called *pa kua* and referred to in English as circle of harmony. Emperor Fu His, in 2900 BC, is credited with its origination. It is a symbol representing all the conditions of interior-exterior, hot-cold, deficiencies-excesses, yin-yang. This emperor's works are the most ancient upon which traditional Chinese medicine is based.[1]

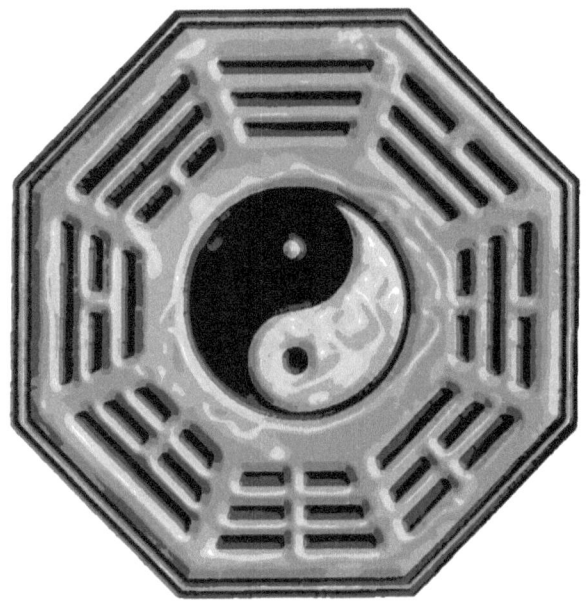

Figure 23. Pa Kua (circle of harmony).

Another emperor, Shen Nung, in 2800 BC, compiled a text *pen-tsao*, which was the first medical text for the use of herbs. It contained 365 drugs, which he had tested on himself.[2]

The most celebrated ancient medical text in China is called the Nei Ching. It was written in 2600 BC by the Yellow emperor, Hwang Ti. This text garnered information that gives us insight into the early approach to Chinese medicine and its orientation.[3]

---

[1] Lyons, Albert S., Petrucelli, R. Joseph II; *Medicine: An Illustrated History*, Harry N. Abrams, Inc. Publishers, NY (1978), p. 125.

[2] *Ibid.*, p. 124.

[3] *Ibid.*, p. 124.

January 1, 1912, Sun Yat-sen, a Western-trained physician, was inaugurated president of China following the revolution and overthrow in 1911 of the Imperial Dynasty. Shortly following, he initiated improvements in hygiene practices in China such as having garbage cleared from the streets and installing running water in major urban centers. A bureau to combat epidemics was established, and Western-style medical schools were developed by a few Western-trained Chinese physicians. The old practice of traditional Chinese medicine was discouraged and, in 1929, outlawed. This caused a great furor from the traditional Chinese medicine doctors who banded together to fight the new restrictions. The masses of China were on the side of traditional medicine, and the attempt to eradicate the old style practice failed primarily because of the belief of mostly uneducated Chinese masses in Taoism and the philosophy of chi with its yin-yang divisions. That attempt to modernize China failed.

The changes initiated by Sun Yat-sen were almost insignificant compared to the size and degenerate condition of the country. From 1916 until 1949, China suffered great political turmoil and instability, with minimal progress made in hygiene and health of the nation. Following Mao's rise to power under Communism in 1949, public hygiene was made a priority. Eradicating the vectors of parasitic diseases, closure of open sewers, immunization programs, and clean water were measures taken to combat a deplorable health status, as documented by Paul Bailey in his book, *A History of Chinese Medicine*. He tells us of epidemics continuously of cholera, plague, black fever (five hundred thousand afflicted in 1949), and ten million were infected by a parasite called bilharzia. One million died each year from tuberculosis, epidemics of scarlet fever, and typhoid; untold millions were infected with malaria. The average life span was thirty-five years. This health status was a result of the mind-set of Taoism and the other Eastern religious concepts. The medical approach to illness was based on such beliefs which allowed these conditions to exist. Traditional Chinese medicine is based on Taoism ("the way"). Three basic beliefs of Taoism are:

1. The creative principle (or universal energy) is called chi and is composed of two parts—*yin* and *yang* (dualism);
2. *Five basic elements* are involved in transformation in creation: *metal, air, earth, fire, water*. Each name represents a "creative" spirit from a specific planet.
3. Man is the "microcosm" of the universe the "macrocosm."

In contrast, the biblical account of creation tells us how God created:

For He spoke and it was done and He commanded and it stood fast (Ps. 33:9)

Man was created by God, forming the dust of the ground into man's form; God breathed into it "the breath of life," and man became a living "soul." Early on in the history of the world, Satan's counterfeit changed this story in such a way that left out the Creator, Jesus Christ the Son of God. This formed the myth of a great power, energy, voice, breath that existed throughout space which was of two parts, good and evil, that when it became properly balanced, creation occurred. The Greeks called this *pneuma*, the cosmic spirit that they believed pervades and enlivens all things and produces change; this equates with the Hindus' *prana*, those of the South Seas mana, and the Chinese chi.

The Chinese explanation for origins is that with the proper balance of yin and yang (which are divisions of *chi*), transformation occurred, which brought the cosmos, earth, and man into existence. Fundamental to traditional Chinese medicine is the astrological concept of the planets being closely associated with earth and man, with the sun and moon having the strongest influence. They had a belief in a "cosmological correspondence" between the houses of the Chinese zodiac and "chinglo channels" (now called meridians) that are said to be in man. Sheila McNamara, in her book, *Traditional Chinese Medicine*, makes the following statement:

> To the Chinese, the human body is the cosmos in miniature. The universe is an organism, and man is a microcosm of the universe . . . Yang is masculine: sun . . . .Yin is feminine: moon.[4]

This belief gives expression in the saying "as above, so below." This concept was prevalent throughout the ancient world but often expressed in different terms. A statement was made by Gregor Reisch (c. 1467–1525) in *Margarita Philosophica*, published in 1503:

> The pagans believed that the zodiac formed the body of the grand man of the universe. This body, which they called the macrocosm (the great world), was divided into twelve major parts, one of which was under the control of the celestial powers reposing in each of the zodiacal constellations. Believing that the entire universal system was epitomized in man's body,

---

[4] McNamara, Sheila; *Traditional Chinese Medicine*, Basic Books (Perseus Books) New York, NY (1996), p. 26.

which they called the microcosm (the little world), they evolved that now familiar figure of "the cut-up man in the almanac" by allotting a sign of the zodiac to each of twelve major parts of the human body.

These beliefs led to "astrological medicine" which was dominant in Europe up until the seventeenth century. The physicians of that time used special "tables," called ephemerides or Alfonsine tables to make predictions based on astrological conjunctions, alignments, and angle between planets. These predictions were then used to perform various healing acts, such as drawing off blood from the body (venesection, cupping, causing great blisters to form), cauterization, surgery, and to choose herbs for medicines with special astral powers. Disease, they believed, came from an interruption of the free flow of "pneuma" or "prana," as well as an imbalance of four body fluids called humors. Each humor was believed to be connected to a planet by correspondence.

To correct a supposed imbalance of "humors," bloodletting (bleeding) was instigated and used by European and early American practitioners and is still done by some Muslims today.

> The practice of lancing, bloodletting, and cupping (*hijama*) to affect specific organs or to mitigate specific diseases based on a postulated relationship between the internal organs and points on the surface of the skin is still prevalent amongst the Muslims worldwide, and nowadays, video instructions for it are available, even on YouTube. It is plausible that the same principle is at the origin of acupuncture channels in China because the distribution of the regions of astrological influences and the related venesection points portrayed in medieval Islamic and European manuscripts significantly resembles the allocation of master, command influential, and other key points.[5]

The Chinese followed a similar concept and saw disease as being a result of disharmony in the balance of yin and yang. This imbalance can occur for many reasons, such as lifestyle. It is believed that some physical disorders are caused by "winds." Foods are considered yin or yang, and the balance of such will influence so as to maintain health or imbalance to allow illness. The beliefs of what causes imbalance in the yin and yang

---

[5] Kavoussi, Ben MS, MSOM, Lac, *Science-Based Medicine*, Astrology with Needles, pp. 5, 6; http://www.sciencebasedmedicine.org/?p=583.

of the body are complex. I will not go into the causes of imbalance but rather will direct our attention to the practices that are said to be capable of restoring balance.

In Ayurveda, *prana*, universal energy, is said to be centered in whirling vortexes of energy referred to as chakras. The flow of energy through the body is said to be facilitated by meditation, yoga exercises, diet, herbs, aromatherapy, and cleansing therapies. In *traditional Chinese medicine* (TCM), the energy is described as flowing through the body in "meridians" which are (imaginary) channels perpendicular to the body. Many smaller channels branch from the meridians and distribute the energy throughout the body. Here too, meditation, exercises, food-drink, moxibustion, acupressure, acupuncture, and other *sympathetic remedies* are used to facilitate the flow and balance of chi.

All creation depended upon *correspondence, association,* and *sympathy* between the various phases outlined above and yin-yang balance of chi. *All disease* of animal and man is considered to be an *imbalance of yin-yang.* Correcting the imbalance is believed to restore health; therefore, methods to balance chi and treat disease were developed over millennia of time.

Diseases are classified according to four different states of disharmony and make up eight syndromes, which include all varieties of disease. These previously mentioned conditions are: imbalance of yin-yang; interior-exterior; hot-cold; and deficiencies-excesses.

The customary way to diagnose an imbalance of energy in traditional Chinese medicine was to observe the tongue and feel the pulse. The tongue was felt to demonstrate changes in energy (chi) distribution throughout the body. Taking the pulse was done not to check the rate and rhythm of the heart but to find where an imbalance of chi existed. One ancient author of Chinese traditional medicine wrote ten large volumes on *pulse diagnosis*. From the pulse and observation of the tongue, those physicians determined the imbalance of chi (qi), where it existed, and then prescribed to balance it.

DISEASE TREATMENT METHODS

This chapter presents those methods of treatment most commonly known and accepted by Western society. These include the use of herbs, martial arts, and acupuncture. The Chinese practice disease prevention, with special emphasis on exercise and diet. Disease prevention is directed toward maintaining a balance of body energies.

In traditional Chinese medicine, herbs and foods are considered to have a "signature" and "like cures like." For instance, walnuts resemble the brain; therefore, walnuts are especially nourishing to the brain. For a child to eat the pig's tail is to assure a straight, strong spine as he or she grows (in China pigs have straight tails). If an herb looks like an organ of the body, then it is considered to have special healing powers for that part of the body.[6]

Ginseng root can resemble the body and its limbs and is therefore considered good for all bodily ailments. The horn of an animal represents a phallic symbol and so is used as an aphrodisiac. Consumption of animal parts, such as a tiger's heart, will give courage. This type of belief has resulted in a large number of herbs being used because of their appearance rather than from their biochemical properties. Many animal parts are likewise used in this way. I visited a very large Chinese pharmacy in Vancouver, British Columbia, Canada, and was amazed to see dried parts of animals, fish, and many other products I could not identify. The store had a thousand or more different substances, some in bottles and some in open boxes.

The idea of "like cures like" is an *association-sympathy* concept and not at all because of the chemical action of our systems. The Chinese found many herbs and substances that really do have significant biochemical action which are used worldwide. Herbal books will often label herbs as either hot or -cold and/or yin or yang. The herbs may then be chosen for medicinal use accordingly so as to influence a sick person's balance of yin-yang and or hot and cold.

MARTIAL ARTS: QIGONG

> Qi gong is the forerunner of traditional Chinese medicine, since *qi*/chi, the subtle breath or life energy is at the heart of everything.[7]

Qigong or (chi kung) means manipulation of vital energy (psychic energy) and is also the precursor of martial arts. Qi is comprised of yin and yang, each contributing to health when in proper balance. Gong refers to achieving the ultimate balance of the two parts. Qigong is a variety of physical exercises and actions practiced to facilitate the harmony of yin and yang. If one is able to superbly balance these parts of qi, he will be able to accomplish extraordinary feats with his powers and will be a *master* of qigong. Qigong is a system of body-mind discipline of traditional Chinese medicine and is the foundation of martial arts.

---

[6] McNamara, op. cit., p.117
[7] *Ibid.*, p. 130.

Fundamentally, qigong is a method of *meditation exercise* aimed at the cultivation of physical and spiritual perfection.[8]

Meditational forms involve stillness, standing, sitting, or lying motionless. More physically active forms will involve breathing exercises in order to inhale the *"vital essence of life."* Physical activity is frequently a slow, smooth, and rounded movement (tai chi chuan). Concentrating on breath and emptying the mind are very important. These activities are *"always with a spiritual element."*[9]

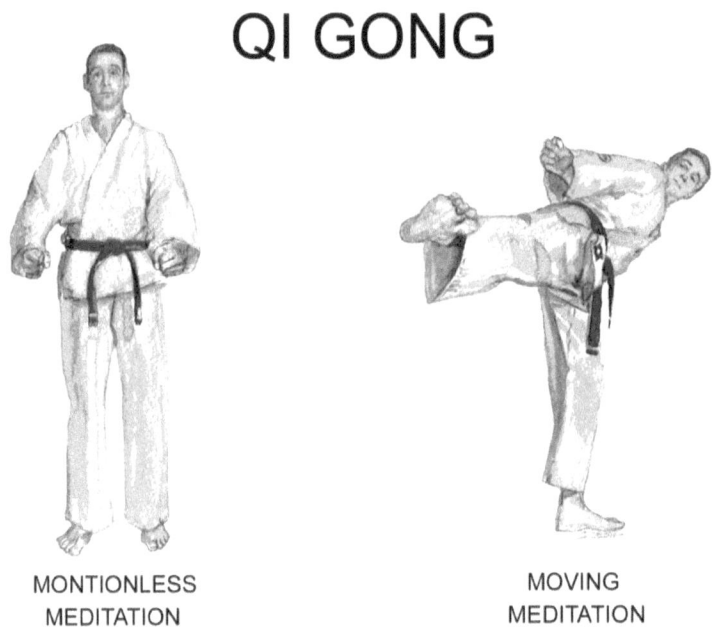

Figure 24. Martial arts

The exercises can be performed alone or by a qigong master for another person, which involves exercising around the other person's body, without making any physical contact. This is supposed to activate the qi within another's body so that the person can be brought into the qigong state. Balancing the qi is the objective, for too little qi is equivalent to illness.

---

[8] *Ibid.*, pp. 127–128.

[9] *Ibid.*, p. 128.

When people do their own exercises or when masters do the exercises for them, qi, it is said, can be directed toward different areas within the body.

> One of its main precepts concerns finding the center of the body to attain perfect balance as a prerequisite to health. Students will be taught to visualize the soles of their feet reaching hundreds of yards deep down into the earth or a rod passing down their spine via entering of their head and penetrating deep into the ground. Once they achieve perfect balance, no one will be able to knock them off-balance. It proves that the qi is perfectly centered, neither too weak in one part of the body nor too strong in another.[10]

In mid-fifth century, an Indian Buddhist monk, Bodhidharma, came from India to the Shaolin Temple (Hall of Three Buddhas) in the Hunan province of China. He had revised Hinduism (referred to as Chan Buddhism), and he brought yoga to the Shaolin Temple monastery. "Legend tells that it was he who taught the monks the methods of physical movement combined with their meditation to enhance spiritual (occult) abilities. Through certain breathing, visualization techniques, and acts of worship, the monks were said to develop almost supra-natural psychic and physical powers." Bodhidharma had written a small book (*The Muscle/Tendon Change Classics*) found at the temple following his death which outlined spiritual and physical exercises which would enable the Buddhist to reach "enlightenment." Thus, from Indian yoga developed the *martial arts* of the Buddhist. The practice spread to Japan, Okinawa, and Korea. Each country brought forth additional styles and names for the practice.

This book by Bodhidharma is given great respect by martial artists worldwide. It outlines the foundation of all martial art forms including qigong. The book presents meditation, attention to breathing, and visualization practices which have great similarity to a book written in 1522–1524, *The Spiritual Exercises of Ignatius Loyola*. The philosophy of Ignatius's book has very close similarity to those of Hinduism, Buddhism, and Taoism.

I once presented this information to an assembly, and a gentleman came to me afterward. He spoke of taking *karate*, one of the disciplines of qigong, and how he and two other students tried to push their instructor off balance and were unable to do so. The question to ask is, what power held him to the ground?

---

[10] *Ibid., p. 128.*

A delegation of Chinese physicians traveled to the United States to present to American doctors this particular aspect of traditional Chinese medicine. They desired to convince the American doctors of the scientific basis of this therapy for which they made great claims. They described studies showing that the power associated with this life force showed up as making changes in electrical brain wave potential, in the molecular rotation of liquid crystal molecules, and in cancer cells, bacteria, and viruses. The following was reported in *The Medical Tribune:*

After the Chinese qigong scientists described their research, Dr. Li Xiao Ming, a qigong master at the Qigong Research Institute at the Beijing College of Traditional Chinese Medicine, demonstrated his art on Dr. Alfonso Di Mino. As Dr. Li did his exercise around Dr. Di Mino, Dr. Di Mino shouted for Dr. Li to lower his hands as he said that he felt as if he "were ready to fly." Later, he said that it felt as if he had an "electric magnetic power inside his body." "My mind was not aware of my body." Dr. Di Mino, a biophysicist, described this "life force" as "the medicine of the future."[11]

Robert Leeds, the vice chairman of the Sino-U.S. Qigong Center, then told the audience that Dr. Li was able to:

> manipulate energies we allegedly are not sensitive to or do not understand. He added that for four thousand years, the Chinese have been able to map out this energy field and manipulate it to such an extent that it can heal.[12]

All across China in the early morning, people can be seen outside practicing various exercises of qigong. All qigong methods are supposed to produce equal flow of energy through the body and thereby promote health. Remember, there is a *spiritual aspect* connected to qigong exercises.[13]

Tai chi is one of the popular styles of qigong. Many people believe that it can be practiced totally free of any spiritual association, but is that so? Sheila McNamara in her book, *Traditional Chinese Medicine,* says of the different qigong exercises:

---

[11] *Medical Tribune,* February 5 (1986) by Elizabeth Mechcatie (medical newspaper)

[12] *Ibid.*

[13] McNamara, op. cit., p. 128.

But they all spring from the same ancient root, and all are based on the meridians which interconnect the internal organs and viscera with the exterior of the body, through which the qi flows.[14]

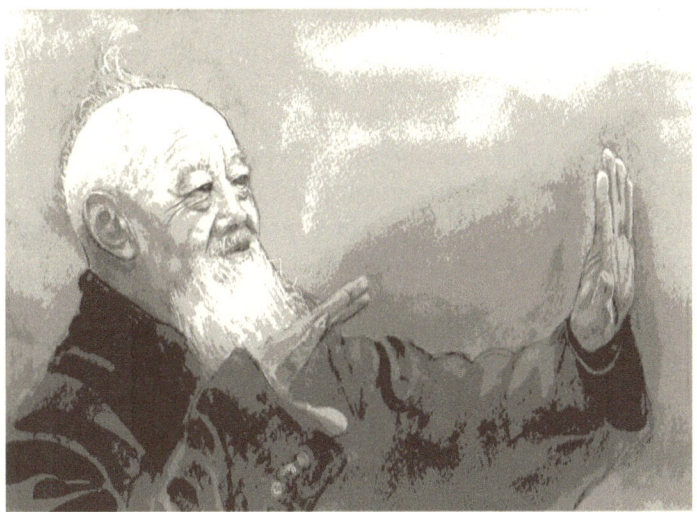

Figure 25. Tai chi chuan.

The martial arts are organized in a hierarchal system with a grand master at the top level of the tenth dan, and the novice at the bottom. The new student finds him or herself at the bottom of the ladder of hierarchy and so is stimulated to begin the trek of attaining the next step in this ladder. The higher the steps on the ladder, the greater self-pride grows.

> Ye know that the princes of the unbelievers exercise dominion over them, and they that are great exercise authority upon those who are weaker. But it shall not be so among you: but whosoever will be great among you, let him be your servant! (Matthew 20:20–28)

A vital part of growth and progression in the arts is to not only improve in physical action and skill but to give the highest respect, honor, and

---

[14] *Ibid.*, p. 128.

[15] *U.S. News and World Report*, Opiate of the Masses, by Bay Fang, February 22, (1999), p. 45.

obedience to the head of the martial arts family. A failure to comply will impede advancement in rank. This aspect of martial arts training may be desired by some families as they believe their youth are being taught discipline, but discipline and allegiance under what flag or worldview?

A question needs to be asked: what is the instruction, attitude, worldview being transferred down through the organizational ladder to reach the novice at the bottom? Let us move up the ladder several steps to the level of fifth dan, the black belt. The power to be attained in martial arts involves more than just physical strength and skill in strength and motion; it is through a *martial spirit*. This is where the super human power is obtained to do super human feats; it is passed down from above in the martial arts hierarchy (page 4 of ***https://secretdangersofmartialarts.wordpress.com/home/5-the-spiritual-hierarchy/***).

> The Shaolin teaches that once a man achieves the title of *disciple* (black belt), he is 'bound' to his master for life, by a spiritual tie not easily broken. The black sash/belt ceremony is very much like a wedding ceremony. For it is only then that the student can begin his training as a true disciple of the art, under the personal instruction of a master. The new disciple receives a very special certificate, which bonds him/her to the master in a tie that can be greater than that of most husbands and wives (same reference as above).

In the reference above, we are informed that whatever spirit possess, the grand master will be passed down to the disciples and instructors below them and on to the lower levels, finally to the novice at the bottom. The higher the level of attainment in these martial arts, the higher the hold of the *spirit* on the person, and the more difficult to separate from it.

When a master of a system attains the level of "grand master" tenth dan and also experiences "enlightenment," he is considered *infallible*. This applies to the spiritual and physical aspects of the art. Thereafter, he communicates and is taught direct from the spirit world, at times from spirits guised as masters and founders of the martial arts long dead. "His training takes the form of secret kata, meditation, and self-awareness in disciplines such as qigong, yoga, nei-gong, baua, hsing-yi, and other esoteric arts. This level of instruction is revered in the martial arts world as the path of the enlightened ones or *Arhat masters*" (*https://secretdangersofmartialarts.wordpress.com/home/5-the-spiritual-heirarchy/* p. 3, 4).

> For we do not wrestle against flesh and blood, but against principalities, against powers, against the rulers of the darkness of this age, against spiritual host of wickedness in the heavenly places. Therefore take up the whole amour of God, that ye may be able to withstand in the evil day, and having done all, to stand (Ephesians 6: 12, 13).

This is where the real power of the martial arts is derived and then passed down the hierarchy ladder, even to the novice. There is more than physical strength involved; additional power from the spirit world (martial spirit) is imparted. When feats of great strength and power are displayed such as breaking great blocks of ice with the head, breaking many thickness of boards with the hand, it is not just physical prowess obtained by exercise; it is enhancement by demonic power.

In the martial arts, there is an even deeper relationship formed by identifying with certain symbols. In this system, the symbols stand for "spiritual powers" imbued to the master. "In the art of kung fu, karate, tai chi, and yoga, these various symbols are used to connect the practitioner to the spirit world. One of the primary ways a symbol is used in eastern mysticism and the occult is as a 'talisman', a means of which to channel an evil spirit. These doorways or *gates* are drawn, painted, written, carved, and/or tattooed on the person's body or property. They (symbols) stand in the sight of the spirit world and the initiated few as marks of affiliation and 'brotherhood'" (https://secretdangersofmartial arts.wordpress.com/home/5-the-spiritual-hierarchy/ p. 6, 7).

Important questions arise upon exposing the roots and core principles involved in the martial arts. Can I participate in them yet stay free of their pagan worldview and just take the good out? My instructor in martial arts is a born-again Christian, and should that not protect from any spiritual concerns and danger? "I have been practicing karate for several years, and I have not experienced anything that would suggest to me that there are spiritual dangers involved." Is it not probable that you are on a witch hunt and have exaggerated the Eastern worldview and spiritual concerns from association in martial art practice? What possible harm or spiritual danger comes from participating in the gentle moves of *tai chi chuan*, even the elderly in rest homes benefit, and no one has seen evidence of demons?

In looking for answer to the questions posed, it is helpful to understand that martial arts are classified as "external/hard" and "internal/soft." *Hard* refers to intensive physical conditioning, powerful strikes with hand and/or feet applying strong force, i.e., as kung fu, karate, and judo. "Internal/soft" forms emphasize *mystical Taoist and Buddhist spiritual concepts*, i.e., tai chi chuan and aikido. *The chi/qi/ki concept or universal force is central.* The emphasis is on balance, physical form of soft, slow-moving movements and seeking control of chi force so as to become *attuned with the universe.* Tai chi chuan originally involved 108 rounded smooth movements (108 planets in Chinese zodiac), but in USA has been simplified to thirty-seven.

Linda Nathan, author of *Dangers and Deceptions of the Martial Arts,* walked away from a championship career in martial arts following conversion to Christianity and, in her booklet, shares with us comments and beliefs of many of the masters in the arts. That "Eastern religious concepts and techniques are key to mastering karate and the martial arts." And "Eastern philosophy should be central to all martial arts instruction." Also "that the martial arts really are training in Eastern meditation" (page 10).

The above-mentioned concepts and techniques that are central to Eastern mysticism and martial arts encompass manipulating the chi/ki force by meditation (mind empting), physical discipline (which of itself may not conflict with Christianity), attention to breathing, or breath control which is more than a physical act; it is an attempt to master the chi/ki/qi force "to gain immortality and to control the universe" (page 13).

Linda further advises us: "Bowing, specific methods of concentration, meditation and breath control, emptying the mind, visualizing yourself doing the kata, calling your teacher 'master', centering in the ki, and trying to 'flow' with the 'oneness of nature' and your 'inner self' are all part of Buddhist and Taoist philosophy. Doing the arts without absorbing at least some of those influences is like *trying to swim in a river and not get wet*" (page 10).

A recent article appeared on the Internet, *"Just Exercise? Former Yogi Says Spiritual Effects of Yoga Occur Spontaneously,"* which gives great insight as to whether we are able to practice the physical techniques of the Eastern religions, taking the good out, and not being spiritually influenced by their religious dogma (*http://womenofgrace.com/blog/?p=29077*).

Connie Fait, a former Tibetan nun and yogi, was head of a Tibetan Buddhist temple and for forty years practiced and studied yoga Traditions. Then she had a Christian conversion and writes to warn the uninformed of the dangers of participating in Eastern yoga practices. *The martial arts are out of yoga.*

Fait makes it clear that whether or not one desires to receive a spiritual influence from practicing the physical aspects of yoga, influence will occur. Here is her quote: "The knowledge of the yogic tradition is deeply hidden in mystery and only understood by accomplished yogis who have passed on those secrets orally to one another for five thousand years. Yoga asanas (postures, positions) are recognized as the main tool to realizing these secrets and is accomplished only through a process of experience. Anyone who is doing yoga asanas is in that same process—*whether or not they are aware of it or intend it*" (emphasis added).

> As with all martial arts, the real power comes through, only through "*spiritual*" training. And all of these mystical eastern practices find their roots in the *Indian Hindu* religion and yoga breathing/meditation techniques. "The very spiritual DNA of a martial style can never be separated or severed from its practice and physical manifestation (*https://secretdangersofmartialarts. wordpress.com/home/4-the-image-of-the-beast/* page 4).

> For "out of the heart, the mouth speaks," and through the physical life, the spirit is made manifest. The fruit of our actions bear witness to the God or powers which we serve and obey (*https://secretdangersofmartialarts.wordpress.com/home/4-the-image-of-the-beast/* page 19).

> You cannot drink the cup of the Lord and the cup of demon; you cannot partake of the Lord's table and of the table of demons (1 Corinthians 10:21).

ACUPUNCTURE AND CHINESE PHYSIOLOGY

Chinese physiology has astrology as its foundation. All qigong exercises are based on the Chinese concept of physiology which teaches that there are fourteen meridians. Qi is believed to circulate through these meridians—the invisible lines of energy channels which are said to travel through the system—six on each side, one in the middle of the front, and one in the middle of the back. They run perpendicular on the body and have multiple small channels which connect to various organs of the body. Acupuncture is performed by needling these meridians at specific points in order to balance the distribution of energy (qi) to organs. Those who are proficient in qigong can bring about this same balance simply by mind power and without needles.

The Chinese describe the distribution of *chi* (life energy) in a manner different from the Ayurvedic system. It is believed that the energy comes close to the skin in various places and can be influenced in those areas to alter its flow.

Stephen Basser, MD, did a very extensive review of studies evaluating acupuncture. His report, "Acupuncture: A History," appeared in the spring/summer issue of *The Scientific Review of Alternative Medicine, 1999*. He learned from his research that in the early 1970s, manuscripts dating from 168 BC, describing medicine as it existed in the third and second centuries BC, were discovered in China at the Ma-wang-tui graves. From these manuscripts, descriptions of all procedures used in Chinese medicine during that period of time were obtained. Acupuncture was not mentioned. It first showed up in the Shi-chi text in 90 BC; however, there are descriptions of sharp stones being used to drain blood from veins prior this date.[16]

> The Ma-wang-tui texts describe eleven "mo," or vessels, that were believed to contain in addition to blood a life force known as chi or pneuma.[17]

It was not appreciated at that time that blood circulates in a closed system. The most important text of the end of the first century BC was the Huang-ti nei-ching. It describes twelve vessels (mo) instead of eleven and gives different courses for the vessels from those given in the earlier descriptions. The vessels are called conduits (ching) or conduit vessels (ching-mo); by this time, it was understood that blood flows through a system where the vessels interconnect. The text also tells of a large number of holes located over the body of these vessels. At the time of this text, there was no distinction made between vessels on the basis of content and no explanation as to how the blood and chi circulated in the vessels. The texts reveal that the belief later developed that chi flowed through a separate system of vessels (today called meridians), which did not contain blood.[18]

Early in the history of Chinese medicine, disease was attributed to imbalances of chi and was caused by demons (hsieh-kuei), and demons were carried by winds, and winds dwelt in caves or tunnels. The demons (evil spirits) were believed to lodge within the vessels carrying chi and disturbing the flow. To dislodge the demon which was clogging the flow of chi, needles were inserted in the holes (tunnels) over the vessels, allowing escape of chi and relieving the congestion.[19]

---

[16] Basser, Stephen MD; Acupuncture: A History, *Acupuncture Watch*; http://www.acuwatch.org/hx/basser.shtm Feb. 22 (2005).

[17] Epler, Jr., DC, "Bloodletting in Early Chinese Medicine and Its Relation to the Origin of Acupuncture." Basser, op. cit. p. 1

[18] Bassar, op. cit., p. 2.

[19] Epler, Jr., DC. "Bloodletting in early Chinese medicine and its relation to the origin of acupuncture." Bull Hist Med. 1980154L357-367; Reported in Basser, *Ibid.*, p. 2

The vessels, and not the openings, were the central feature of "ancient" acupuncture, whereas in modern practice, the points appear to be of prime importance. The vessels have, over time, lost their association with the vascular system and in the West are now viewed primarily as functional pathways lining the openings. The term "meridian" rather than "vessels" merely serves to aid in clouding the issue.[20]

Pulse diagnosis was developed during the time that chi was believed to flow through blood. It was believed that the location of blockage of chi could be determined by feeling the pulse.

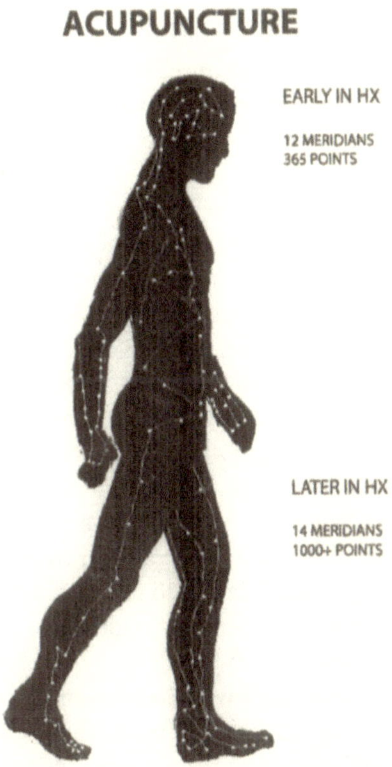

ACUPUNCTURE

EARLY IN HX

12 MERIDIANS
365 POINTS

LATER IN HX

14 MERIDIANS
1000+ POINTS

Figures 26. Acupuncture points.

---

[20] Unschuld PU. *Medicine in China: A History of Ideas*, Berkeley, CA: University of California Press; (1985), Reported in *Acupuncture Watch;* Basser, op. cit., p. 2.

Over time the connection between needling and chi, which formed the basis of acupuncture, was described in the context of an emerging cosmological view of the world, not evident in the earlier descriptions of medical bleeding. Organic medicine was subsumed under this emerging system of *cosmological correspondences*.[21]

Early in the history of acupuncture, there were twelve meridians and 365 points, one point for each day of the year. This has changed, and now many more points and fourteen meridians are said to exist. The body is supposed to have twelve organs. The Chinese day is considered to be twelve hours, which covers the twenty-four hours we have in a day. One hour of Chinese physiology time equals two hours of our time. The chi is claimed to flow around through the twelve organs, on schedule, where one organ will have the dominance of chi for one Chinese hour (two hours) and then another organ, so covering all organs in twelve divisions of the day. This is analogous to the zodiac and the planets and reflects the belief that man is a small cosmos.

Acupuncture at specific points is believed to cause a change of the energy (chi) flow running through that specific point to bring a desired balance of the yin and yang. This method is used for all types of illnesses, even for overcoming habits such as smoking. Some people claim to have experienced great relief from pain. Others have stopped smoking. What are the believed causes of the presumed imbalance of energy which results in disease? Lifestyle, different foods, and many other things are believed to influence the balance of energy. Winds are also believed to be a source of over one hundred different diseases.

Treatment entails balancing the energy (chi) or using like cures like therapy. Prevention involves meditation and/or meditation in exercise and balancing the yin-yang of food. It is also important to have balance in the home, such as the proper placement of furniture.

As mentioned previously, energy balancing techniques of Chinese traditional medicine are as follows: meditation, meditation in exercise, breathing exercises, qigong, tai chi and martial arts of all types, diet, drugs, minerals, herbs, moxibustion, acupressure, and acupuncture. Acupuncture is by far the most popular healing methods of traditional Chinese methods in the West. Today the proponents of acupuncture commonly use the term *energy* in referring to chi; however, this is misleading as

---

[21] Unschuld PU. Nan-ching: *The Classic of Difficult Issues.* Berkeley, CA: University of California Press (1986), p. 5; Reported in Basser, op. cit., p. 2.

> The core concept of chi bears no resemblance to the Western concept of energy (regardless of whether the latter is borrowed from the physical sciences or from colloquial use).[22]

This is true in Ayurveda (prana) as well as traditional Chinese medicine.

The Christian believes in the God of Creation who, by the power of His spoken word, created the heavens and the earth. The universe and man are sustained by His power, as is healing. And salvation of man is obtained through faith in the belief in the life, shed blood and death, and resurrection of Jesus Christ

The pagan denies the living God (Trinity), yet he recognizes there is a power that created and sustained the universe. We learned in chapter 4 of his explanation for creation, of the vital force believed to sustain us, and of the balancing of the supposed force's two (yin-yang) divisions to heal. This power was considered a *spiritual* force; therefore, a system was devised whereby man believed he could manipulate and influence this power to sustain well-being, to heal, as well as to obtain eternal life.

The creative power of God is not measurable or demonstrable by mechanical measuring instruments and is not under the control of man. This power, which paganism separated from God, had many names, such as vital force, prana, chi, qi, and more recently, universal energy. The term *energy medicine* is commonly used to refer to the various techniques used in holistic health therapies. Scientists who are believers in these theories desire to show that this power (chi) is truly in the field of modern science and attempts to measure and demonstrate such. It is most likely that the common use of the term *energy* in reference to the "vital force" power has come from this desire. To the established believer in Hinduism or Taoism, the term *energy* may be an insult to his beliefs. The words *prana, chi or qi, mana*, etc., are not true synonyms of the word *energy*.

DOES ACUPUNCTURE WORK?

Acupuncture seems to do something for some people but nothing for others. Could it be a placebo effect? Why have we not had studies that really determine if it works by the placebo effect or not? Part of the confusion and lack of solid "yes" or "no" answers rises out of the difficulty of doing quality scientific studies on this procedure. It is difficult to do a "mock" acupressure or acupuncture procedure. However, hundreds of

---

[22] Unschuld PU. Nan-ching op. cit., p. 5; Reported in Basser, op. cit., p. 2.

studies have been done to test the effectiveness of the procedure over the past thirty-five years.

In 1981, the Academy of Sciences of the German Democratic Republic produced a statement regarding the effectiveness of acupuncture. Their summary, written by Rudolph Baumann and published in *Zeitschrift fur Experimentelle Chirurgie* (14:66–67, 1981), concluded that acupuncture points are unknown to science and have not been demonstrated; not all acupuncture point charts match. All methods attempting to prove acupuncture points have failed, and equal effects of acupuncture when specific points are not needled. Acupuncture is not used by anyone on infectious or true organic disease such as diabetes. Equal results are to be expected from hypnosis, suggestion, and autosuggestion. The conclusion of the article did not recommend research to teach the subject to medical students or physicians.

Dr. Basser reported in 1999 that:

> Carefully designed and conducted scientific studies have so far failed to demonstrate that the Chinese acupuncture is associated with more effective pain relief than either placebo or counterirritant stimulation such as TENS (transcutaneous electrical nerve stimulation).[23]

TENS has been used for many years for mild to moderate chronic musculoskeletal pain. Basser has concluded that from a scientific viewpoint, it can now be said with confidence:

1. The concept of chi has no basis in human physiology.
2. The vessels, or meridians, along which the needling points are supposedly located, have not been shown to exist and do not relate to our current knowledge of human anatomy.
3. Specific acupuncture points have not been shown to exist—as noted earlier; different acupuncture charts give different numbers and locations of points.[24]

For the past thirty years, science has not been able to explain the physiologic actions from acupuncture or to detect any true lasting value from the use of acupuncture. Many proponents of this technique will rise up in alarm by this statement, but this is what I have found.

---

[23] *Ibid.*, p. 6.
[24] Basser, op. cit., p. 8

In November 1997, the National Institute of Drug Abuse held a consensus conference on acupuncture. The meeting was arranged by a Dr. Trachetenber, who is reported to be a strong advocate of acupuncture. Wallace Sampson, MD, FACP, presents a critique of the conference in *Acupuncture Watch*.[25] He mentions that the first question that arose was: why investigators who had previously made studies on acupuncture, which showed no measurable effect from acupuncture, were not a part of the presenting scientists? There seemed to be present only proponents of acupuncture. Prior analyses of research of acupuncture (1986, 1988, 1990) had revealed that the best quality of research showed negative effects, and the low-quality studies were mostly positive.

Dr. Sampson makes the following comment:

> The lack of critical, scientific thinking was apparent in the panel's report which was sixteen pages long. It obviously was composed before the conference and changed somewhat after the presentations. Despite the uneven literature and the lack of firm evidence to support the conclusions, the consensus statement panel recommended acupuncture for musculoskeletal pain, some headaches, and nausea . . .[25]

Dr. Sampson's article comments that the consensus conference did not show evidence of true scientific reasoning and had rejected the more obvious cause of believed effects. That of the natural history of disease, regression to the mean, expectation, Stockholm effect (identifying with and aiding the desires of a dominant figure), habituation, fatigue, and other known mechanisms. He concluded that strong bias would be needed to agree to the conference conclusions.[26]

Why would physicians make a consensus statement labeling acupuncture as being scientific if there is really no hard data confirming it? There could be several reasons, among which is the desire to place it in an acceptable light with patients and the scientific community. Those physicians who believe in Eastern mysticism and practice its techniques do not enjoy being considered as on the fringe of scientific medicine, so when an organization such as the National Institute of Health puts out a consensus opinion that

---

[25] Sampson, Wallace I. MD; *Acupuncture Watch*, Critique of the NIH Consensus Conference on Acupuncture, March 2005, p. 2; http://acuwatch.org;

[26] *Ibid.*, p. 2.

acupuncture is science-based, this elevates its status. Also, if there is a consensus from an influential medical body that a particular procedure is science-based, it is easier to persuade insurance companies to pay for its use. Acupuncture is cheap to perform; the risks are low. It is popular, and the financial returns are very good. Never underestimate the financial interest.

Reports of studies testing acupuncture, some with positive results as to benefit over and above more conventional methods, continue to appear. Most of these studies are dealing with discomforts and disorders that have strong subjective type complaints. These include headaches, a variety of aches and pains, etc. To do true double-blind studies with acupuncture is almost impossible. There have been some sham acupuncture studies where the patients cannot detect if the needle is inserted or not and other studies that place needles anywhere but on the acupuncture points. The results of the sham and wrongly placed needles compared to the correct acupuncture procedures are almost the same. Do they work? Yes, many times, as do the fake procedures. I have never seen a study done using acupuncture for pneumonia, diabetes, coronary heart disease, meningitis, or other serious disease. We have had studies going on for forty years, and still the results are questionable. If it is so good, should it not be easy to show a difference, a large difference, using acupuncture versus not using it?

There was a positive report on a review of fifteen studies made by Duke University Medical Center in North Carolina of the use of acupuncture for postsurgical pain and which was reported on the Internet by Reuters Health Service on October 17, 2007. Acupuncture was done before and after surgery. There was less pain on those receiving the acupuncture than the controls but not freedom from pain. There was less nausea, dizziness, and also of urinary retention. Urinary retention often occurs with abdominal surgery because of reflex from pain.

Remember, surgery has been done on people using acupuncture as the anesthetic; so too was surgery done without pain in years past in India by use of hypnotism.

In the report by Reuters Health, a comment is made that doctors at the National Institutes of Health do not understand how acupuncture works. Many proponents of acupuncture will claim that the case is settled and may give you answers as to how they believe it works. In the following paragraphs, I will share with you information as to that which is known about possible physiologic actions of acupuncture. This information comes from the New England Journal of Medicine (July 17, 2010/363:454–61). I obtained a report of a study done in 2008 and reported in *Science Daily*, January 21, 2009. The report concluded that headache sufferers can receive some help from acupuncture even if needles are not inserted in the acupuncture points. In two separate reviews, Cochrane researchers showed benefits for headache sufferers with migraine patients benefitting most. However, fake procedures were as effective.

In these studies, it was attempted to establish as to whether acupuncture would reduce the frequency of headaches. The study involved 6,736 patients in thirty-three separate trials of tension and migraine types. Over an eight-week period, there were less headaches with treatment in comparison to pain meds only. In the migraine studies, acupuncture was superior therapy to drugs, but fake treatments were as effective. In tension-style headache, acupuncture therapy was slightly superior to fake treatment.[27]

Why are we so hung up on using something that is so difficult to prove as to whether it has true benefit? If this procedure is what I understand it to be, then if I choose to use it, I have subjected myself to the influence of Satan's counterfeit healing system, with little chance of true lasting benefit above that of a fake procedure. We know that it has been used as an anesthetic wherein people undergo surgery and are wide awake and even can eat during a surgical procedure. Is there power in acupuncture? Yes, but whose power? The results of applying acupuncture may well be as dependent upon the connection of the therapists to the powers of the occult as the theosophy society states that radiesthesia is in radionics (see Divination chapter). Studies on acupuncture never consider this factor.

In 1893 and 1958, the British Medical Society and the American Medical Society, respectively, made a consensus statement on hypnosis as being based in science, even though there were no explanations as to how it worked. That it worked no one disputed, yet the Christian may recognize the source of its power as of the occult (see chapter on hypnosis). I have observed reports on acupuncture for more than forty years, waiting for the definitive evidence that this technique works in the hands of anyone (not just sensitives), that it works consistently on all people, and that it convincingly produces lasting benefits. I am still waiting. I recognize that there has been an occasional person who had severe pain of the back or in some other location and experienced dramatic relief, or someone stopped

---

[27] Linde, K., Allais G., Brinkhaus, B., Manheimer, E., Vickers, A., White, A.R. "Acupuncture for tension-type headache." Cochrane Database of Systematic Reviews, Issue 1. Art. No.:CD007587 DOI: 10.1002/14651858. CDO07587

Linde, K., Allais, G., Brinkhaus, B., Manheimer, E., Vickers, A., White, A.R. "Acupuncture for tension-type headache." Cochrane Database of Systematic Reviews, Issurue 1. Ar. No.: CD001218 DOI.

smoking easily, etc. Such testimonies can be persuasive but in no way add up to conclusive evidence.

When we choose to receive medical treatment from an acupuncturist, a serious concern is that of placing oneself in the hands of a person who has poor or no understanding as to proper diagnosis and treatment, thus allowing serious disease to continue without identification and proper care. Many diseases are difficult to recognize even by highly trained and experienced physicians.

Steven Barrett, MD shares the story of a forty-year-old individual who was examined by several different practitioners of acupuncture for the same chronic back pain. The patient visited seven different acupuncturists over a two-week period. The diagnosis of qi stagnation was given by six examiners, blood stagnation by five, kidney qi deficiency by two, yin deficiency by one, and liver qi deficiency by one.

Therapy recommendations varied even more. Points to receive needling varied between four and sixteen. Number of needles to be used in a treatment varied from seven to twenty-six. Only 14 percent of same points were prescribed for needling by more than two practitioners.[28]

One would think that with the lack of studies reporting positive effects of acupuncture, interest in its use would subside, but just the opposite has happened. More young physicians who have embraced the Eastern philosophy have matured into experienced physicians and, by their numbers alone, have considerable influence. Many of them have been promoted to positions of leadership in medical institutions and schools. Public pressure to try these "wonderful methods" has caused many hospitals to offer some type of alternative therapies. A scientific investigational study on acupuncture and its potential for being physiologically therapeutic to certain disorders continue.

A physician is faced daily with common ailments that are difficult to treat, such as fibromyalgia, migraine headaches, and osteoarthritis of back, hips, knees, and fingers. The medications used in an attempt to control the ever present pain are of themselves fraught with problems and danger. So physician and patient alike are always looking for an effective and safe way to bring relief. The physical risks of using acupuncture are low, and many feel that if it is not helpful, what have they lost? When pain is unrelenting, a person is driven to try anything suggested, and this is why "testimonials" as to the great benefit received by some type of therapy have ready followers. I will present three short summaries of studies using acupuncture as therapy done recently on fibromyalgia, migraine headaches, and osteoarthritis.

---

[28] Barrett, Stephen, MD; *Quackwatch Home Page*, Be Wary of Acupuncture, Qi Gong, and "Chinese Medicine," p. 7, Jan. (2004).

In the *Annals of Internal medicine*, July 2005, Dr. Dedra Buchwald of the University of Washington in Seattle reported a study on fibromyalgia using acupuncture. Acupuncture was administered twice a week for twelve weeks. The final report was that people with fibromyalgia were no more likely to report decrease of pain than people who received acupuncture wherein needles were inserted into random locations rather than specific acupuncture points, or they received simulated acupuncture but without needles.[29]

Reuters Health Information (2006-03-02) reported on a German study using acupuncture for migraine headaches. Nine hundred patients were randomly selected to receive Chinese traditional acupuncture, sham acupuncture, or drugs—all showed equal effectiveness. Drug therapy for migraine is far from satisfactory, so this comparison does not reflect as much benefit for acupuncture as it may seem.[30]

The British medical journal *Lancet*, July 9, 2005, carried an article by Dr. Claudia Witt from Charite University Medical Centre in Berlin in reference to a study she and her colleagues conducted on osteoarthritis. This study involved 294 patients, ages fifty to seventy-five years of age with osteoarthritis of the knee. The average pain intensity of the group was forty. (The higher the score, the greater the pain.) The final analysis reported 149 patients were assigned to acupuncture, 75 to minimal acupuncture (inserting needles in distant nonacupuncture points), and 70 to a waiting "control" group. The treatment groups received twelve treatments over eight weeks. At that point, average scores on a standard osteoarthritis scale were 26.9 for the acupuncture group, 35.8 for the minimal acupuncture group, and 49.6 for the controls. At twenty-six weeks and fifty-two weeks, there were no differences between any group.

> The editorialists, both from the Churchill in Oxford, UK, conclude: "We are still some way short of having conclusive evidence that acupuncture is beneficial in arthritis or in any other condition, other than in a statistical or artificial way.[31]

Some might say, "But there was benefit for the migraine sufferer, and drugs were not needed." Allow me to speak of another factor not considered in any of these studies, that of the power of Satan. If a practitioner of acupuncture is a believer in the Eastern thought or Western occultism and the patient has allowed him or herself to participate in this technique that comes from

---

[29] Reuters Health, eline, 7-05-2005 (archived)

[30] Reuters health, eline, 3-2-2006, (archived)

[31] Reueters Health, eline, 7-8-2005 (archived)

Eastern mysticism, is it not possible that the power of Satan can cause apparent benefits? Are we not told in Revelation 13:13, 14 that miracles will be manifest to deceive and in Revelation 16:14 that these are spirits of devils/demons?

Have there been studies showing a benefit from acupuncture? Yes, there have been. It seems that almost all the studies I read have been on conditions that involve pain, nausea, or various types of discomfort. For these symptoms, the studies will often show a positive benefit; however, those benefits are usually only mildly better than sham or no acupuncture. After a few weeks to three months, the difference between those tested and the controls usually have returned to being equal.

Let us consider a study where acupuncture was used for control of nausea and vomiting caused by receiving chemotherapy, also a study of patients receiving radiation for cancer treatment of the throat and neck area and receiving acupressure therapy for the resulting xerostomia (dry mouth) reported in *CA: A Cancer Journal for Clinicians* (volume59/no.9/September/October 2009). The studies used acupressure bands which caused pressure to be applied to a specific acupressure point on the wrist. Previous studies have shown acupressure bands to be beneficial for control of nausea. Peter Johnstone, MD and William A. Mitchell, professor and chair of radiation oncology at the Indiana University School of Medicine, report the study for chemotherapy nausea.

The study was divided so that there were controls not receiving therapy with acupressure bands as well as those wearing the bands. Rigid record taking was instituted of the time of nausea symptoms, the amount of medications taken to control nausea, and the number of times vomiting occurred for those receiving therapy as well as the control group.

At the conclusion of the study, those receiving acupressure therapy had a reduction of nausea and associated symptoms of 28 percent and the controls a reduction of 5 percent. However, when the records of how much antinausea medication was taken and the number of times vomiting occurred, there was no difference between those taking the acupressure treatment and the controls.

Investigators at University of Texas MD Anderson Cancer Center in Houston tested acupressure on patients having received radiation to the neck area that resulted in xerostomia (dry mouth). They had patients record the degree of dry mouth and the amount of time it caused distress. They also tested the amount of increase of saliva in the mouth that occurred from the acupressure treatment.

The conclusion of the study was that there was very significant difference in relief of symptoms of those taking the acupressure treatment versus those not taking. However, there was no difference in the amount of saliva produced between the two groups.

In the final evaluation of the two groups, it was clear that those receiving acupressure therapy reported beneficial (subjective) results, yet the measurements in each of the two studies did not reveal a difference in physiological changes between therapy and no therapy (objective results). Dr. Johnstone states the following: "We have evidence now *proving that a disconnect* often exists between a patient's reported symptoms and objective evidence of those symptoms" (emphasis added).

In June 2010, the Center for Inquiry Office of Public Policy located in Washington DC presented a paper titled "Acupuncture: A Science-Based Assessment," a position paper from this center authored by Robert Slack, Jr. This report brings an up-to-date assessment of the scientific status of acupuncture as revealed by improved testing techniques in the past several years. The optimistic conclusions about the effects reported by use of acupuncture in past research during the 1970s to the 1990s was due to the placebo effect but was not recognized because of not having a *placebo* in testing. This new and changed understanding is a result of the development of "sham" acupuncture technique which has caused a "complete unraveling of nearly all acupuncture claims." The 1997 National Institutes of Health report on acupuncture as being effective for nausea, headache, and dental pain now carries the following disclaimer:

> This statement is more than five years old and is provided solely for historical purposes. Due to the cumulative nature of medical research, new knowledge has inevitably accumulated in this subject area(. . .), thus some of the material is likely to be out of date and, *at worst, simply wrong*[32] (emphasis added).

The Cochrane Collaboration, one of the world's most trusted evaluator of medical literature, undertook a recent systematic review of the research concerning acupuncture. The results of this analysis were included in an article presenting recent acupuncture research by Edzard Ernst in *The American Journal of Medicine*. He states:

> During the past ten years, however, researchers have begun to take a more rigorous look at acupuncture, designing studies that are properly randomized and adequately controlled for placebo effect. Though research is ongoing, an increasingly robust body

---

[32] www.csiop.org/uploads/files/Acupuncture_Paper.pdf

of literature has accumulated *showing that acupuncture has no intrinsic clinical value.*[33]

After discarding reviews of only three or fewer primary studies, there emerge only two evidence-based indications: nausea/vomiting and headache. Interpretation of this evidence must be done with caution. Quality placebo testing has been developed, and using these methods, recent trials suggest that *acupuncture has no specific effects in either of these conditions* (Ernst, 2008, 1027).[34]

In "Acupuncture: A Science Based Assessment," Robert Slack, Jr., pointed out that there are many articles to be found that do conclude that there has been "encouraging effectiveness" from the use of acupuncture. For individuals that are not acquainted with scientific testing, it seems that these types of articles present solid evidence of benefits of acupuncture. Truth in science is better demonstrated by studies that test by use of a double blind, randomly selected, and having (1) test group, (2) placebo group, (3) control group, and (4) with a large number (hundreds) in each group. The evaluation of results will also be double blind, that is, the individual doing the acupuncture treatments will not be the person to do the evaluation. The person evaluating will not know which test group of individuals he is evaluating. This helps reduce bias and comes closer to revealing truth.

Slack further states that with this development of an effective sham—placebo technique of acupuncture—there has been much better evaluation, with the results indicating: (1) that real acupuncture is not more effective than when a placebo procedure is done; (2) for many conditions there is no benefit for either acupuncture or sham procedure.

In this same review by Robert Slack, Jr., he mentions that there have been leading proponents of acupuncture and other alternative therapies, such as Andrew Weil, MD, that emphasize that these therapies have far less potential to cause harm than many conventional treatments. Therefore, they should be judged by a "sliding scale" as to their value of effectiveness. The less the risk of side effects of therapy, the less strict should be the criteria for effectiveness. This is not science; it is bias of the highest order. One cannot use two standards to evaluate therapeutic effectiveness decided

---

[33] *http://www.csicop.org/specialarticles/show/acupuncture_a_science-based_assessment/   p. 1*

[34] *Ibid.*

upon the degree of potential side effects. It does, however, often enter into the decision as to whether to use a therapy or not.[35]

A study (638 patients) of the use of acupuncture and its effectiveness for chronic low back pain was reported in May 2009. This research study was conducted by Daniel Cherkin, PhD, senior researcher with the Group Health Research Institute in Seattle, Washington. Patients were divided into four groups: (1) standard acupuncture; (2) individualized acupuncture; (3) placebo acupuncture using toothpicks to touch the skin; (4) standard medical treatment without acupuncture.

The patients treated with any of the three styles of acupuncture were reported to fare better than no acupuncture. Dr. Cherkin concluded that acupuncture was beneficial in treatment of low back pain and that the study had stimulated the question as to how acupuncture works. Other scientists reviewing the study conclude that this study does not prove that acupuncture works but that it shows the results are equal to use of a placebo; hence, the obvious is that acupuncture itself does not work. However, the lay press and proponents of acupuncture accept and voice the opinion that the study proved acupuncture is effective and does work.[36]

The New England Journal of Medicine (July 29, 2010, 363:454–61) contained an article that reviewed recent research on acupuncture. In this scientific article, the studies mentioned in the above paragraphs were included in its evaluation of acupuncture. This article in the NEJM originates from the Center for Integrative Medicine, University of Maryland School of Medicine, and the University of Maryland Dental School; also from Department of Neurology and the Program in Integrative Health, University of Vermont College of Medicine, Burlington; and the Institute for Social Medicine, Epidemiology, and Health Economics, Charite University Medical Center, Berlin.

Integrative health programs seek to bring together therapies of Western scientific medicine and alternative (nonscience-based therapies such as Ayurveda and traditional Chinese medicine) therapy. Thousands of offices and clinics across America and several medical schools have combined these methods. As seen by the names of the organizations behind this particular article, one recognizes the potential bias to be expected; however, I found the article to be quite scientific with an obvious attempt to avoid bias.

---

[35] Slack, Robert, Jr., Acupuncture: A Science-Based Assessment: *A Position Paper from the Center for Inquiry Office of Public Policy*, June (2010).

[36] Acupuncture for Chronic Low Back Pain, *The New England Journal of Medicine*, Boston, MA, July 29 (2010); 363:454–61.

In this article, a short explanation is presented of the Chinese theory of chi and yin-yang, meridians, and Chinese traditional medicine's concept of physiology that was presented earlier in this chapter. Then this statement is made on page 3:

> Efforts have been made to characterize the effects of acupuncture in terms of the established principles of medical physiology on which Western medicine is based. These efforts remain inconclusive, for several reasons . . . .[37]

These reasons are given in the following summary of findings from studies testing for physiologic changes from acupuncture performed mostly in animals:

- Acupuncture will activate peripheral nerve fibers of all size.
- Acupuncture experience is dominated by a strong psychosocial context, including expectation, beliefs, and therapeutic milieu.
- Injecting the skin at the spot of presumed acupuncture point with a local anesthesia will block the analgesic effects of acupuncture.
- Endorphins are released by the brainstem, subcortical, and limbic parts of the brain.
- In rats, electrical acupuncture has shown release of hydrocortisone from pituitary (adrenal) gland which, in turn, results in anti-inflammatory responses.
- MRI studies have revealed changes in the limbic and basal forebrain areas when prolonged acupunctures stimulation is done.
- Positron emission tomography has shown that acupuncture increases u-opioid-binding for several days in the same brain areas as stated above.
- Acupuncture has mechanical stimulation effects on connective tissue.
- Adenosine is released at the site of needle stimulation.
- There is increase blood flow at the local site of acupuncture.

In spite of what may look like to some as powerful positive proof of the physiological action of acupuncture, the article in the *New England Journal of Medicine* (July 29, 2010) states the following: .

---

[37] *Ibid.*

However, the various observations that have been made are not sufficient to permit a unified theory regarding the effect of acupuncture on mechanism of chronic pain.[38]

The article tells us of a meta-analysis study (information of many studies placed into one study and analyzed) in 2008 which included 6,359 patients with low back pain. *The real acupuncture treatment was no more effective than sham treatment.* However, with real or sham treatment, there was *subjective* improvement over conventional treatment without acupuncture. This same finding was reported in the previously described *Cochrane Collaboration Study*. This information is to be found in the Supplementary Appendix available with the original article in the *New England Journal of Medicine* (July 29, 2010).

Two additional studies are referred to in this article in *NEJM*, July 29, 2010, they come from German investigators. One study with 1,162 patients over eight years compared real acupuncture versus sham procedure for chronic low back pain. There was little difference between the groups, and at six months, they were identical yet somewhat better than the control group that did not receive acupuncture. The other German study involved 3,093 patients over seven years, and this study on low back pain was measured by use of a *questionnaire* concerning reduced back function. Two groups were tested, one with conventional therapy and one with acupuncture. The acupuncture group had significant improvement above the nonacupuncture group, as revealed by *questionnaire*. The results are taken from subjective responses of the patient.

Your attention is now directed to the setting in which acupuncture is delivered. In the traditional practice, the insertion of the needle may be accompanied by a variety of other procedures, such as palpation of the radial artery in the wrist, as well as pulses in other locations. The tongue may be inspected in detail, recommendations as to use of herbs, etc. All these actions are based on the application of the principles of traditional Chinese medicine in contrast to Western scientific physiological medical concepts.

To the credit of the authors of this article, we are not left at this point with the conclusion that acupuncture functions on a physiologic basis; actually, they suggest its function may well be explained from a *psychological* standpoint, and more research is needed in that direction. There is continuing debate in the medical community regarding the role of the placebo effect in acupuncture. See quote below:

---

[38] *Ibid.*

> As noted above, the most recent well-powered clinical trials of acupuncture for chronic low back pain showed that sham acupuncture was as effective as real acupuncture. The simplest explanation of such findings is that the specific therapeutic effects of acupuncture, if present, are small, whereas its clinically relevant benefits are mostly attributable to contextual and *psychosocial* factors, such as patients' beliefs and expectations, attention from the acupuncturist, and highly focused, spatially directed attention on the part of the patient. These studies also seem to indicate that needles do not need to stimulate the traditionally identified acupuncture points or actually penetrate the skin to produce the anticipated effect . . .[39]

In the closing part of this extensive article, recommendation is given for additional studies to further evaluate the efficacy of sham (placebo) acupuncture without skin penetration, since it *may be possible to achieve the same benefits by not doing invasive needle punctures*. The master of qigong tells us he can accomplish feats and healing equal to using needles in acupuncture simply by performing qigong about a person. Light beams shined on the skin are said to work as well as needles; on and on it goes.

Wow, this reminds me of the experience of Mesmer. First, he used magnets to affect healing, and then he learned he did not need magnets as he could accomplish the same simply by his hands. From there, he moved on to the use of only the mind in bringing apparent healing; Mesmerism—hypnotism. In this chapter on traditional Chinese medicine, I have not had the motive or desire to prove that the therapies are simply—fake. I believe, at times, quite remarkable changes may occur, and apparent healing takes place, yet I ask the question: By what or whose power does it work? That is the concern.

For the past three thousand plus years, the power of Eastern healing has been accepted and referred to a *spiritual power*. It is only in the last seventy-five to one hundred years has there been an attempt to describe its action in terms of modern physics. There is only one source of spiritual power, God Almighty, the Creator of the universe, and then God has allowed Satan a certain amount of power by which he can deceive.

Why do I warn against using therapies of traditional Chinese medicine if one does not believe in the astrological concepts upon which acupuncture is based but only wants to take of the "good" of the method? I believe that as a person understands traditional Chinese medicine's origin and

---

[39] *Ibid.*

theory of man being the *microcosm* of the *macrocosm* (universe) and that a balance of a two-sided universal energy referred to as chi when rightly balanced created the universe and man and when out of balance creates illness and malfunction; it would be impossible to participate in these so-called healing methods without acceptance of that power. Is it a treatment method that will cure infectious or chronic diseases or increased life span? Thus far, no evidence has been presented to support such.

In China, for at least three thousand years, traditional Chinese medicine was part of medical care (acupuncture for two thousand). What was the health status under this system? It was dismal. Neither public nor personal hygiene was practiced. Chairman Mao attacked these conditions head-on in the 1950s, and a national movement to improve hygiene personally and publicly was instituted. By the end of the 1950s, great progress had been made in reducing infectious diseases. This was done by making changes that were scientific, not by practices based on astrological concepts of unbalanced energy. Clean water, closed sewer systems, cleanliness of body and homes, controlling vectors of infectious disease and parasites, and immunization brought improvement.[40] Life span doubled in fifty years; it was one of the most remarkable medical feats of the twentieth century.

As infectious diseases in China came under control and living habits along with diet changed to include use of more animal products, the degenerative diseases of the West began to replace infectious disease. Today, the number 1 cause of death in China is vascular disease, followed by cancer.

This has been a very brief glimpse of the most commonly used healing methods of traditional Chinese medicine, which have been practiced in China for at least two thousand or more years. The end result has been abysmal, and it took the introduction of scientific medicine to improve health and increase life span in China, doubling in fifty years. None of this can be attributed to traditional Chinese medicine.

What is so attractive about a system that has no proven track record of improving health? What causes us to flock to it as if it was something new and wonderful? Could it be we have accepted its *spiritual philosophy* and have chosen to partake of the "tree of knowledge of good and evil?"

In the next chapter, we will look at the emergence from the West of other energy balancing therapies.

---

[40] Dominique and Marie-Joseph Hoizey; *A History of Chinese Medicine*, UBC Press University of British Columbia, Vancouver, BC, Canada (1993), pp. 173–174.

10

VISUALIZATION AND GUIDED IMAGERY

I was a visitor at Christmas time in a large church filled to capacity. A young man home visiting his parents had been asked to offer prayer prior the sermon. When he came to the podium, he asked the audience to join him in a special form of prayer. He explained that some years before while in a Christian college, a teacher in the theology department had taught him a special way of praying. He asked us to follow him in our minds through imagination as he, by imagery, took a walk down a beautiful country path lined with trees, the leaves on the branches hanging low as we walked through them. We journeyed into a pleasant meadow with a stream running through; here, we were asked to kneel and present our prayer. As we knelt, in this imaginative endeavor, we were advised that a beautiful little bird might fly to our shoulder singing a melodious song of praise. The young man then proceeded to pray a proper prayer for the occasion.

As he was leading the congregation in this imaginary walk prior his prayer, I wanted to stand up and shout, *"No, no,* just get on your knees and ask forgiveness for what you are doing." It was an extremely strong impulse that came to me, being timid, and a visitor I did not do what this impression was suggesting I do. "No one would understand," I reasoned, and probably I was right, but I was concerned about what he was doing even if he was not. He had received direction by his college professor in "guided imagery." Well, so what? He had made a beautiful prayer and presentation, so why all the fuss in my mind?

Within the past year, I received an e-mail message from an alarmed mother of a college student telling me of her daughter's recent experience in a nearby Christian college. A guest speaker was featured at an evening vespers who, during his sermon, asked the students to get out of their chairs and walk to some location within or just outside the auditorium in which they were meeting. At their selected location, they were to put away all outside thoughts and begin to visualize—in their minds, placing themselves on some distant planet. In this imagery, they were to find a bench or place where two could sit. Continuing, they were to conjure up Jesus Christ in their mind and then invite him to sit and join in conversation.

The following story was shared with me by a participant in a church-sponsored seminar. In 2010, a special seminar was conducted at a church conference's convention center. In one of the classes, at the later part of the seminar, the subject of handling stress and burnout was presented. The participants were asked to get comfortable, put feet flat on the floor, close the eyes, and relax. Music began to play that was without melody and played continuously in the back ground. A man's monotone voice, friendly and welcoming, was heard coming through the music asking that each one go deep down inside themselves to find any negative energy. Again, to go deep, deeper down, pushing out through the arms, legs, hands, feet, fingers, and toes the bad energy.

Once the bad energies were pushed out, then in imagination, they were to conjured up in their mind a forest scene with a path lined with golden stones. The invitation came to wander down this path, observing the birds and listening to the noise of the nearby stream. When coming to a small clearing, the invitation came from the voice to choose a "spirit guide" to assist in the rest of the journey. This guide could be anything of our choosing—bird, dog, an angel, whatever. Next on the path, a fountain of water was observed, and the voice suggested taking a cup and to drink in positive energy from the water. Then the voice said, "Let us take time now and thank the spirit of the earth." To close, the voice suggested that positive energies could be sent out from each one to others who might need it.

The participant, who shared this story with me, said that when it was all over (twenty-two minutes), he expressed his concerns to the instructor and the class about the practice and mentioned that the only time he could remember a *creature* guiding in a decision led to the fall of our first parents. Then came the accusations from some of the class—"narrow minded."

Recently, I was reading a book written by a Christian psychiatrist who had gained my attention and admiration in a very convincing way. I believed God had impressed this author with wisdom from on high. Suddenly I came up short in my reading as I looked at the next sentence in the book. The doctor was commenting on the value and benefits of a technique referred to as guided imagery. I had a feeling of concern as to how he might be using guided imagery; does he use it in a way that points to power of the Creator God or to a power that is supposed to be immanently within *self*, the counterfeit of the power of God? What is it with me that trigger these responses to words and phrases naming certain techniques that others may consider proper and even valuable? Allow me to share with you why I have these feelings when encountering the word and the expression—"visualization" and "guided imagery." You will need to make your own decision concerning the appropriate use of such nomenclature and the techniques in their use after you read the explanation of why I am affected so, as I choose not to make the conclusion for you.

In the past forty years, I spent thousands of hours reading and studying the topic of this book, looking for answers to questions I had as well as questions of others concerning many popular healing techniques that are herein presented. While reading about many different techniques of alternative-style healing, I frequently encountered the word *visualization* and the expression "guided imagery." It was obvious that I needed a better understanding of the origin, history, use of, and the meaning of these terms. Let me share a little of what I learned.

First, the following is what I understand these expressions to mean as I have seen them used. The two terms *visualization* and *guided imagery* are used synonymously. I have found them to be used that way in many writings. A definition of *visualize, guided imagery* follows: by imagination, in one's mind forming a picture, an action, a change of something, etc. As one repeatedly forms and thinks upon the imaginary mind picture, a happening, etc., there is the belief that doing such will actually cause it to come about or to form. Is it analogous to being a creator, by the power of your mind?

A definition, from another source, of *visualization* and *guided imagery* is given:

> Creative visualization is the technique of using one's imagination to visualize specific behaviors or events occurring in one's life.[1]
>
> Advocates suggest creating a detailed schema of what one desires and then visualizing it over and over again with all of

---

[1] Fink, Ronald A., *Creative Imagery: Discoveries and Inventions in Visualization*, Routledge Publishing, (1990), ISBN 0805807721 reported in Wikipedia/visualization.

the senses (i.e., what do you see? What do you feel? What do you hear? What does it smell like?).[2]

What is its origin? Michael Harner, the leading shaman of today, claims it is ancient with the shamans. He points out that holistic medicine of today is trying to reinvent many of the old techniques of shamanism. He cites *visualization*, altered states of consciousness, aspects of psychoanalysis, hypnotherapy, meditation, positive attitude, mental and emotional expression, etc.,[3] as some of these techniques.

We know that Hinduism was formed more than three thousand five hundred years ago and that visualization or imagery is a fundamental doctrine and practice. The goal in Hinduism is to bring the latent *divinity of man* into full godhood and then to leave this world of reincarnation cycles and join the spirit world of nirvana. This is done by raising the latent *kundalini* (mother serpent god power) at the base of the spine up through the seven chakras to meet the male serpent god *Shiva* at the crown chakra (top of head) where they (male and female) meet in sexual embrace, and thus immortality and full godhood are achieved. *Meditation, visualization, and chakra clearing or cleansing are necessary to achieve such*.[4] This information comes from a book that was dictated by a spirit calling itself, "the Tibetan master" or "Djwal Kul," the same name given by the spirit that channeled through Alice Bailey the information in the books that are the "Bible" for the New Age Movement. The thought comes to me perhaps this channeling spirit is Satan himself.

From the book *Milarepa: Tibet's Great Yogi*, we have the following comment in regard to entering the state of "tranquil rest":

> In realizing the nonexistence of the personal ego, the mind must be kept in quiescence. On being enabled by various methods to put the mind in that state as a result of a variety of causes, all thoughts, ideas, and cognition cease, and the mind passeth

---

[2] Roeckelin, Jon E., *Imagery in Psychology: A Reference Guide*, Greenwood Publishing Group (2004), ISBN 0313321973 reported in Wikipedia/visualization; Fezler, William, *Creative Imagery: How to Visualize in All Five Senses*, Published by Simon and Schuster (1989), ISBN 0671682385.

[3] Harner, Michael, *The Way of the Shaman*, Harper Collins Publishers, New York, NY (1990), p. 136.

[4] Prophet, Elizabeth Clare, *Djwal Kul Intermediate Studies of the Human Aura*, The Summit Lighthouse, Inc. Colorado springs, Colorado (1974) p. 78, 114, 121.

from consciousness into a state of perfect tranquility, so that days, months, and years may pass without the person himself perceiving it; thus, the passing of time hath to be marked for him by others. This state is called shi-ney (tranquil rest). Thus, by *thought process* and *visualization*, one treadeth the path[5] (emphasis added).

John Ankerberg and John Weldon in their booklet, *The Facts on Holistic Health and the New Age Medicine,* present additional insight to the subject of visualization:

The practice of visualization is ancient and claims to work in a variety of ways. For example, by using the mind to contact an alleged inner divinity or "higher self," practitioners claim they can manipulate their personal reality to secure desired goals such as optimum health and the acquisition of wealth. Visualization is often used as a means to or in conjunction with altered states of consciousness, and it is often accompanied by occultic meditation. It has long been associated with pagan religion and practice such as shamanism and shamanistic medicine. It is frequently used to develop psychic abilities and in *channeling* to contact "inner advisers" or spirit guides.[6]

Dave Hunt and T. A. McMahon make the following statement:

Paul Yonggi Cho declares: "Through *visualization* and dreaming, you can incubate your future and hatch the results."[7] Such teaching has confused sincere Christians into imagining that "faith is a force that makes things happen because they *believe*." Thus, faith is not placed in God but is a *power directed at God*, which forces Him to do for us what we have believed He will do. When Jesus said on several occasions, "Your faith has saved (healed) you." He did not mean that there is some magic power triggered by believing, but that faith had opened the door *for Him to heal* them. If a person is healed *merely because*

---

[5] *Milarepa: Tibet's Great Yogi:* Oxford University Press (1971), p. 141

[6] Ankerberg, John, Weldon, John, *The Facts on Holistic Health and the New Medicine*, Harvest House Publishers, Eugene, Oregon, 1992 pp. 45, 46.

[7] Cho, Paul Yonggi, *The Fourth Dimension* (Logos, 1979) p. 44; Reported in Hunt, Dave, Weldon, John, *The Seduction of Christianity: Spiritual Discernment in the Last Days*, Harvest house Publishers, Eugene, Oregon (1992), p. 24.

he believes, he will be healed, then the power is in his mind, and God is merely a placebo to activate his belief. If everything works according to the "laws of success," then God is irrelevant and grace obsolete.[8]

As stated previously, *visualization* and *imagery* are fundamental core concepts of Hinduism and have spread into many holistic healing techniques, such as crystal healing, biofeedback, and most self-healing methods. Elmer Green, in his book *Beyond Biofeedback,* states that visualization seems to be the quickest way to program the body. He feels that the body will follow *"command visualization,"* and the whole body will respond to this directive given by thought and imagery. He explains:

> Instead, we visualize what we want to have happen globally, and body converts the command visualization into the individual neural process for execution. The body seems to know what to do if the person knows what is desired.[9]

Green further explains his use of visualization in therapy relating to biofeedback (self-hypnosis, see chapter on biofeedback).

> *In attempting to make a physiologic change through the focus of attention, it is important to realize that it is not accomplished by force or active will. It is done by imaging and visualizing the intended change while in a relaxed state* (mind in passive or neutral state). *We call this* passive volition (passive will). *Relaxation is important because* it is easiest then to have the casual, detached, and yet expectant attitude that is useful in bringing about the desired change.
>
> It has been found helpful to try to visualize clearly the part of the body that is to be influenced while using the autogenic phrases (which means "self-regulating phrases"—mantras) that I will give you. In this way, a contact appears to be set up with that particular body part. This seems to be important

---

[8] Ankerberg, op. Cit., pp. 24, 25.
[9] Green, Elmer and Alyce, *Beyond Biofeedback,* Knoll Publishing Co., Inc (1989), p. 168.

in starting the chain of psychological events that eventuate in physiological changes.[10]

Elmer Green is telling us it takes a *mind in an altered state of consciousness* to effectively respond to visualization. *Stilling* the mind is done by meditation. And then, by using visualization, healing that is said to come from *within* is "tapped" into.

Visualization has gained great popularity and is presently used as a way to bring about success in many endeavors and enterprises, business, sports, education, psychology, religion, military, and even health and healing. This worldwide popularity can, to a great extent, be credited to the efforts and writings of Shakti Gawain. In 1978, she wrote *Creative Visualization;* and by 2002, six million copies had been sold, and the book translated into thirty-five languages. It truly has had a worldwide impact. Other authors had written on visualization prior but without the popularity and extensive circulation that Shakti's writings have gained.[11]

In the following paragraphs, a short summary of the information contained in Shakti's *Creative Visualization* will be presented. The principles she presents as to the source of power of visualization, methods of utilizing such, and application to life experiences are shared by other authors.

Ophiel wrote the text *The Art and Practice of Getting Material Things through Creative Visualization* in 1967, Ronald Shone wrote the book *Creative Visualization* in 1988, and there have been many others with the same basic concepts. The purpose and goal of visualization is to create what one desires or feels need of. To make use of visualization in our own life, Shakti tells us *it is not necessary to "have faith" in any power outside of our own selves*; we need only utilize the *principles* that govern the working of the universe.

> Creative visualization is magic in the truest and highest meaning of the word. It involves understanding and aligning yourself with the natural principles that govern the workings of our universe and learning to use these principles in the most conscious and creative way.[12]

---

[10] *Ibid.*, p. 33.

[11] Gawain, Shakti, *Creative Visualization*, Nataraj Publishing, a division of New World Library, Novato, California (2002) p. xi.

[12] *Ibid.*, p. 6.

Let us review the principles that writers, who give support to creative visualization, tell us are the forces that govern the universe. The concept of universal energy, life force, chi, etc., is foundational. Every material thing is energy turned into solid matter. Energy is said to vibrate at various frequencies having different qualities, from lighter to denser. *Thought* is considered a light form of energy and is easily changed and transformed into something else. Creative visualization is the act of *thought* being transformed into what we have imagined or image in our minds; it is proclaimed to be a simple act of rearranging the form of energy by the power believed to be within our mind—*self.* In reality, it is the attempt to mimic the creative power of God.

To effectively perform visualization, one has to experience a mind-altering status, by bringing the brain wave pattern from beta to alpha rhythm. This is done using the same procedures and acts as is done in meditation. Actually, it is a form meditation.[13] The mind comes to the attitude of "letting go of attachment" which is really *passivity of the mind*, allowing the opening of channels to the soul and causing creative energy to flow.[14] Shakti tells us that only good can be produced from creative visualization; how is it that if there is power to transform energy by the power within man's mind, it can only form that which is good? Behind this concept is the belief that man is inherently good, that there is no sin, and that man will judge himself.

Another point presented in how to be successful in visualization is to have a feeling of being connected to "your inner spiritual source." What is this inner spiritual source? We are told it comes from the infinite supply of love, wisdom, and energy that roams the universe. In her book, Gawain gives several names by which she feels one may identify his or her source, such as "God, goddess, universal intelligence, the Great Spirit, the higher power or your true essence, the higher self, the wisdom that dwells within, etc. This power is identified by those writing on this subject as coming *innately* from within *self.* Simply stated, it is the *pagan's god*. Shakti expresses it in the following comment:

> Almost any form of meditation will eventually take you to an experience of your spiritual source or your higher self. If you are not sure of what this experience feels like, don't worry about it. Just continue to practice your relaxation, visualization, and affirmations. Eventually you will start experiencing certain

---

[13] *Ibid.*, p. 43.

[14] *Ibid.*, p. 37.

moments during your meditation when there is a sort of "click" in you consciousness, and you feel like things are really working; you may even experience a lot of energy flowing through you or a warm, radiant glow in your body. These are signs that you are beginning to channel the energy of your higher self.[15]

We can agree with comments made in Gawain's book concerning the positive effect of our thoughts relevant to our health—that of entertaining thoughts that are positive, happy, of gratitude, appreciative, etc., instead of negative, constrictive, accusative, and other similar moods. Our expressions of appreciation and gratitude are to be directed to the Creator God, Jesus Christ the Son of God as the source of our strength and well-being, not some power that is lying latent within oneself which is said to be a part of the universal mind and just waiting to be found and put into service. We also are aware that as we express thoughts of praise and gratitude to others, it can in turn be positive in their lives. This truth is counterfeited by the adversary of God in the following way.

The teaching in the Eastern and pagan dogma is that the universal energy throughout the cosmos of which our mind is a part is interconnected to everything in the universe and also to other people's minds. By creative visualization, one is able not only to influence oneself toward healing; but by visualization, one is able to affect someone else's health, even if at a far distance by the visualization act. This is said to bring "instant cure" many times even without the other person being aware of your act on their part. This healing by visualization and at a distance, unknown to another, is believed to occur by having universal energy flow through that person doing the visualization and on to the person chosen to receive this energy. One's *higher energy is* connected to another's *higher energy.*[16]

Remember in the chapter on Ayurveda, we learned that the goal of the Hindu is to move the flow of universal energy through the chakra system so efficiently that the connection with the energy of the universe is so strongly connected as to cause one to be "one with all," "as above so below," "one is all and all is one," and that this status brings a person into "nirvana," connected with the "spirit world" of bliss. Visualization combined with meditation is taught to be a necessary and an integral part of this ascension to godhood by opening the energy centers, the chakras.

The beginning of this chapter presented the story of a young man asking the church congregation to join him in a visualization experience

---

[15] *Ibid.*, p. 53.
[16] *Ibid.*, p 83.

during his prayer. He had received guidance in this style of prayer from his religion teacher in a Christian university; he had been guided to create a sanctuary in his imagination. The *sanctuary* was the meadow through which a small steam flowed, and therein a bird singing its song of praise flew and lit on his shoulder. This sanctuary is promoted (falsely) to be a place of retreat, a place of rest and relaxation, of safety, that one can go to when weary and tired.

Shakti Gawain, as well as other teachers of visualization, present the way to meet our "inner guide" after we have created the "sanctuary" in our imagination. The inner guide has many names, such as counselor, spirit guide, imaginary friend, master, etc. To meet this guide, place yourself in meditation; and by visualization, walk down the path to your personal sanctuary. As you come down the path into the sanctuary, your guide will come from the opposite direction to meet you. This guide may be a bird, squirrel, rabbit, or any type of animal as well as a human being. You then begin a conversation with this guide and show it around the sanctuary. You ask the guide what advice it has for you, express your appreciation for its presence and assistance. Invite this entity back; thereafter, the guide is there for you to call on anytime you have need of counsel, wisdom, knowledge, support, love, or guidance of any type.[17]

Ronald Shone is senior lecturer at Sterling University in the United Kingdom and author of *Autohypnosis*, *Advanced Autohypnosis*, *First Steps to Freedom*, and *Creative Visualization: Using Imagery and Imagination for Self-Transformation*. While Sakti Gawain has gained vast popularity with her book and lectures over many years, Shone presents a more intellectual expose of his understanding and belief in imagery and visualization. Although Shone is in agreement with Gawain on this subject of visualization, he does add to her explanations in several areas. These additional points will be presented in the following paragraphs.

A most fundamental precept to visualization is to be in a *relaxed state*. This, he tells us, is best achieved by the use of autohypnosis; he actually refers to it as a *"hypnotic state."* One needs to arrive at a condition wherein the eyes are closed, breathing is slow and regular, and muscles totally relaxed, words or phrases are verbally being repeated. This state can be accomplished either in a lying position or sitting. To arrive at this situation, practice is necessary, and eventually it will happen almost suddenly as one chooses to place himself in this deeply relaxed or hypnotic state. To illustrate to the reader the depth of "relaxation" of which Shone is writing,

---

[17] *Ibid.*, pp. 94–97.

I take a quote from page 139 of his book *Creative Visualization: Using Imagery and Imagination for Self-Transformation*.

> One final observation: before you *awaken*, you should picture yourself totally free from pain and doing all the things you want to do (emphasis added).

Shone teaches that this act of visualization is carried out in the brain; it is a "right brain" function. What does he mean by the expression "right brain"? He teaches that the left side of the brain has to do with logic, reason, mathematics, reading, writing, language, and analysis; while the other, right side, functions for such acts as recognition, rhythm, visual imagery, creativity, synthesis, dreams, symbols, and emotions. Why is it important to form an image in one's mind? Shone tells it this way:

> Why are visual images in the mind so important? The most important things about visual images is that they can influence the body... A strongly formed image will lead to an emotional response or some other bodily response. *It does not matter whether the image is about reality or something totally imaginary.* Both will create changes in the body that are consistent with the image...
>
> But it is not only the body that is influenced by images. Behavior, too, is influenced by them. Again, the result is similar. *A strong image leads to behavior consistent with the image being formed in the mind's eye.* It does not matter whether the image is one of reality or unreality. What matters is whether the image is *strong* and whether you have *belief* in the image.[18]

He makes reference to the *power of the will*. He refers to such as a force which belongs to the *inner self* and which gives direction and purpose to our actions. There is no outward manifestation of this entity; it simply directs or makes the choice of our actions. It is a force which in our use will command, stimulate, regulate, and direct all activities.

Elmer and Alyce Green, in their book *Beyond Biofeedback*, frequently refer to the use of visualization with biofeedback therapy. In the preface of their book, they comment that the principles of psychophysiologic

---

[18] Shone, Ronald, *Creative Visualization: Using Imagery and Imagination for Self-Transformation*; Destiny Books, Rochester, Vermont (1988), p. 6.

self-regulation has been known for two thousand five hundred years but primarily used by shamans (witch doctors). They have attempted to translate the writings of a shaman into modern language as follows:

> (1) We can more easily understand how involuntary process of body and mind, the major part of the "internal cosmos," are continuously influenced and controlled by *visualization,* and (2) we begin to understand that the "external cosmos," outside our skins, also responds to visualization—though only shamans and occultists seem to have known much about the latter . . . From our viewpoint, the development of full human potential starts most easily with mastery of *body* energies through internal control of images, emotions, and volition (the will), and the process can be extended to energies which influence the outside world. It is striking that in yogic theory, ten pranas (ten kinds of energy), which can be self-regulated, control the world inside the skin—and the *corresponding* pranas affect the outside world. "As below—so above!"[19]

The "will-volition," not "will-power," is the governing power in our minds, and through its proper use, a change can be made in one's life. We yield it up to Christ and place ourselves under divine influence. We will receive strength from above to develop a pure and noble life, a life of victory over our habits and lusts. Everyone has this privilege to unite our will with the unwavering will of God.

That which is critical to the use of the will is to whom do we yield it? Christ or Belial? As I understand the use of visualization as outlined in the books I have read, I believe that to participate in imagery and visualization as taught, I would be yielding my will to Satan. Later in this chapter, I will write about the proper use of imagery and visualization wherein we give our will to Christ, not to Satan, for his direction and guidance in our lives.

The subject of "Self" is frequently written about in most disciplines in alternative healing techniques. Ronald Shone expands beyond the usual explanations of the beliefs behind the term *self.* It is important to have an understanding of this term to better comprehend the subject of "inner guides" which are, in truth, fallen angels, workers for Satan—demons.

The Eastern mind-set considers that there are the following divisions of self: the conscious self; the unconscious self; the true self; superconscious

---

[19] Green, op. cit., p. xix.

Self; and the collective unconscious self. Explanation of each division is not needed for the point I wish to make.

The author, Shone, presents to us the idea that each of the above unconscious entities has an "inner guide" that we can call upon to assist us in life and gain wisdom and advice from. Within Eastern thought and Western occultism concepts, the unconscious levels of the mind have available, latently, the entire wisdom of the universe. To access this wisdom, "inner guides" are contacted; discussion ensues, and the information or understanding which we wish to know is obtained.

The technique of contacting an inner guide necessitates a deep state of relaxation, a quieted mind (*hypnotism*), or the attempt will not be successful. Notice the following quotation:

> In this section, I wish to discuss how you can use creative visualization to call on your own inner guides. The technique itself is straightforward, but it does require a little practice. First, get yourself into the deepest relaxed state that you can ... For this particular use, it is important to get as deep as possible because your inner guides reside in those layers of consciousness not so easily accessible while conscious thoughts "cloud" the mind. Only when the mind is quietened can you even begin to approach an inner guide, or earlier attempts will be wasted.[20]

Shone goes on to explain that we not only have a guide for each of the unconscious selves but a male and a female guide as well. We are said to have the privilege to contact whichever guide we wish to speak to and be able to talk and ask questions. The guides are to help us reach "our other selves." We are to invite the guides to return and thank them for their service. In this way, they are available whenever we desire their presence and service. It is also important to express to the guides that we desire to be able to contact them in the future. Visualization is commonly used as a healing modality.

The basic principle is that your body and mind are inseparable. The whole person must be treated—mind and body. In holistic medicine, prevention is also important. First and foremost, one must obtain a deep relaxed state, a *hypnotic state*, to be able to use visualization in healing. In an infection, one will image white blood cells attacking the germs and destroying them. In a broken bone, imagine repair cells lying down bone, restoring intact bone, etc. An additional practice for which some may use

---

[20] Shone, op. cit. p. 28.

visualization is the diagnosing and detecting of a disorder in the system. It is done in the following way:

An Inner Body Search: Start with very deep relaxation, and then the body must be changed into a very small entity, and then enter yourself through the blood stream, through the nose, through the throat, through a sweat gland, etc. Once inside, you may make your way around the body inspecting all regions. You find a tumor in the brain, you clear it away with a laser, and then you leave via the tear duct.[21] There seems to be no level to which visualization cannot function. If you think the above-mentioned beliefs and practices are a bit out of the ordinary, then consider the next proclamation that author Ophiel makes as to our origin.

Ophiel has written several books which, by the titles alone, a person can gain an appreciation as to the belief system he supports. Titles: *Art and Practice of Astral Projection, Art and Practice of the Occult, Art and Practice of Clairvoyance, Art and Practice of Caballa Magic*, etc., and also *The Art and Practice of Getting Material Things through Creative Visualization*. I present his answer as to where we came from:

> We created ourselves, for ourselves, and by ourselves, by our own mental powers!
>
> Naturally, we did this creating ignorantly, but we did it nevertheless. As I said before, the time can come that you can take and will take your own personal divine powers into your own hands and direct the right use of the power. And then only will you begin to use your divine powers as they should be used and as you should use them—in the right way and for your own benefit.[22]

And the Buddhist says: "We have created our own bodies."[23] Think back to the incident I spoke of in the opening paragraph, the prayer imagery. After walking down a path covered with foliage, a bird appeared as you knelt to pray. I read of such a scenario occurring after repetition of the imagery, the bird, the squirrel, the rabbit, or whatever creature appears in this guided imagery appears quickly and may even dialogue with you. It may become your "guide," appearing even without imagery initiation.

---

[21] *Ibid.*, pp. 147, 148.

[22] Ophiel, *The Art and Practice of Getting Material Things through Creative Visualization*, Samuel Weiser, Inc., York Beach, Maine (1967) p. 12.

[23] Govinda, *Foundations of Tibetan Mysticism*, Samuel Weiser, NY, p. 159.

I wish to share with the reader comments and information relevant to guided imagery and visualization presented by Richard Gerber, MD in the book he authored, *Vibrational Medicine*. He is considered one of the outstanding scientists and writers in New Age scientific writing. He is an internal medicine specialist yet governed in his thoughts by his deep belief in the pantheistic Eastern belief system. In his book, he states that he and his wife are "clairvoyant," and that much of the information in the book has come *from channeling*. I quote:

> I would like to point out to the readers of *Vibrational Medicine* that I believe this book is the result of a cooperation between healers and researchers on the the physical plane and beings who exist on the higher spiritual planes. This cooperation has made possible the transmission of a wealth of information that is much needed on the planet at this time. Many of the sections of this book are actually *"messages from spirit"* that I have accumulated over the years, *channeled* through various sources.[24]

In a discussion of the value and use of a type of meditation which Dr. Gerber labels "active meditation," which involves use of visualization combined with imagery, he gives an illustration as to how they can be used to obtain advanced knowledge. A person will imagine himself enrolling in a school of higher education, one that grants advanced degrees. Continue by imagining yourself attending classes in a school of higher learning:

> Oftentimes, the *advanced meditator*, when visualizing him or herself attending classes in a school of higher learning, may actually be working with *inner teachers* (spirits) and learning on an *astral* level.[25]

Gerber adds another illustration of visualization and guided imagery. The individual *stills* the mind and body by various *relaxation techniques* and then turns their consciousness to their *"higher selves"* (innate inner knowledge) concerning aspects of the past, the present, and the future. The person then listens for meaningful information which may come in the

---

[24] Gerber, Richard, *Vibrational Medicine: The No. 1 Handbook of Subtle—Energy Therapies*, Bear and Company, Rochester, VT (2001), p. 37.

[25] Ibid., p. 397.

form of *words, images, or feelings*. An additional illustration gives us added depth in the use of imagery in a spiritistic manner.

This example has to do with *dialogue* with "higher self" (a spirit) while being dedicated to higher learning. This dialogue will be combined with various types of visual *imagery exercises* which involve cleansing the *auric field* and the *chakras*, as well as creating a greater alignment of the *physical* and *subtle bodies*. An example of an imagery exercise is as follows. Take a crystal in each hand, hold your hands in front of the third eye center (forehead), and visualize subtle energy in the form of colored and white light entering into the body through the crystals. The energy taken into the body causes a rising of the vibrational rate of the body and raises the consciousness to a higher frequency level. The person can see oneself shrinking and entering into the crystal. You can then decide to enter a hall of knowledge within the structure of the crystal:

> This hall of knowledge can be set up like a library. Only this unique library allows one access to information about oneself in present and past lives, as well as allowing one to obtain general information about any number of historical subjects. The visual metaphor of the library allows one to use imagination to tap into higher levels of cognitive processing. The technique of visualization itself, when used in conjunction with the meditational process, allows human beings to not only reprogram their own bio computers (as in biofeedback and autonomic control) but also to access levels of inner potential not ordinarily available to waking consciousness. Visualization and imagery holds the key to unlocking the hidden reserves of human thoughtpower.[26]
>
> Behind imagination lie the doors to higher levels of reality. The ability to use symbolic imagery also holds the key to tapping into vast inner sources of creativity and insight.[27]

The deception of imagery and visualization has entered the church like a "Trojan Horse" according to Hunt and McMahon in *The Seduction of Christianity*. How did it get there? Let's follow the trail as authors Hunt and McMahon unfold the story.

---

[26] *Ibid.*

[27] *Ibid.*, pp. 397, 398.

To understand our present society and our world, it is important to understand the influence that secular psychology has had on its formation. The great expansion of this influence took place following World War II. In 1946, U.S. Congress passed a National Mental Health Act, establishing a federally funded program to expand the study of psychology in universities, including seminaries throughout the nation. This was new to seminaries. Hunt and McMahon tell us that by 1950, nearly 80 percent of these seminaries were offering advanced studies in psychology. Paul Vitz, in the 1980s, a professor of psychology at New York University, wrote the following:

> Psychology as *religion* exists . . . in great strength throughout the United States . . . (It) is deeply anti–Christian . . . (yet) is extensively supported by schools, universities, and social programs financed by taxes collected from Christians . . . But for the first time, the destructive logic of this secular religion is beginning to be understood[28] (Italics by author).

In 1951, Carl Rogers, one of the foremost proponents of secular psychology, spoke of *"professional interest in psychotherapy,"* as being the most rapidly growing subject in social sciences of that time. Hunt and McMahon comment that by the mid-1980s, psychology had attained the status of a "guru" and "who's who." "Scientific standards of behavior" are relieving consciences of obedience to God's moral laws. In this way, as well as through introduction of sorcery as science, psychology is the major change agent in transforming society.

> Humanistic and transpersonal psychologies have now embraced the entire spectrum of sorcery. For example, the twenty-second annual meeting of the Association for Humanistic Psychology held in Boston, August 21–26, 1984, was heavily flavored with Hindu/Buddhist occultism. The official daily schedule included early morning yoga, tai chi, meditation. About half of the "preconference/postconference institutes" involved blatant sorcery, with such subjects as *visualization* and healing . . . Trance states and healing, operation of alchemy, *guided imagery*,

---

[28] Vitz, Paul Clayton, *Psychology as Religion: The Cult of Self-Worship*, Eerdmans (1997), p. 10: Reported in Hunt and McMahon, *The Seduction of Christianity*, p. 29.

shamanic (witchcraft) ecstasy and transformation, being the wizard we are[29] (emphasis added).

Dr. Beverly Galyean, consultant to the Los Angeles school system, wrote in an article in *The Journal of Humanistic Psychology* the following:

> Human potential is inexhaustible and is realized through new modes of exploration (i.e., *meditation, guided imagery*, dream work, yoga, body movement, sensory awareness, energy transfer (healing), reincarnation therapy, and esoteric studies).
>
> *Meditation* and *guided imagery* activities are the *core* of the (confluent/ holistic education) curriculum[30] (underline emphasis added).

Is it any wonder that *visualization* and/or *guided imagery* have entered the church? Few religious or science leaders have perceived that this sorcery is not neutral and is in fact anti-Christian. To partake of the use of visualization is to partake of the worldview out of which it has its origin, pantheistic concepts, the belief that within ourselves divinity exists which can be articulated to actually *create*. At the root of modern and humanistic psychology is "self," while the Bible teaches us to die to self.

> I have been crucified with Christ: it is no longer I who live; but Christ lives in me: and the life which I now live in the flesh I live by faith in the Son of God, who loved me, and gave Himself for me (Galatians 2:20).
>
> I can of Myself do nothing. As I hear, I judge: and my judgment is righteous, because I do not seek My own will, but the will of the Father who sent me (John 5:30).

What about visualization, imagination, imagery, which I do in my mind and that I use to plan my future, to do work for today, to invent, to solve problems? Has the author of this book lost his judgment, his common

---

[29] Hunt and McMahon, *The Seduction of Christianity, Spiritual Discernment in the Last Days*, Harvest House Publishers, Eugene, Oregon (1986), p. 30.

[30] Galyean, Beverly-Colleene, Guided Imagery in Education, *Journal of Humanistic Psychology, Fall 1981, Vol. 21, No. 4*; Reported in Hunt and McMahon, op. cit., p. 30.

sense by incriminating any imagination or originality? What may seem like an unbalanced attack on visualization and guided imagery by careful analysis will reveal a distinct difference between Satan's counterfeit and God's true gift of imagination and use of imagery. God, in creating man, gave him a mind that has attributes, making it capable of reflecting upon the mind and character of God; he was given the ability to reason, to imagine, and to use imagery to grow in mind and wisdom. These activities are to be guided by God and under His influence.

When we allow the influence of Satan to be our guide, accepting his concept that we have divinity within ourselves and by using the techniques of visualization and guided imagery, we are led to believe that we are able to use that divinity to achieve certain accomplishments. Remember from previous paragraphs we learned that those activities are part of the Hindu's trek to reach the supreme self—godhood.

> And whatever ye shall ask in My name, that will I do, that the Father may be glorified in the Son. If you ask any thing in My name, I will do it (John 14:13, 14).

The proper use of imagery has value. The Bible contains imagery throughout the Old Testament and the New Testament. The sacrificial system pointing to the future death of the Son of God as a substitute for sinful man was initiated by God Himself. This ceremony was to help man realize that sin resulted in death of the sinner, but through accepting by faith, the merits of the shed blood and death of Christ the Divine Son of God, as man's substitute, man could regain paradise and eternal life. The entire tabernacle service was imagery and teaching God's plan of salvation for man. The parables Jesus told used imagination and imagery to teach saving truths. They were written to stimulate the mind of man to seek for eternal truths stored in the Bible. The prophecies of Daniel and Revelation are filled with imagery.

Imagery has a place in our thoughts and minds, but it is imperative that we have chosen the Holy Spirit to guide our imagination and not the power of Satan. If in prayer we rely upon God, the Holy Spirit will open our minds to Bible imagery to learn and be able to teach eternal truths of hope and salvation.

11

REFLEXOLOGY AND OTHER ENERGY-BALANCING THERAPIES

At the heart of alternative medicine therapies is the doctrine of correspondence or sympathies between the cosmos, earth, and man. This concept is central to the term *life force energy*. This energy in theory is emanating from the cosmos, from which all things are said to be made and within which all are *one* (pantheism).[1] Let us look at some popular therapies for health disorders developed from this theory.

Early in the development of the astrological system in Europe, the twelve houses of the zodiac were assigned to various parts of the body starting at the head with Aries the ram and ending at the feet with Pisces, the fish. The organs of the body were then assigned to the remaining individual houses.[2] The Chinese divided the body in a vertical manner, believing that a special universal cosmic energy they (referred to as chi) ran through the body following twelve vertical divisions called meridians. These meridians had side channels to distribute the energy to the various organs of the body. In contrast, the Hindus described the distribution of vital energy as being concentrated in seven centers in the body called chakras. The chakras utilized nadis (small channels) to distribute energy to the tissues surrounding each chakra. When the energies of the chakras were combined; an aura was believed to surround the individual.

---

[1] Levington, Richard; *East-West Journal of Natural Health and Living,* The Holographic Body, August 1988, Kushi foundation, Brookline, MA, p. 46.

[2] Bessy, Maurice; *Magic and the Supernatural,* Spring Books, NY (1970), p. 73.

As previously explained, the cosmos was considered the macrocosm and man, the microcosm. Man was then divided into micro-microcosms. Specific locations on the body were believed to have developed association in such a way as to represent the entire body. It was believed that cosmic energy influenced man by correspondence, association, and/or sympathy.[3]

One of the first body locations considered to reveal this sympathy, or correspondence, was the hand. It probably began in the Sumerian civilization. Birth omens were obtained by inspecting a newborn infant for any sign which would predict the child's future. Palmistry likely had its origin in this manner.[4]

> Palmistry, or Chiromancy, had roots in the ancient Vedas of India 4,500 years ago.[5]

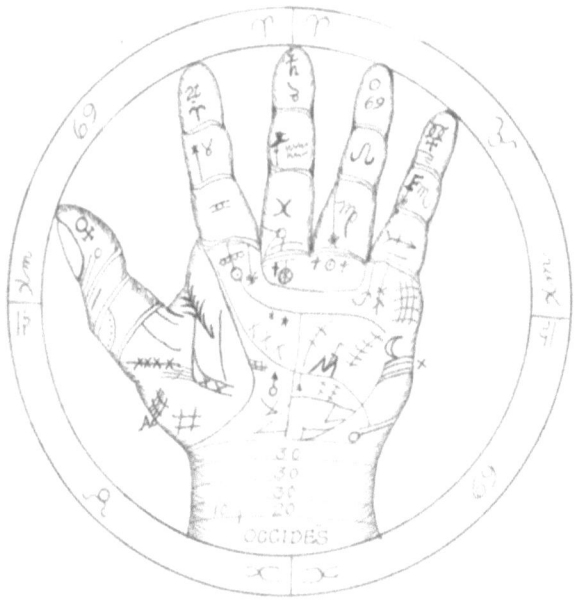

Figure 27. Palmistry and zodiac

---

[3] Levington, op cit., pp. 36–47.
[4] Garrison, Fielding H. A.B., MD; *History of Medicine*, W.B. Saunders and Co. Philadelphia, PA. (1929), p. 63.
[5] Levington, op. cit., p. 38.

Additional areas of the body that were believed to have correspondence with all other areas of the body were added over time. Now, a total of eighteen areas on the body are considered to be *holograms* of the whole.[6] The most common locations are ear, hand, foot, the web between thumb and forefinger, tongue, etc. Apart from the hologram locations, the musculature and fascia (membranes, tendons, ligaments) of the body are also believed to have many points that may impede the flow of universal energy so as to influence the function of body, mind, and spirit. Pressure or some type of physical stimulation to those points is said to affect—to correct the flow of universal energy.

Why so many types of therapies if the treatments are effective? Because none of them are based on physical science but on the paranormal or psychic; the actual physical method used matters little in medical treatment. It depends on the mental attitude and acceptance of the theory of *universal energy* or *cosmic intelligence*.

Zone therapy—now called reflexology—Rolfing and similar massage—shiatsu, Reiki, craniosacral therapy, polarity, and applied kinesiology—are techniques used by various holistic healers. These methods are collectively referred to as body therapy or soma therapy. Martial arts, tai chi, and qigong are body or soma exercise-type treatments also providing *life force medicine*.

Since it is believed that physical disease is a condition of unbalanced life force, universal energy, or chi within the body because of congestion or blockage of flow, and then correction of the imbalance would be achieved by manipulating points of correspondence. This is the foundation of acupuncture, acupressure, reflexology, and several other techniques collectively labeled "soma" (body) therapies.

REFLEXOLOGY

In 1913, an American doctor, William H. Fitzgerald, MD, initiated a method of applying pressure to localized areas on the body to effect anesthesia for performing ear, nose, throat, surgery. By 1923, it had been expanded to treat most all medical disorders and was very popular with self-appointed healers.

---

[6] Levington, op. cit., p. 43.

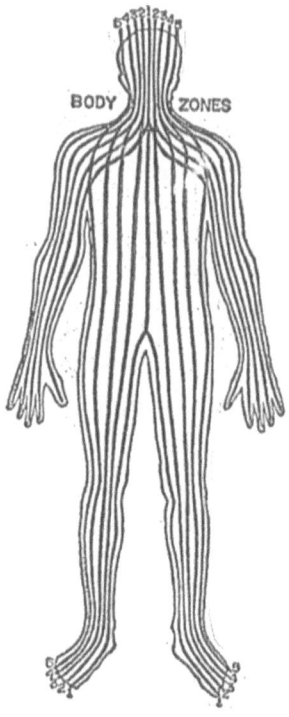

Figure 28. Zone therapy.

Dr. Fitzgerald was an admirer of and influenced by Swedenborg, the famous Swedish spiritualists of the 1700s. Fitzgerald believed in *universal energy* or, as it was called in those times, vitalism. He was not the absolute originator of using pressure to areas on the body to affect healing; rather, he borrowed this concept from the Chinese and Egyptians. An issue of *East-West Journal* (March 1990) relates that a form of reflexology was in use in China during the earliest period of China's history. In addition, a hieroglyph depicting reflexology was found in a physician's tomb in ancient Egypt. Fitzgerald was "determined" from his own reasoning that the body was divided into ten specific zones, five on each side (not substantiated by science), believing that each zone carried its own bioelectric energy which made direct connection to the brain. He applied pressure to specific points on the body and then proceeded with operative procedures to the ear, nose, or throat area without the patient experiencing pain. Fitzgerald further theorized that such pressure would treat disorders of body organs that he had allocated to correlate with the ten zones.

Eunice D. Ingham, an American, took up this therapeutic approach (zone therapy) in the 1930s and carried it further, making it popular. She mapped out specific points on the feet and hands that she determined were sympathetic to specific organs. By rubbing those points on the hands or feet, beneficial effects or cures could be accomplished. A lady in England, Doreen Baylay, called Fitzgerald's and Ingham's zone therapy, *reflexology*, and it is now very popular and practiced around the world.

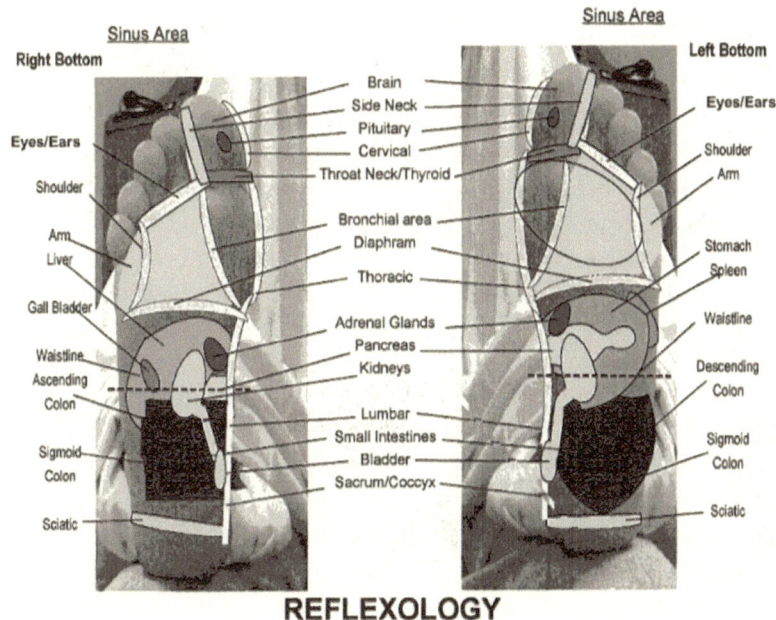

Figure 29. Reflexology chart of foot.

Reflexology is the discipline of massaging the hand, foot, or ear to diagnose, predict future disease, and effect healing of present disease. It is founded upon belief in universal energy, vitalism, prana, chi, etc. Reflexology is also a variant of acupressure and/or shiatzu, which are based on body correspondences and the meridian concept of Chinese traditional medicine. Reflexology has a similar philosophical background.[7]

---

[7] HYPERLINK *"http://emedicine.medscape.com/article/324694-overview"* (access on Internet by entering massage, traction, manipulation: eMedicine Clinical Procedures); Levington, op. cit., pp. 36–47.

However, the theoretical Western explanation of reflexology contends that there are nerve connections directly from the feet or hands to the brain from whence connecting to various organs of the body. By rubbing a very specific point on a hand or foot, the nerve impulse is said to travel to the brain and is transferred on to a particular organ, thus correcting any abnormality of that organ.[8] Reflexologists may or may not teach that there are *crystals* of calcium or uric acid and/or other substances on the nerve endings in the hands or feet. These crystals are supposed to have caused congestion of universal energy flow about and through nerves, which are purported to connect directly with organs of the body. Massage is said to break up the crystals, which will relieve nerve or energy blockage; the nerve can then impart health to the area of affliction.[9] No one has ever found these crystals by anatomical dissection or by any other method.

Reflexology purports the ability to diagnose, as well as to treat, by massaging either the hand, foot, or ear. Foot therapy in reflexology is the most common area for performing therapy, but hand treatment is supposed to be just as effective. Reflexologists proclaim that there are seven thousand two hundred nerve endings on the bottom of a foot. I have never seen an anatomy or neurology book that said such, and even if it did, that does not mean the proclaimed point has specific connections to the various organs. There is no evidence that rubbing nerve endings would correct abnormal function of tissues elsewhere in the body.

If a person looks on the Internet for information relevant to *reflexology*, there will be found 6.5 million Web sites. It is a worldwide phenomenon. What disorders are claimed to be improved by use of reflexology? Some reflexologists speak only about relief from stress, while others make no limits as to types of problems that can be treated and will be benefited. Have there been any studies of scientific quality? There can be found on some Web sites studies that claim to show benefit to many various medical disorders. Quality studies are another thing. It is very difficult to design a study for testing reflexology that uses randomly selected, double blind, placebo, and a control group.

William T. Jarvis, PhD, a professor at Loma Linda University, teaches research methods to aspiring scientists. He often challenges a new group of students to devise a study design to test reflexology. I will share with you some of the studies done using designs created from his classes.

---

[8] Bergson, Anika; Tuchak, Vladimir; *Zone Therapy*, Pinnacle Books, Inc., New York, NY, p. 2; Levington, op. cit., pp. 36–47.

[9] Levington, op. cit., pp. 40–41.

Using questionnaires, seventy subjects were asked to record any health problems they had encountered on any of forty-three anatomical locations in the past two years. A reflexologist then examined each of the individuals in a blinded manner. The feet were exposed, but a sheet covered the individual, and no voice contact was allowed. From this test, the results of determining a diagnosis by reflexology were no better than guessing.

In another study, three practicing reflexologists examined eighteen individuals that had at least one to six different conditions identified by physicians. The end results were that there was no correlation between the reflexologists' findings and those identified by a physician.

A third study dealt with thirty-three women with premenstrual syndrome (PMS) which were randomly selected and assigned to either ear, hand, or foot reflexology or a placebo group which had sham reflex points massaged. The women selected their personal symptoms from a list of thirty-eight symptoms which are commonly associated with this syndrome. They then received reflex therapy. The results were that the treatment group had a modest reduction in symptoms compared to the placebo group. The placebo group complained that their treatment was rough and with discomfort. The group with improvement had thirty minutes of pleasurable relaxing treatment. This study suggested there may be some reduction of symptoms from PMS. There was no proof of a connection between reflex points and body organs.

A fourth study was done on patients with asthma, a disorder that is frequently claimed by many Web sites to be benefitted by reflexology. Ten weeks of therapy was given to a treatment group and to a control placebo group. Lung function studies were conducted on both groups which did not change on either group. The conclusion was that no evidence of improvement beyond placebo was shown.[10]

Dr. Jarvis, in an article found on the Internet, shares with us his experience over several years as he did studies on reflexology. In the classes, he conducted for postgraduate studies in methods of research at Loma Linda University. He would bring a registered reflexologist to the class and have this individual present the theory and demonstrate the practice of reflexology. As previously mentioned, he would challenge the students to design a method of testing the theory presented by the reflexologist. Eventually the reflexologist confided in Dr. Jarvis that even as he believed in reflexology, he would like to see a study testing it.

---

[10] *http://www.quackwatch.com* post¬ed Sept. 16, 1997. (Reflexology: A Close Look by Steven Barrett M.D.) accessed 3-30-11

Since reflexology claims to be able to prevent and to predict future disease, how do you test for that status? You cannot. Dr. Jarvis decided to test whether reflexologist could detect a present disorder of an individual, and if the reflexologist failed that test, then there would be no reason to try to design a test that determines whether or not future disease can be detected. This study was the one reported above on seventy people. At the conclusion of the study, the reflexologists agreed that it was not possible to diagnose present problems by reflexology, thereby accepting the conclusion that reflexology would not be able to predict future disease or even to be therapeutic.

> From that time on, his practice would involve simple foot massages for people who wanted them with no diagnostic or therapeutic claims.[11]

A good foot rub is relaxing and without ill effects and no one should avoid such if they enjoy it. Just do not expect it to be diagnostic or correct health problems. Do not get caught up in such thinking, for if we do, we are then venturing into a system that is founded upon the doctrine of universal energy which leads us away from God's system of health. The danger of accepting this type of therapy is that if people feel they have gained help in their personal discomforts from such a therapy, they begin to believe the philosophy by which the benefits are explained. This allows acceptance of the *vital energy* concepts and leads in to accepting Satan's counterfeit health system, the "right arm" of his false message of salvation.

In a subset of reflexology, the ear is believed to represent the entire body by reflex. When the ear is used in therapy, it is termed *auricular therapy*. In the *East-West Journal of Natural Health and Living* (August 1988, page 43), the claim is made that there are at least eighteen known locations on the body, labeled holograms, wherein a specific point is claimed to influence a specific organ. The hand, the thumb, a tooth, the tongue, and many other areas are said to be micro-microcosms of man and of the cosmos.

An abstract from the Med J., August to September 7, 2009: *Is reflexology an effective intervention? A systematic review of randomized controlled trials.*

Objective: Evaluation to determine if reflexology is effective or not for any medical condition.

Date Sources: Six data bases searched for randomized trials.

---

[11] *http://www.ncahf.org/articles/0-r/refelexology.html*

Disorders Studies: Anovulation, asthma, back pain, dementia, diabetes, cancer, foot edema in pregnancy, headache, irritable bowel syndrome, menopause, multiple sclerosis, the postoperative state of premenstrual syndrome.

Conclusion: The best evidence available to date does not demonstrate convincingly that reflexology is an effective treatment for any medical condition.[12]

Reflexology is practiced around the world. It is a sympathetic remedy based on the concept that man is the microcosm of the macrocosm (the cosmos). Again, reflexology can be considered a variant of acupressure or shiatzu.

MASSAGE

Body massage combined with hydrotherapy will result in a marked increase in circulation of blood and body fluid. The delightful sensation of a good massage to the muscles is beneficial for anxiety, mood, and happiness. Massage for a bed-ridden patient is refreshing and restful.

Today, there are several forms of massage being used by New Age healers, using different names, but based on the same basic dogma, that is, a physical disorder is the result of an imbalance of cosmic energy forces. Their form of massage is directed at correcting the flow of these supposed *cosmic forces* within an individual. Massage treatment itself is appropriate, but often, it is *hi-jacked* and used by the devil to insert his doctrines through medical therapeutics into the mind of man. His methods are "spiritually" based and are not dependent upon the physical laws of God.

Let us review several of these modified massage methods whose therapeutic effects are explained by "balancing of energies" or relationships to earth's forces.

ROLFING

In the mid-1940s, Ida Pauline Rolf initiated a form of massage therapy to correct a physical disorder that she postulated existed, that of an imbalance of structure and movement of the entire body. Rolf presented a theory that "bound up" fascia (connective tissue) often restricts opposing muscles from functioning in concert with one another. Her special massage method was aimed at separating her hypothesized bound-up fascia by deeply separating the fibers manually to loosen them and allow effective movement patterns.

---

[12] *http://www.ncbi.nlm.nih.gov/pubmed/19740047*

She called her method *postural release* and later, *structural integration of the human body* and presently the *Rolfing method of structural integration*. The *Rolf Institute of Structural Integration* states that Rolfing is

> a form of bodywork that reorganizes the connective tissues, called fascia, that permeate the entire body.[13]

Such a physical condition has not been recognized by science, and there is no literature to support value in use of Rolfing in a disease group.[14]

Rolfing therapists believe that their techniques facilitate flow of *universal energy*. The pagan worldview of astrology, of association, of correspondence, and of sympathy of man with the cosmos is base doctrine. They look to a counterfeit creation power and teach this dogma as they apply and explain therapeutic measures. Even as some therapy might have beneficial aspects in and of itself, this worldview may be presented as the source of healing. This in turn initiates a change in the recipient's worldview as a result of the treatment. It is not just the therapeutic modality that can influence us but the very concepts of the therapist and the explanation given, crediting the movement of universal energy for healing. By partaking of these therapies applied by "healers" with this pagan worldview, we place ourselves on Satan's ground.

It is also taught that this type of treatment brings a higher level of *consciousness* through mind/body rejuvenation.

> Rolfing is based upon Wilhelm Reich's theory of "character armor"—that the "consciousness" can be found in the body as well as the brain, and that energy blockages cause lots of problems. "Because mind and body are interconnected, the results of past traumatic experiences show themselves in a person's posture . . ." Through deep muscle massage—which may be painful, even torturous, these blocks can be broken down and a harmonious mind-body system achieved. (The physical massage causes emotional release; hence, it is an emotional as well as physical treatment).[15]

---

[13] http://www.rolf.org

[14] Jones, T.A., "Rolfing," *Physical Medicine and Rehabilitation Clinics of North America*, 15 (4):-799–809. Doi:

[15] Weldon, John, Wilson, Clifford, *Occult Shock and Psychic Forces*, Master Books, San Diego, California (1980), pp. 229, 230.

In 2007, Dr. Mehmet Oz, while on the Oprah Winfrey TV show, endorsed Rolfing and likened it as someone doing yoga for you; Christian beware.

SHIATZU

Shiatzu (finger pressure) is another form of mind/body energy-balancing therapy in the massage group. It is considered diagnostic as well as therapeutic. Skilled fingers are said to be able to detect energy imbalances and, in turn, correct such. It claims to be able to stimulate the immune system, thereby benefiting the whole body.

A large variety of shiatzu therapy disciplines exists in Japan and throughout the world. It has similar basis in the meridian concept as acupressure and acupuncture. This massage is gentle and is done close to the diseased organ.[16] It, too, is a treatment based on the correspondence or sympathies of the body to the cosmos—man as the microcosm of the macrocosm. It has its origin from Japan.[17]

The book *Shiatzu* assures us that shiatzu therapy can equal the results of acupuncture without use of needles. The book also lists the following disorders that one can expect to see improved from its therapeutic use.

> Ankle sprains, appetite, asthma, bedwetting, blood pressure, chills, constipation, diarrhea, eyestrain, fevers, hangovers, headaches, heart pain, hemorrhoids, hiccups, indigestion, insomnia, knee pains, leg cramps, nervousness, neuralgia, nosebleed, numbness, menopause, menstrual cramps, morning sickness, nausea, motion sickness, nasal congestion, common cold, neck cramps, nervousness, neuralgia, rheumatism, sciatica, sexual problems, sinusitis, swelling, toothache, whiplash, and much more.[18]
>
> Acupuncture uses needles, zone therapy (reflexology) concentrates principally on applying pressure to the hands and feet, and shiatzu employs its own type of pressure. It does not matter much that the key points might be called by different names—reflexes, acupuncture points, or shiatzu points. The seed of thought, basic to all, is the same. The history of shiatzu

---

[16] Bergson, Anika, Tuchak, Vladimir, *Shiatzu*, Pinnacle books (1976), pp. 1–3.
[17] *Ibid.*
[18] *Ibid.*, face cover back side.

then goes back to this deeper understanding of its essential nature. Thus, we owe our thanks not only to Namikoshi but also to the ancient Chinese and to the American pioneers of zone therapy as well. [19]

The difference among the various treatments seems to lie in the kind of pressure treatment recommended by each method, yet in all methods, results are obtained. To this day, no one quite knows why.[20]

POLARITY THERAPY

Polarity therapy is a combination of ancient Eastern and Western holistic health-care ideas, adhering to the energy field hypothesis, and formed by Randolph Stone in the 1940s. Universal energy is described as becoming unbalanced when unequal distribution occurs to the poles of the body's energy field, divided into the body's right and left side. The right side is charged with "positive sun heat energy" and the left with "cooling moon receptive energy."

Balancing techniques used are: (1) touch (massage or acupuncture); (2) stretching and exercise; (3) diet, and (4) mental-emotional process. They correct the disturbance of balance of the "etheric electric."

There is no scientific basis for this belief or any reproducible measurements of this system. Stone referred to the unproven energy as "breath of life," ki, chi, prana, and or life force.

REIKI

Reiki is a popular "body-mind-spirit" therapy imported from Japan. It is a soma therapy, and which the next chapter will deal with at length.

CRANIOSACRAL THERAPY

Craniosacral therapy is another body-mind-spirit therapy quite like Reiki in its application, with a very soft touch to the head and neck area. It could be considered a continuation of phrenology with therapy directed more to the body than to the mind. This therapy too will be presented in depth in the next chapter.

---

[19] *Ibid.*, p. 2.

[20] *Ibid.*

APPLIED KINESIOLOGY

Kinesiology is a true science of muscles and body movement and is not to be confused with *applied kinesiology*. Applied kinesiology is another method of energy manipulation, *diagnosis by divination*, and treatment that has become popular with some chiropractors, naturopaths, an occasional dentist and physician, and with many in the public sector. The practitioners of this technique say they are more interested in prevention of illness than with treatment. It is their claim that they can evaluate five body systems—nervous, lymphatic, vascular, cerebrospinal, and meridian. (No meridian system has been demonstrated to exist.) They do not separate the systems in testing. It is a test of a specific muscle for strength and is done by pushing and/or pulling against a muscle group, with the patient resisting. The test is supposed to reveal the chi or universal energy flow through specific areas of the body.

> Applied kinesiology claims to induce proper structural and chemical-nutritional organization in the body, as well as "left and right brain" hemisphere balance. It claims to evaluate and correct problems of the nervous, circulatory, lymphatic, skeletal-musculature, and "meridian" systems, thereby maintaining health. Its practices are believed to permit the even flow of *cosmic energy* throughout the body, thus nurturing individual organs and systems with the proper supply of chi energy.[21]

This same technique is claimed to detect vitamin and/or mineral deficiency. There are supposedly specific points at various places on the body which will correlate with these deficiencies. If a finger is held on one of these points, that is said to correlate with a specific vitamin or mineral, testing of the correlating muscle group is believed to reveal a deficiency or normal level. If a person wishes to test for allergies to a substance or food, then this substance can be held in one hand or in the mouth, and again the muscles are tested. If a weak response occurs as judged by the examiner, the diagnosis of an allergy is made. This is a form of *divination*.

> There shall not be found among you any one that maketh (makes) his son or his daughter to pass through the fire, or that uses divination, or an observer of times, or an enchanter, or a witch (Deuteronomy 18:10, KJV).

---

[21] Ankerberg, John; Weldon, John; *Can You Trust Your Doctor?* Wolgemuth and Hyatt, Brentwood, TN (1991), p. 154.

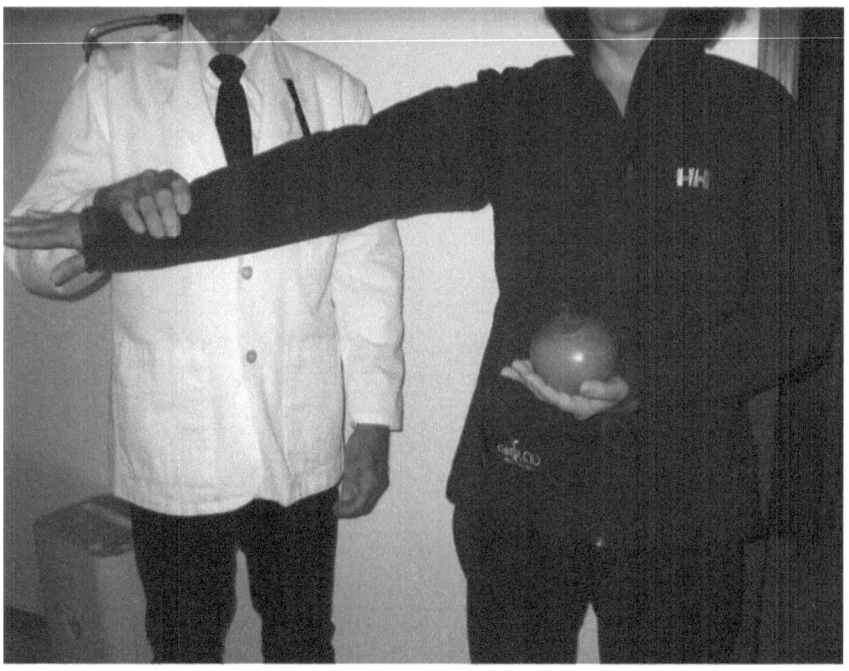

Figure 30. Applied kinesiology.

BI-DIGITAL O-RING TEST

A method quite similar to *applied kinesiology* but not so well known is the *Bi-Digital O-Ring test* (BDORT). This test has its origin from Yoshiaki Omura, MD, ScD, of the USA. Dr. Omura's Web site opens with the statement seen below:

> Through the methods and materials presented here, you may witness a revolution in medicine, dentistry, and technology because Dr. Yoshiaki has discovered a way to test which materials (pharmaceutical or "natural" medicines, drugs, hormones, vitamins, minerals, supplements of any type, anesthetics, herbs, dental restorative materials, food, clothing, cell phones, chemicals, etc.) are potentially health-giving and life-promoting for a person and those which are potentially harmful.[22]

---

[22] http://www.bdort.org

Dr. Yoshiaki's Web site states that Dr. Yoshiaki's special diagnostic test will, within an hour, diagnose and begin treatment on early phases of vascular disease, Alzheimer's, autism, cancer, etc. Positive tests identify such disorders before any other physicians or test can. Makes a claim that the test may be the ultimate in preventive medicine. What is the test that this article refers to says is the ultimate?

It involves the testing person holding his thumb and forefinger of one hand together to form an "O-ring," and then he places a finger from his other hand on the patient, or he may use a wand to touch the patient at acupuncture points or over an organ, etc. Another person will attempt to pull apart his thumb and finger. If the finger and thumb circle is weak at any time when the probe or finger is placed at a location on the body, it signifies disorder in this area. The wand/probe can be placed anywhere on the body or on any medication, herb, etc., and the test tells the practitioner the diagnosis, chooses the therapy, etc. It is essentially the same as *applied kinesiology*. It is simply another form of *divination* performed by "hands on."

TOUCH FOR HEALTH

Touch for health is another variant therapy and is explained on the same concept as for acupuncture, i.e., the flow of chi through *meridians*. Instead of using needles or massage, this form of therapy involves determining approximately which meridian is involved, then running the hands up and down the meridian, to correct the energy imbalance. Gentle massage is applied by the practitioner's finger to the same energy centers as pierced by the tiny acupuncture needle. This finger massage is known as acupressure.

THERAPEUTIC TOUCH

Another practice in the West that is similar to qigong, or falun gong of Chinese traditional medicine, is *therapeutic touch*. It is not an exercise but a technique of (supposed) energy transfer which does not involve touching the patient. It is done by placing the hands a few centimeters above the body and traversing the body to determine the balance of *life force energy*. This technique has swept through the nursing profession in the UK and America. The *British Medical Journal* (April 4, 1998, page 1042) reported that over one hundred thousand people have been trained in this modality, with forty-three thousand being professionals. How many today?

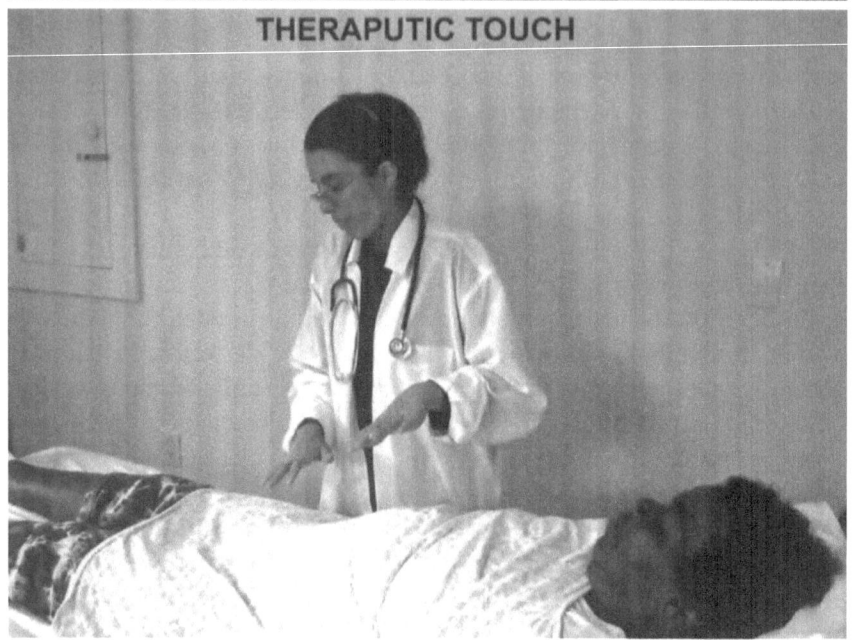

Figure 31. Therapeutic touch.

I have read that in Russia, this treatment method has been standard training in medical schools for years.[23] It has gained great popularity because it claims to get results without adverse side effects. It has gained acceptance in the highest academic centers for training nurses. Many hospitals have had teams of nurses who administer this *touch*. The practitioners of therapeutic touch say that they can improve a wide variety of medical conditions, such as decubiti ulcers (pressure sores), Alzheimer's disease, and thyroid disorders, etc., by correcting the energy-field disturbances, which they are able to feel and *repattern*

> by passing their hands over a patient's body at a distance of 5 to 10 centimeters.[24]

---

[23] Swain, Bruce; *East-West Journal of Natural Health and Living*, Shushi Foundation, Brookline, MA, May (1989), p. 30.

[24] McCarthy, Michael; Therapeutic Touch Fails Child's Test, *The Lancet*, April 4, 1998 (A British Medical Journal).

The originator of this type of energy medicine is Dora Kunz, a past president of the theosophical society.

> Dora Kunz is herself a "spiritualist'" who looks to "invisible intelligences," "angels," and theosophy's "ascended masters'" for inspiration and guidance.[25]

Delores Krieger, RN, credits Dora Kunz for her knowledge of this practice. Krieger also had additional training in occult healing techniques. She studied yoga, Ayurvedic medicine (Hindu occultism applied to medicine), occultic Tibetan medicine, and Chinese traditional medicine.[26] Delores Krieger has been a leading promoter of therapeutic touch in the nursing profession. Therapeutic touch is an example of the Hindu concept of *prana* (vital energy, chi) under a new guise. Krieger stated that the Hindu version of universal energy is the basis for healing energy that is said to be transferred. She comments that the practitioner of this so-called art is the *conduit*, not the generator, of the energy believed to be present.

> Prana may be transferred from one individual to another and may not be so readily apparent to us unless we have gotten into the practice of and literature of hatha yoga, tantric yoga, or the martial arts of the orient.[27]

The therapeutic touch technique is based on four steps:

a. Centering – meditation of therapists prior to applying treatment.
b. Assessment – scanning the patient's energy fields with the hands, feeling for energy imbalances.
c. Unruffling the field – checking for stagnant energy and sweeping this energy away with the hands.
d. Transfer of energy – moving energy via the hands to the patient so as to correct energy imbalance.

---

[25] Kunz, Dora; *The American Theosophist*, December (1978), Viewpoint, reported in Ankerberg, *Can You Trust Your Doctor?* op. cit., p. 393.
[26] Ankerberg, op. cit., p. 393.
[27] Krieger, Delores, *The Therapeutic Touch*, p. 13; Reported in Reisser, Paul C., MD, Reisser, Teri K., Weldon, John, New Age Medicine, Global Publishers, Chattanooga, TN, 1088), p. 45.

Whatever their initial appeal, energy therapies inevitably beckon the budding healer into more hard core "new consciousness" thinking since these systems are in essence profoundly mystical.[28]

In April 1998, three medical journals, *Journal of the American Medical Association*, *British Medical Journal*, and *Lancet* (also a British medical journal), reported a study done by Emily Rose, a nine- year-old girl testing the ability of practitioners of therapeutic touch. In her test, the therapeutic touch practitioners put their hands through a small hole in a shield that prevented them from knowing if anyone was on the other side or not. Then a person's hand would be put very close to the therapist's hand, and the therapist was asked to tell when a hand was near his or her hand. The results were no better than guessing. This was done as a school project, and the quality of the experiment was such that when written up by adults, it was accepted and placed into three prestigious medical journals. The conclusion of the journals editors were:

> Twenty-one experienced therapeutic touch practitioners were unable to detect the investigator's *energy field*. Their failure to substantiate therapeutic touch's, *most fundamental claim*, is unrefuted evidence that the claims of therapeutic touch are groundless and that further professional use is unjustified.[29]

As we close this section concerning various massage methods, a little should be said concerning various mechanical apparatuses that are sold to effect massage. Swedish-type massage by hand or by machine can and may be a desirable experience and should not be considered as "spiritualistic." It is when the therapist may describe or explain benefits and actions of the massage as being a method of unclogging, diffusing, or imparting "energy" we know we have a therapist that is connected to the power of Satan. Therapy from this person then becomes of concern.

MASSAGE MACHINES:

There are many machines, chairs, and/or beds sold to effect massage. I see no concern here. However, if in purchasing for my own use or going

---

[28] Reisser, op. cit., pp. 47–48.
[29] Linder, Rosa, BSN; Rosa, Emily; Sarnor, Larry; Barret, Stephen, MD; *The Journal of American Medical Association*, April 4 (1998), pp. 1005–1010.

to a place to receive treatment from such an instrument and its benefits are explained as coming from a manipulation of universal energy to impart health and I accept that concept, then I believe one is on Satan's ground.

I am often asked about a particular machine as to whether it is a part of the above-described occultic pseudoscientific electronic gadgetry. One such machine is the "chi machine." There are several close copy duplicate machines with changed names and selling for a lesser price. I opened the Web site for the original chi machine" and found that the site makes comments about the "me-too" machines and how one will not receive the real therapy from these copycats.

The chi machine was imported into the United States from Japan where its originator received a Japanese patent. It is a device that moves the legs in a figure eight motion. One lies down, with legs together and outstretched, with ankles on a holder; the holder then moves the ankles and legs side to side in a smooth figure of eight motion one hundred forty times a minute. The motion is not more than four inches in width. It does cause some motion of the pelvis and extension into the spine, similar to the motion of a fish swimming.

The Federal Drug Administration has given it a class III status. It has been shown to lessen swelling in the legs when edema is present. Therefore, there is some physiologic action but very minimal. It was not compared with the benefits for reduced swelling in legs by lying down with legs elevated.

But what about the questions as to its spiritualistic influence? I read through the Web site of the "original chi machine," and there seemed to be nothing I could find that gave a hint that spiritistic ideas were incorporated into its use. After a long list of attributes of the proclaimed physiological benefits of using the apparatus, I found what I suspected from the beginning—that it was a machine developed to promote the movement of the Eastern dogma of chi—universal energy. The Web site advances the concept that exercising internal organs increases chi, a force proclaimed by Chinese to be the basis of life and well-being. It is proclaimed to exist throughout the universe and is the source and power of healing. The chi machine, by moving a person's legs in an elliptical cycle, is said to elevate and facilitate the flow chi in the body for well-being.

> These Eastern traditions emphasize healing and good health based on a life force energy, which flows in channels through all living forms. The chi machine aids in unblocking the "chi"

pathways and ensures a maximum flow of healing source throughout your body and organs.[30]

This is another example of a pagan healing method presenting itself under the banner of science and proclaiming all sorts of nonproven benefits from a scientific standpoint, when in reality the whole objective is to introduce the Eastern pagan dogma. In the chapter on "Mystical Herbology," I write about a book on aromatherapy which made the statement that twenty years earlier, the introduction of aromatherapy was done through strict promotion as if its value was only physiological benefits. But now the acceptance of the spiritual nature of aromatherapy is so accepted there can be direct comments on its spiritual power.

What about receiving therapy from a person who has definitely accepted the universal energy—spiritualistic doctrine but gives me regular physical therapy as the doctor prescribed? Should I look elsewhere for a therapist that is not tied into such beliefs? I will leave that to you; I cannot answer for you. It is between you and God. However, with the understanding I have obtained in researching this topic, I am convinced that eventually that therapist will exert influence in accordance to his beliefs, and it can make it easier to accept pantheistic dogma.

I wish to share with the reader concerning a particular massage table that is sold around the world coming out of Hong Kong and perhaps marketed in many countries that does give some concern. There are a number of Web sites on the Internet advertising this massage table under the name Nuga Best. It is widely promoted and very popular throughout the countries of Ukraine and Russia. In my investigation of this table, I once went to a treatment center in Ukraine that had several tables and where the therapist was treating up to forty patients each day. Because of lack of an interpreter at the time of the visit, I was not able to hear what a new patient would be told about the machine and its benefits. The price for a treatment was expensive. While visiting the therapy center, I did read the machine's manual from the manufacture. There were no comments made anywhere as to the effectiveness or improvement of disorders that one could expect from therapy. It totally avoided any comments as to its use. This is a customary pattern for machines that are not shown to be of true therapeutic value. The manufacture avoids any legal conflict. However, the agents who sell machines and those directing treatment may have a story to tell which may not be bound to reality or truth.

---

[30] http://www.energywellnessproducts.com/chimachine.htm

I am going to share with you what information I obtained on a Web site promoting the Nuga Best Therapeutic Thermal Massage Table. I printed out the four-page article about the Nuga Best massage table and its description the following is the opening paragraph:

> The special genius of Nuga Best, the result of extensive research and development, lies in the *marriage of the ancient Eastern healing arts of acupressure, massage, and moxibustion (heat therapy) with modern chiropractic theory,* far-infrared light therapy, and modern technology. Thus, through our products and services, we contribute to society and to the health of the human race (emphasis added).

The Web site contains four pages of written comments; it intermingles the pantheistic Eastern thought and healing traditions with the comments on the value and benefits of the machine. This intermingling is careful, however, to never really say directly that the machine influences the power that those Eastern healing traditions proclaim. It lets the reader assume so but has protected the author from being accused of teaching that the machine accomplishes such. This is a technique I have frequently run into in the subject of alternative healing. The article talks about chi, life force, power, the universal life energy that is said to run through everything. It is written so as to appear that the machine will aid the movement of this imagined energy. See the quote below:

> Nuga Best automatically massages the muscles and tendons around the spine, relaxing hardened nerve roots, relieving tension, and improving the flow of *chi.* Lie back, relax, and enjoy[31] (emphasis added).

As one lies on the massage table, the "highly therapeutic" heated jade rollers emit far-infrared light beams as they roll up and down the spine. A comment is made about a massage phase and an acupressure phase. Massage from the table is said to stimulate major acupuncture meridians along the spine, causing powerful bioelectric impulses to course throughout the nervous system. Massage from the machine is said to increase circulation of the blood and of *vital force energy*—(chi).

---

[31] http://bigskywellnesscenter.com/ The article about nuga best machine is no longer on this web site. I called the center and they said the machine caused to much pain so they stopped using it and removed the article quoted.

We are told that Nuga Best massage does the same as acupuncture yet without the needles or the focused pressure of acupressure. The physiological benefits are widely known, so says the article: relaxed muscles and tendons, reduced anxiety, less insomnia, increased circulation, and over all, improved flow of chi. Let the Christian beware.

MAGNETS

A longtime patient of mine, a retired nurse and institutional church worker, sat on the exam table in my office. He complained of pain in the feet. I removed a shoe and found magnets inserted in various places in the shoe. This patient and his wife informed me that that day, they were to have delivered to their home a mattress and pillows filled with magnets. Earlier that week, they had attended a special retreat for retired church workers. A demonstration of the supposed health benefits of magnets had been made at the retired workers retreat by a member of the church who was in the business of selling magnets. I shared with these friends my concern and gave them some references to study and urged them to rethink their choice. The mattress and pillows were sent back.

The use of magnets has become popular in the treatment of pains and aches and a variety of other distresses. It is a billion-dollar industry. Magnets are being used in sports, and housewives have also been convinced of its value. Magnets are applied to various places on the body and left for hours or days. They are placed in shoes, in pillows, in mattresses. This practice is supposed to make one stronger, increase circulation, and generally restore health. There is not a shred of scientific evidence to support these claims, but that does not seem to matter as long as someone testifies as to how much it helped them. There seems to be no concern that the magnet might create some abnormal function. The belief is that it can only do good.

What seems silly and harmless, except for the money transferred into someone else's hands, is really a technique quite like the others we have been studying. There may be no talk of balancing energy, yet it is implied that the application of magnets at various places on the body corrects unbalanced polarity. There may be claims made that the influence of the earth's magnetic field has been altered in some way, and by use of magnets, this imbalance will be corrected. Consider this statement from a magnetic healer:

Magnet therapy focuses on electromagnetic energy surrounding and infusing the body and works with this energy in as much as the subtle energy practices work with subtle energy.[32]

A study was done on the use of magnets in treating plantar fasciitis of the heel by Mark Winemiller, MD, at the Mayo Clinic. Ninety-six people with heel pain participated in the study. Fifty percent were treated with magnets in their shoes, and 50 percent were given fake magnets. At the end of three months, there was no difference between the two groups. There was improvement in both groups but no difference one from the other.[33]

In September 25, 2007, the Canadian Medical Association Journal carried an abstract reporting a meta-analysis study done on the use of static magnet therapy by Max Pittler, MD, and colleagues at the Peninsula Medical School of the University of Exeter and Plymouth. This meta-analysis contained twenty-nine studies and found "no convincing evidence to suggest that static magnets might be effective for pain relief." The studies looked at foot pain, fibromyalgia, lower back pain, carpal tunnel syndrome, diabetic peripheral neuropathy, or delayed onset muscle soreness. Results were mixed for osteoarthritis, so no conclusions were made for this disorder.

History tells us of the use of magnetism millennia ago. Probably the first electrified substance (static electricity by rubbing) used in treatment was amber, and then lodestone—ferrous oxide—was found in Magnesia (Western Turkey) as a natural magnet. Magnetic substances were carved in the shape of body organs and placed over the organ as therapy. At various times in the past, magnetic therapy became popular and then faded. In the sixteenth century, a historically famous physician, Paracelsus, used magnetism in his treatments. Magnetism was believed to be the same power as in hypnosis.

Franz Anton Mesmer (1733–1815) is known as the father of modern hypnotism. He graduated and received his degree in medicine from the University of Vienna in 1766. In his book, *On the Influence of the Planets*, he proposed that:

> Stroking diseased bodies with magnets might be curative.[34]

---

[32] *New Age Encyclopedia*, Gale Research, Detroit MI (1990), p. 28.

[33] Reuters Health Information (2005-09-21): *Magnetized insoles don't appear to relieve foot pain*, http://www.reutershealth.com/archive//2005/09/21/eline/links/20050921/eline/links/eline003.html (archived)

[34] New Age Encyclopedia, Gale Research, Detroit, MI (1900) p. 29.

He affected his first cure by passing magnets over the body.

> Like Paracelsus, Mesmer believed that the microcosm of the human body reflects the macrocosm of the universe; he also believed that the corresponding parts are tied together by a universal magnetic fluid.

> In 1776, Mesmer met Gassner and became convinced that all of Gassner's cures (passing hands across a body without magnets) could be explained by his own theory of animal magnetism. Before this meeting, Mesmer had achieved cures (by passing magnets over the patient's body), but the fact that Gassner achieved the same results with his bare hands led Mesmer to wonder whether the healing power might reside in the human body itself rather than in the magnets; dispensing with the magnets, he too began to pass his hands alone over patient's bodies.[35]

When these practices eventually progressed on to hypnotic trances and psychic experiences, magnets were discarded.

The above comments are not to be confused with the use of magnetism such as the MRI diagnostic machine and the use of pulsating electromagnetic field about a fractured bone to promote healing. These methods work on known laws of science. It is interesting to note that no one has ever heard of a person being healed of a disorder by being placed for an hour in an MRI diagnostic machine, although it is one the most powerful magnets on earth. Powerful magnets that are electrically pulsated are used occasionally to treat the most severe forms of depression. There can be benefit from this treatment. It is not to be confused with the popular use of magnets in shoes, pillows, mattresses, etc.

IRIDOLOGY

An alternative method of making a medical diagnosis for the present and predicting disorders in the future is *iridology*. This is a *divination* method which involves examining the iris of the eye and inspecting the color, texture, and location of various pigment flecks in the iris. The practitioners say they can detect *imbalances* in the body's system which in turn can be treated with vitamins, minerals, herbs, and in other ways. Iridology is practiced around the world. However, the technique is rarely accepted by a conventional

---

[35] *Ibid.*

medical doctor. Some chiropractors and naturopaths utilize it, and there are many nonmedical people who present themselves as iridologists.

Modern iridology had its start from Ignatz von Peczely, a Hungarian physician who, in his youth, had broken a leg of an owl and noticed a black stripe in the lower part of the owl's eye. He theorized that the broken leg caused the black stripe. However, this does not happen.

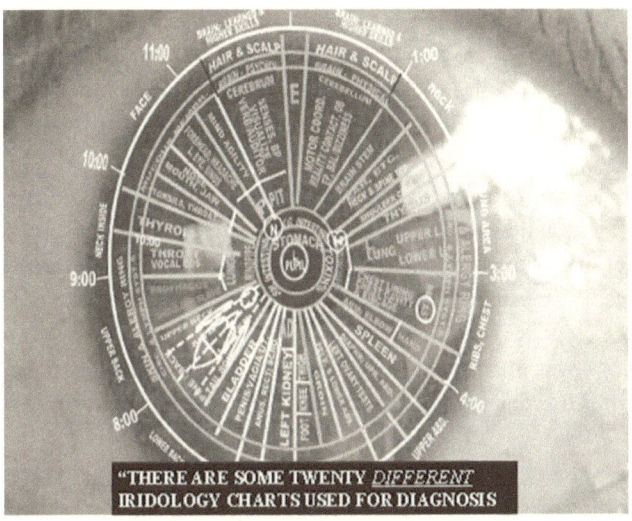

Figure 32. Iridology chart.

The right side of the body is said to be represented by the right iris and the left side by the left iris. The iris is divided into ninety sections with each section supposedly representing relationship to a specific part of the body. Disease or disturbances in those areas of the body are said to present changes in the iris which can be seen by the skilled examiner. Jessica Maxwell, in her book *The Eye-Body Connection*, claims that:

> The basis for iridology is the neuro-optic reflex, an intimate marriage of the estimated half million filaments of the iris with the cervical ganglia of the sympathetic nervous system. The neuro-optic reflex turns the iris into an "organic etch-a-sketch" that monitors impressions from all over the body as they come in.[36]

---

[36] Maxwell, Jessica; *What Your Eyes Tell You about Your Health*, Esquire, January (1978). Reported in Ankerberg, op. cit., p. 340.

Ophthalmologists have not found the above statement to be true. Only a rare optometrist will accept it. The technique has been scientifically tested a number of times, and each time it has failed to support the claims of its adherents. The iridologist might make claims as to the accuracy and scientific basis for iridology, such as that it is based upon a neuro-optic reflex, a connection between the optic nerve and the iris and the rest of the body. The problem here is that the signals of the optic nerve only go to the brain. There is no signal traveling from the brain back up the optic nerve to the eye. In spite of the lack of scientific proof for a basis by which it can work, or of true accuracy in its use, iridology is still very popular.

> Iridology can be traced to ancient Chinese astrological practices; however, according to Dr. Carter, the first precursor published on iridology was Phillippus Meyen's *Chiromatica Medica* (Germany, 1670).[37]

Iridology was introduced to America in 1904. The most recent leader of iridology in America was the late naturopath, Bernard Jensen (1908–2001).

> Jensen is not a scientist but is a New Age healer, a fact revealed in his various works, such as *Iridology: Science and Practice in the Healing Arts*. In this text, he discusses his belief in reincarnation, astral travel, psychic development, and other occultic practices and philosophies.[38]

He claims that:

> Iridology can be used in conjunction with any other form of analysis and diagnosis.[39]

The iridologist believes he can:

> Determine the inherent structure and the working capacity of an organ, detect environmental strain, and tell whether a person is anemic and in what stage the anemia exists. He can determine

---

[37] Ankerberg, John; Weldon, John; *Can You Trust Your Doctor?* Wolgemuth and Hyatt, Brentwood, TN (1991), p. 341.

[38] *Ibid.*, pp. 343–344.

[39] *Ibid.*, p. 343

the constructive ability of the blood. He can determine the nerve force, the responsive healing power of tissue, and the inherent ability to circulate the blood.[40]

The same belief says that the iris of the eye can show acute, subacute, chronic, and destructive stages in the body.

> Many other factors are also revealed such as organic and functional changes . . . It foretells the development of many conditions long before they have manifested into disease symptoms.[41]

We are told that:

> No other science tells so accurately the progress from acute to chronic states. Only iridology is capable of directing attention to impending conditions; only iridology reveals and evaluates inherent weaknesses.[42]

> In using iridology, you need ask no questions, yet you can tell where pain is, what stage it is in, how it got there, and when it is gone.[43]

There is no truth to these claims, as emphasized by the following test of iridology. In 1979, Bernard Jensen and two other practitioners of iridology were given 143 photographs of irises of patients eyes to view and determine which individuals had kidney impairment. (Forty-eight had a diagnosis of kidney disease as revealed by standard blood tests; the rest had no kidney disorder.) These iridologists were not able to separate the diseased from the normal. One iridologist had picked out 88 percent of normal patients as having kidney disease; another examiner found that 74 percent of those patients that had severe kidney disease were identified as

---

[40] Jenson, Bernard, *The Science and Practice of Iridology: A System of Analyzing and Caring for the Body through the Use of Drugless and Nature-Cure Methods,* Provo, UT, Bi-World Pub. Inc. (1952), pp. 10, 21, 26. Reported in Ankerberg, op. cit., p. 344.

[41] *Ibid.*

[42] *Ibid.*

[43] *Ibid.*

normal. This test was reported in the *Journal of American Medical Association* (242, 1385–1387, 1979).

The *British Medical Journal* (297:1578–1581, 1988) carried an article of a test given to five leading Dutch iridologists. They received a stereo color slide of the right iris of seventy-eight people, half of whom had a diagnosis of gallbladder disease, and the other half were free of any disorder. The five practitioners were not able to differentiate the diseased from the normal and were not able to agree among themselves as to who were diseased or not. This typifies the results of many tests given to iridologists.

Another problem that exists in iridology is that there are no standards in the charts used to represent the eye, from which the diagnosis of the health condition of the person being examined is made. The following quote presents this problem:

> For example, there are some twenty *different* iridology charts that a practitioner may choose from in his practice.[44]

Does iridology have an astrological basis for existence? Does it have its base in the "universal energy" concept? Like much of New Age medicine, iridology makes use of the concept of mystical energy. In fact, the pupil of the eye is held to be a repository of sorts for the body's "energy," according to many iridologists.

> Most iridologists agree that the integrity of the body's energy is reflected by the quality of energy in this (pupil) hub or core.[45]

As to astrology, iridologist Brint sums it up this way:

> From an Eastern point of view, the eye may be viewed as a *mandala* . . . The mandala links the microcosm and the macrocosm. Through the mandala, man may be projected into the universe and the universe into man. In iridology, the macrocosm and the microcosm are linked in our eyes. Iridology may be summed up as the observation of the change that arises from the interplay of various levels of consciousness and results in one's unique evolution into greater [occult] truth and light.[46]

---

[44] Ankerberg, op. cit., pp. 346–7.

[45] Berkeley Holistic Health Center, *The Holistic Health Hand Book*, Berkley, California Press; Berkley, CA (1978), p. 159.

[46] *Ibid.*, pp. 155, 162.

12

REIKI: CRANIOSACRAL THERAPIES

Reiki is a popular "body-mind-spirit" therapy performed by the application of hands. The palms of the hands will gently touch the body, or might not touch, in various anatomical areas for three to five minutes and in a set of up to twenty locations for a full treatment. There is no massage; the treatment will last from sixty to ninety minutes. Treatment schedule may be weekly with two to four visits. With use of Reiki, no diagnosis is needed or made. Any type of physical or mental disorder is considered as a disturbance of a *universal energy*, believed by Eastern neo-pagans and Western occultists to permeate and flow through our bodies. (Note: there are more than one million American Reiki therapists.)

The name *Reiki* is defined by the following synonyms: Spiritual power, mysterious atmosphere, intelligence, divine, miraculous force, etc. *Rei* refers to ghost, spirit, soul, supernatural, miraculous, divine, etc.; while *ki* refers to spiritual energy, vital energy, life force, etc. It is the same meaning as qi, chi, prana, mana, vitalism, and the other hundred names used to refer to this imagined force. Reiki has been defined further as a nonphysical healing energy made up of "life force energy" that is guided by a higher intelligence or spiritually guided life force energy. This is not referring to Jesus Christ, the Divine Son of God that the Christian follows.

The *Oxford English Dictionary* adds to our understanding of the alternative healing method of Reiki:

> Hence, therapy, apparently based on an ancient Tibetan Buddhist technique, developed in Japan in the late nineteenth or early twentieth century by Dr. Mikao Usui (1865–1926)

in which the therapist channels this energy from himself or herself into the patient by gently laying on of hands to activate the natural healing processes of the patient's body and restore physical and emotional well-being.[1]

Mikao Usui is credited with rediscovering this healing method in 1922. It was believed to have existed in Tibet in the 1800s. Usui made it popular in Japan beginning in 1924 and continued teaching this method to others until his death in 1926. From then on, one of his students, Chujiro Hayashi, carried on the training of practitioners. Hawayo Takata, trained by Hayashi, came to the United States and has been the prime mover of the therapy in this country. She died in 1980. Reiki branched into several divisions in Japan as well as here in the USA.

The difference between Reiki and many other new Age healing techniques is that treatment is not supposed to unclog or balance universal energy. Reiki simply facilitates moving the energy from the cosmos through the therapist and on into the client where it is then said to heal physically, mentally, emotionally, and spiritually. The teaching is that the energy has intelligence which can seek out and heal anywhere there is disorder, making diagnosis unnecessary.[2]

It is reported that the recipient often feels warmth or tingling in the area being treated, even when a nontouching approach is being used. A state of deep relaxation, combined with a general feeling of well-being, is usually the most noticeable immediate effect of the treatment, although emotional releases can also occur.

> What sets Reiki apart from other hands-on healing modalities is that to become a channel to receive the energy, you must be attuned by a Reiki master. The attunement *(initiation into the occult)* opens you to receive and channel Reiki energy to others.[3]

Training to be a practitioner is divided into three levels.

First-Degree Level: This involves four "attunements" by a Reiki master in four sessions activating the "chakras," creating an open channel for the energy. The attunement methods are not made known, and it is a secret to be held by those receiving the attunement. At the end of the four

---

[1] Simpson, J., Weiner, M., Proffitt, et al., Oxford English Dictionary (1989), 2nd ed.
[2] Roberts, Llyn and Levy, Robert, *Shamanic Reiki*, O Books (2008), pp. 2–5.
[3] *Ibid.*, p. 2.

attunements, the new therapist is ready to apply treatment. It is reported to be a very pleasant experience to receive Reiki, as a feeling of warmth and security pervades. It is said that once you become a Reiki therapist, you never lose the ability.

Joyce Morris, in *The Reiki Touch*, carried in the Movement Newspaper, October 1985, tells of a woman who received Reiki therapy. After the first session, she remarked:

> I don't know what this is you've got, but I just have to have it.

Another business lady remarked the following:

> Reiki should be available through every medical, chiropractic, and mental health facility in this country. Your fees are a small price to pay for such impressive results. I don't know how Reiki works, but it works; that's all that counts in my book.[4]

The Reiki Magic Guide to Self-Attunement text by Brett Bevell speaks to the first attunement:

> I have sent a Reiki attunement across all time and space to all individuals who say the Reiki first-degree attunement chant revealed later in this chapter . . . If you say this chant with the intent of being attuned to the first degree of Reiki, you will be attuned in the act of saying the phrase. This works because the attunement has been sent out across time and space to intersect with anyone who says the Reiki first-degree attunement chant while intending to be attuned.[5]

Second-Degree Level: This level of training intensifies the Reiki energy, allowing the practitioner to channel energy at a distance and to affect deeper healing. It also introduces three symbols used to increase the power of the practitioner's healing ability. When completing this level of training, the practitioner can heal over long distances.

Third-Degree Level: (Reiki Masters) In third-degree Reiki, you are attuned and trained with the capacity to attune others to Reiki. Another

---

[4] Barbara Ray, PhD, *The Reiki Factor*, Smithtown, NY: Exposition Press (1983), p. 63.

[5] Bevell, Brett, *The Reiki Magic Guide to Self-Attunement*, Crossing Press, Berkeley, CA 94707 (2007), p. 9.

symbol is learned which is said to add power to the person having attained to this level.[6]

Why so many words and space discussing Reiki? It is a power that can be used to transform another person into New Age consciousness (thinking). It accomplishes what the meditative path does for others; it changes the way people think, and what they believe is reality. They may embark thereafter to learn yoga, meditation, and other spiritual transformation practices. Old values change, and truth is no longer truth.

In many physical therapy clinics, different New Age practices are common, especially with massage therapy. The therapist may be combining Reiki and other energy balancing methods without the patient even being aware. Reiki seems to be the most exciting therapy practiced and appears to be spreading the fastest. A leading Reiki master made the following comment:

> When I looked psychically at the energy, I could often see it as thousands of small particles of light, like "corpuscles" filled with radiant Reiki energy flowing through me and out of my hands. It was as though these Reiki corpuscles of light had a purpose and intelligence.[7]

A Reiki master explains *attunement*:

> Reiki attunement is an initiation into a sacred metaphysical order that has been present on earth for thousands of years . . . By becoming part of this group, you will also be receiving help from the Reiki guides and other spiritual beings who are also working toward these goals.[8]

Again, a Reiki master shares her experience in practicing this modality:

> For me, the Reiki guides make themselves the most felt while attunements are being passed. They stand behind me and direct the whole process, and I assume they also do this for every Reiki

---

[6] *Ibid.*, p. 76.

[7] Rand, William Lee, *The Nature of Reiki Energy*, The Reiki News, Autumn (2000), p. 5.

[8] Rand, William Lee, *Reiki: The Healing Touch*, Southfield, MI: Vision Publishing (1991) p. 48. Reported in Youngen, Ray, *A Time of Departing*, Lighthouse Trails Publishing (2006) p. 95.

master. When I pass attunements, I feel their presence strongly and constantly. Sometimes I can see them.[9]

Is Reiki compatible with Christianity? Isn't it natural healing? Check out this quote:

> During the Reiki attunement process, the avenue that is opened within the body to allow Reiki to flow through also opens up the psychic communication centers. This is why many Reiki practitioners report having verbalized channeled communication with the spirit world.[10]

The foundation of spiritualism (contact with the dead) is to believe the lie told in the Garden of Eden: you will not die, your eyes will be open, and you will be wise like God knowing good and evil (Genesis 3:4, 5). Reiki is a fast track to make that connection with the spirit world. Ponder this next quote from another Reiki master:

> Nurses and massage therapists who have been attuned to Reiki may never disclose when Reiki starts flowing from their palms as they handle their patients. Reiki will naturally "kick in" when it is needed and will continue to flow for as long as the recipient is subconsciously open to receiving it.[11]

Reiki has become popular in several Catholic convents, and some have conducted training in attunements. It has spread throughout Protestant circles as well.

---

[9] Stein, Diane, *Essential Reiki* (Berkley, CA: Crossing Press, 1995), p. 107 Reported in Youngen, Ray, *A Time of Departing*, Lighthouse Trails Publishing (2006), p. 95.

[10] Desy, Phylameana lila, *The Everything Reiki Book*, Avon, MA: Adams Media (2004), p. 144. Reported in Youngen, Ray, *A Time of Departing*, Lighthouse Trails Pub. 2006 p. 97.

[11] *Ibid.*, p. 270.

A systematic review of randomized clinical trials in 2008 assessed the evidence for effectiveness of Reiki. The conclusion: efficacy had not been demonstrated for any condition.[12]

> In March 25, 2009, the Committee on Doctrine of the United States Conference of Catholic Bishops issued Guidelines for Evaluating Reiki as an Alternative Therapy, halting the practice of Reiki by Catholics including Reiki therapies used in some Catholic retreat centers and hospitals. The bishops concluded [rightly] that the procedure was not compatible with either Christian teaching or scientific evidence; it would be inappropriate for Catholic institutions, such as Catholic healthcare facilities and retreat centers, or persons representing the church, such as Catholic chaplains, to promote or to provide support for Reiki therapy.[13]

CRANIOSACCRAL THERAPY

Craniosacral therapy is another body-mind-spirit therapy quite like Reiki in its application, using a very soft touch to the head and neck area. Reiki is said to initiate a flow of cosmic energy through the therapist to the patient; however, therapists of *craniosacral therapy* tell us that they are correcting the clogged, sluggish, unbalanced flow of cerebrospinal fluid about the brain and spinal nerves. The disturbance of cerebrospinal fluid flow is proclaimed by those practicing craniosacral therapy to be the source of most disease and disorders of the human body. Such a concept is not recognized by medical science; indeed there is no evidence to support such a hypothesis.

At the time of the origin of this craniosacral hypothesis and resulting therapy, phrenology was popular. Phrenology was established upon the hypothesis that pressure to areas of the skull would alter the function of the brain and personality. Diagnosis was done by feeling the skull's shape, and in turn therapy for the mind, personality, and character was performed by applying pressure to specific areas of the skull. Large hoods were used

---

[12] Lee, MS, Pittler, MH, Ernst, E., Effects of Reiki in Clinical Practice: A Systematic Review of Randomized Clinical Trials, *International Journal of Clinical Practice* 62 (6): 947.doi:10.1111/j.1742-1241.2008.01729.x. PMID 18410352. (2008) Retrieved 2008-05-02.

[13] Committee on Doctrine of the United States Conference of Catholic Bishops, *Guidelines for Evaluating Reiki as an Alternative Therapy*, March 25 (2009).

Alternative & Mystical Healing Therapies

to cover the head and contained adjustable protrusions (which could be screwed in or out to different lengths) and when worn, applied pressure to selected points on the head for "mind-cure" treatment.

Craniosacral therapy had its origin in the United States through William Sutherland (1873–1954), an osteopathic physician. Sutherland would have been well acquainted with phrenology which may explain what motivated him to do some strange testing. Around 1901, he experimented on himself by placing belts around his head and then tightening those belts in certain positions about the head. He experienced headaches, disorientation, and gastrointestinal distress from these tests. At times when he tightened belts in other positions on the head, he might feel relief and well-being. From this experimentation, Sutherland developed the hypothesis that the cranial bones have motion one upon another; and by pressure, they can be moved. This in turn alters the flow of cerebrospinal fluid flow surrounding the brain, spinal cord, and spinal nerves, thus restoring health. He did not limit his description of disorders caused by improperly flowing cerebrospinal fluid to physical but also included mental and emotional health.[14]

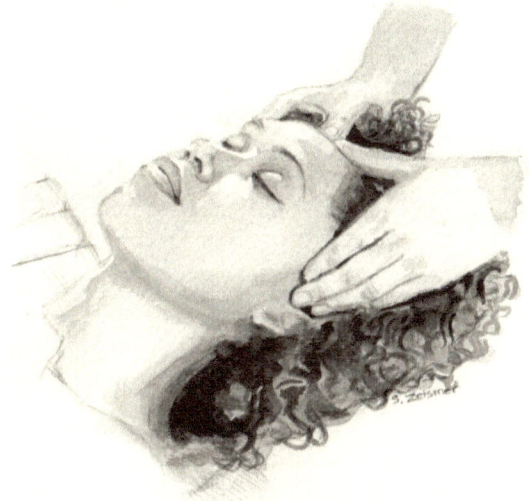

Figure 33. Craniosacral therapy.

Dr. Sutherland eventually sensed a *power*, which he called the the breath of life, that arose from within the patient *without* his touch as the

---

[14] http://www.craniocean.com/what_is_cranial.htm;
http://www.craniosacraltherapy.org/History_02.htm

therapist. He believed that this breath of life carried a basic Intelligence—he capitalized the word *Intelligence*—which the therapist could employ for delivering health. Sutherland and his associates considered the breath of life to carry a subtle yet powerful "potency" or force, which produces subtle rhythms which are transmitted around the body. He believed that this power—breath of life—came from the body's inherent life force itself (chi, prana, universal energy). He theorized that the cerebrospinal fluid distributed the breath of life throughout the body. Dr. Sutherland took his hypothesis to osteopathic schools in the 1940s. This new teaching was labeled "Osteopathy in the Cranial Field."[15]

The concept of cerebrospinal fluid flow being related to all diseases has never been verified by science nor has a soft touch to the head been shown to alter the flow of spinal fluid. It is one man's hypothesis which a few others accepted without verification. This treatment modality does not fit the scientific explanation of the physiology of the nervous system, so how does it fit into spiritualism? How do we explain "the breath of life" that has Intelligence and arises from within the patient? Let us explore further.

In the mid-1970s, another osteopathic physician, John Upledger, who had accepted Dr. Sutherland's hypothesis, began to teach the technique to nonosteopaths. Upledger is actually the one who coined the term *craniosacral therapy*, as he was not allowed to use the term *cranial osteopath* for those who were not osteopaths. Dr. Upledger became the mover behind craniosacral therapy as we know it today.

Dr. Upledger added some techniques to Dr. Sutherland's original method. One contribution is referred to as therapeutic imagery and dialogue. By the use of this contribution, Dr. Upledger may see a response he calls *somato-emotional release*, whereby the patient and therapist can engage together directly with the patient's "inner wisdom" (breath of life) to receive knowledge about the patient that is unknown to either patient or therapist.[16]

Part of the hypothesis of craniosacral therapy is that the body develops what Upledger calls *energy cysts*, which are said to be located at various locations of the body, especially in the connective tissue, such as ligaments, joints, and muscle. These so-called energy cysts are said to be the result of some unresolved physical or psychological trauma of the past, which then allow a variety of clinical symptoms to form. By use of therapeutic imagery and dialogue, these cysts can be resolved, along with whatever clinical

---

[15] http://www.osteohome.com/page16/page30/page30.html

[16] *http://www.larsonwell-being.com/craniosacral-therapy/*

symptoms that are present. Present-day science has not found any of the above hypotheses to be true.[17]

Stan Gerome, an instructor at the Upledger Institute, wrote an article titled "Dialogue, Imagery, Craniosacral Therapy, and Synchronicity," explaining imagery and dialogue. Gerome gives an illustration, and the following is similar: A patient, John, being attended by a craniosacral therapist, complains of pain at a point in his back which has limited his activity for several weeks. The therapist will ask if an image wants to come from that spot. John replies, "Yes, I see a stone." The therapist continues, "What color is the stone?" The patient answers, "It is brown." The therapist asks, "What is its size?" "It is the size of a marble," the patient answers. "What is its name?" the therapist asks. The patient answers, "Anger." Now the therapist asks John's permission to speak directly to the stone. The questions are: how long have you been there, who put you there, and does this person know you are there? Answer: "I have been here for years. Ben put me here, and he does not know I am here." Therapist: "John now knows you are there, and tell us why you are there." Answer from Anger: "I am here so I could protect him from events in life he did not want to admit to." Therapist: "Anger, do you want to be free? Anger: "Yes." Therapist: "What will free you, Anger?" Anger: "For John to see me as his anger."

When John accepts this dialogue as truth, the energy cyst is said to relax and dissolve, and John's problem of back pain heals. This is spoken of as "synchronistic," where both the cyst and the physical problem resolve. What is the origin of such philosophy? Gerome credits Carl Jung (a famous spiritualistic psychiatrist) with the concept of "synchronicity." Jung founded analytic psychology and, while working with people's conscious mind, proceeded to develop the unconscious concepts of psychology. A report of a belief of Jung's is of interest:

> It appears that many of Jung's beliefs were derived from *The Tibetan Book of the Dead*. It had been his constant companion ever since its first publication in England in 1927, and Jung considered its content the quintessence of Buddhist psychological criticism, an initiation process the purpose of which was to restore to the soul the divinity lost at birth. This is a very strong confession of faith in a book, the *Bardo Thodol*, that gives instructions to the dead and the dying and serves as

---

[17] http://www.massagetherapy.com/glossary/index

a guide to the dead during the heavenly and hellish journey of forty-nine days between death and rebirth.[18]

Stan Gerome, a promoter of craniosacral therapy, in his article "Craniosacral Therapy" stated that he believes Jung's concept of "sychronicity" is at work in craniosacral therapy.[19] *Synchronicity* is a word Jung formed to explain connections between events or happenings that seem related. For instance, if a person uses "telepathy" to communicate a message to someone else in a far distant location and the message somehow gets through, etc., this is synchronicity by Jung's definition. Similarly, the illustration continues. If a disturbance of flow of universal energy through the body at some location caused a psychological disturbance in the personality, correcting the flow by whatever method would clear the personality defect. That connection between energy flow and a personality flaw is Jung's *synchronicity*.

Synchronicity is best explained by understanding there are agents of Satan, fallen angels, that can influence, carry messages, and be the power in Jung's sychronicity. Jung was a known spiritualist and also a theosophist; in essence, spiritualism.

In 1999, the British Columbia (Canadian) Office of Health Technology Assessment (BCOHTA) published an article titled, "A Systematic Review and Appraisal of the Scientific Evidence on Craniosacral Therapy." Their conclusion was that the theory is invalid and that practitioners cannot reliably measure what they claim to be modifying.

A physicist, Eugenie V. Mielczarek, emeritus professor of physics at George Mason University in Fairfax, Virginia, presented a paper, with the help of Derek C. Araujo, Adam Magazine, and Lori Sommerfelt, representing the Center for Inquiry concerning the physics proclaimed by distant healers to be involved in Reiki, craniosacral therapy, therapeutic touch, qigong, or any so-called distant healing. The summary of her paper follows:

> Alleged distance healers justify their claimed abilities in terms of an unsubstantiated biomagnetic field of about two milligauss emanating from the hands of certified distance healers. However, a two-milligauss field strength is eighteen

---

[18] Fodor, Nandor, *Freud, Jung, and Occultism*, University Books, Inc., New Hyde Park, New York 11040 (1971), p. 157.

[19] http://www.iahe.com/images/pdf/stan.pdf

orders of magnitude below the energy needed to affect any biochemistry. The postulate of an unknown energy field width eludes all science-based investigations and measurement but nevertheless causes a transmission of energies large enough to affect the chemistry of cell cultures flies in the face of all micro and cellular biology experimentation and well-tested theories of physics. This postulate of a medically healing energy field, which can only be generated by certain individuals, fails all test of medical science.[20]

---

[20] Mielczarek, Eugenie V., *A Fracture in Our Health Care: Paying for Non-Evidenced Based Medicine*, Center for Inquiry, Office of Public Policy, Washington DC

13

MYSTICAL HERBOLOGY

Ever since man was restricted from partaking of the "Tree of Life" in the Garden of Eden, he has been searching for that magic sustainer of life. The plant kingdom has been the main source of his investigation for this "elixir of life," with some additional interest in minerals. In the search for health, the field of *herbs* has had a long history. Winston J. Craig, PhD, gives a cursory review of ancient civilizations' involvement with herbs and minerals in his text *The Use and Safety of Common Herbs and Herbal Teas*. An herb is a plant that is valued for its flavor, scent, medicinal properties, and, often, its perceived "spiritual" values.

Records found from ancient civilizations in Mesopotamia, Egypt, India, and China have revealed the use of various herbs as medicinals. The oldest records date to near 3000 BC. These oldest records show a rational approach to treatment of disease, but by 1500 BC, almost all civilizations had reverted to an irrational and mystical approach. The emphasis for herb use became primarily spiritual and/or mystical combined with *astrology* in application as therapy for disease without understanding of biochemical action. The same combination of spiritual, magical, and astrological relationships is a common belief in herb use today. The belief in a combination of properties of plants has led to a concept that plants have a *personality*, *a spirit*, a *consciousness* on a very high plane, electrical magnetic frequency, and pronounced effect upon the human mind and emotions.[1]

---

[1] Tisserand, Robert B., *The Art of Aromatherapy, Healing Arts Press*, Roschester, VT 05767, (1977), pp. 45–49.

The use of herbs has been a fundamental practice in all ancient health and healing systems. Herbs are considered helpful in "bridging" the cosmic energies, which are said to be internal and external to the body. In Ayurvedic practice, herbs are always to be used in conjunction with meditation, diet, and other Ayurvedic approaches to health. Benefit from herbal therapy in Ayurveda medicine will depend upon its being added to other therapies. Little to no benefit is to be expected when it is used alone.

The herbal remedies of the past were not chosen for medicinal use because of their biochemical properties; but for their supposed ability to influence balancing a vital force, a universal energy said to be in and flowing through mankind. Out of this use, however, it was recognized that certain plants had a variety of effects upon people; and over time, many plants began to be used as a result of their biochemical effects. Many present-day medicines are derived from herbs. More will be found by ongoing research. The use of some herbs in small amounts (such as turmeric) is of value as they contain many powerful chemicals that are healthful.

Ayurveda also used minerals in its treatment methods for thousands of years. Substances such as arsenic, antimony, and mercury were in common use until this past century. Mercury was the most popular mineral used and was given almost as a universal antidote for illness. Mercury, in the Hindu's understanding, is "semen from Shiva," one of their prominent gods.

The ancient apothecary, or pharmacy, had minerals and a variety of plant substances. Some of these pharmacies grew their own plants and prepared minerals for administration. Of particular note in alchemy is the mineral *mercury*, a silver-white element derived from the red cinnabar ore. It is a deadly poison. The use of mercury continued down through the centuries; and in the early 1800s, mercury, in the form of mercurous chloride (calomel), was given for almost all ailments. When I began the study of medicine in 1955, there were several forms of mercury still being used in medical care. It was quite effective as an ointment to treat fungus infections of the skin. Injections of *mercuhydrin* were used as a diuretic. Gradually, physicians began to understand its long-term toxicity, and its use faded.

Plant lore and much of herbal use is based on the doctrine of pantheism: "one is all, all is one"; "as above, so below." The pagan's story of creation is that a blending of a two-part (yin and yang) universal (life force) energy to a point of perfect balance created all material things. It also supposedly gave to living plants a high-level frequency of cosmic energy, "a soul." It is *this teaching* that is believed in the neo-pagan culture to give plants and herbs ability to have an influence upon the mind of man. For millennia, herbologists have believed that there is a spiritual power connected with herbs. In more recent years, this spiritual power has been expressed as electromagnetic energy with a high-wave *frequency*. There is always this attempt to explain *mystical power* and *life force energy* in the terms and concepts of modern physics, making it more acceptable to the nonbeliever of mysticism. Such teaching is also more deceptive to the unwary.

In the chapter "Universal Energy," explanation is given to the teaching promoted in New Age/neo-pagan belief systems concerning seven levels of perceived vibrational frequencies of universal energy. Energy traveling at the speed of light is said to become material substance forming the cosmos, earth, and all that is on it. The higher (hypothesized) frequencies (subtle energies) are said to promote higher levels of consciousness. Herbs are believed to possess high-frequency energy; therefore, herbal treatment is believed to be most effective on the mind of man and is useful for therapy on emotions and mental conditions.[2]

The field of herbalism has much that is good but also opens a *chasm* that many fall into thinking they are following a "natural" method. User beware as one can easily be deceived into accepting a false system of healing and in so doing give homage to another God.

The emphasis in this book's chapter on herbal use will be to expose this counterfeit of God's healing methods. Some of these false aspects are very difficult to ferret out as the explanation of the application and use of certain methods sounds so beneficial and can blend so closely with the truth. This is especially so in aromatherapy.

Most people will make their judgment as to whether a method is proper to use or not by whether they receive apparent benefit. This is never a test to be used to determine if a therapy is free of being Satan's counterfeit. Satan is not going to waste his efforts on a therapy that does not bring changes or *apparent* improvement. The Bible tells us (Rev. 13:14; 16:14; 19:20; II Thess. 2:9) he has power to do miracles—not fake miracles but real miracles.

The greatest use of herbs in the past was guided mainly by a *world view* that saw their influence upon humans not by biochemical action but as substances containing *life forces* by which man supposedly increased his own life force. The New Age movement of today looks to herbs both as a spiritual power—energy—and as active biochemical agents. This will be better demonstrated in the following comments on flower therapy and aromatherapy.

INTRODUCTION TO A PAGAN PHILOSOPHY OF HERBS

> Herbs are "Magick." They have been the primary source of medicines for people of every culture and were considered

---

[2] *Ibid.*, pp. 10–12, 92–103.

"magickal" or spiritual by many of them. An ancient *earth based* spiritual belief system concerning herbs appears in many ancient cultures and civilizations such as Celtic, Chinese, Indian, and Native American philosophies, just to name a few. Their religious beliefs shaped their view and relationship with the "Great Spirit," and the relationships between their citizens.[3]

This belief system involves a holistic view of illness and utilizes herbs according to religious belief. Earth-centered religion still permeates herbalism today. Herbalism is part of the *religion of nature*, the concept of balance of mind, body, and spirit also relying on intuition as well as science.

Exploring what pagans believe about relationships said to exist between plants and man gives us more understanding as to why they have interest in the use of herbs, plant essences, essential oils, and aromatherapy for healing. This relationship is said to be that all plants have *souls* and *spirits* that guard and protect the species. Many plants are said to have also *animal spirits* attached.

> Pagans work with Nature, respecting and worshipping the spiritual forces they observe. Nature is perceived as the domain of the gods and of spirits. Nature religions teach a philosophy of *divine linking* between all of the earth's inhabitants.[4]
>
> Cachora (Indian Shaman) is quite plain about the underlying principle of healing herbs. He says that healing takes place when a person connects into the plant spirit, becoming the plant and understanding its personality. Using spirit as the method of transference, the plant's energy or healing properties are transmitted to.
>
> The person ... healing can take place by calling on the spirit and taking into one's mind the spiritual essence of the plant.[5]

In following paragraphs, we will explore more concerning the belief in and use of plants, their essences, essential oils, and aromas as used by many today for health and healing.

---

[3] http://www.purifymind.com/PhilosophyHerb.htm
[4] *Ibid*.
[5] Worwood, Valerie Ann, *Aromatherapy for the Soul*, New World Library, Navato, California 94949, (1999), p. 9.

Herbs have a proper use for their taste and biochemical properties. I recommend the book *Nutrition and Wellness: A Vegetarian Way to Better Health*—written by Winston J. Craig, PhD, RD, professor of Nutrition at Andrews University—which covers much of the presently known benefits and information on the biochemical properties of herbs.[6] A second book I recommend is *Drugs, Herbs, & Natural Remedies* by Mervyn Hardinge, MD, DrPH, PhD.

FLOWER THERAPY

Flower therapy is a component of herbalism.

> Various flower remedies are also typically involved in the world of the occult, such as the *Vita Florum* and *Bach Flower Remedies* which claim to operate on the basis of cosmic forces and permit psychic diagnosis, prognosis, and other forms of guidance.[7]

The occultist Douglas Baker discusses the underlying theory in the use of flower remedies in his book *Esoteric Healing*. He states that:

> Dr. Bach had discovered that dew which accumulated on the petals of wild flowers before sunrise, was changed dramatically by the presence of sunlight so that it now had an energy potential within it . . . each plant's dew had a quality of its own, a type of energy absorbed into the dew that could be used as a specific remedy. We should not be surprised, after our careful examination of the occult forces, a plan . . . that these could be applied to correct imbalances in the astral and mental auras of Man.[8]

---

[6] Craig, Winston J., Ph.D., R.D., *The Use and Safety of Common Herbs and Herbal Teas, Second Edition*, Golden Harvest Books, 4610 Lisa Lane, 'Berrien Springs, MI, (1996).

[7] Ankerberg, John, Weldon, John, *Can You Trust Your Doctor?* Wolgemuth & Hyatt, Publishers, Inc. Brentwood, Tennessee, (1991), p. 260.

[8] Baker, Douglas; *Esoteric Healing* Vol. 3, part 2, of *"The Seven Pillars of Ancie Wisdom: The Syntheses of Yoga, Esoteric Science and Psychology*, Herts, England, (1976).
Reported in Ankerberg, *Can You Trust Your Doctor?* Wolgemth & Hyatt, Publishers, Inc., Brentwood, Tennessee, (1991), p. 260.

Flower essences are prepared by placing the petals in water and in the sunlight. The water is then said to contain the flower's essence. The water is administered by placing drops of it on the tongue at various times each day over an extended period of time. It may be that the person prescribing the flower essence will make the diagnosis and then choose the proper flower for treatment by use of a pendulum.[9] Applied kinesiology is another method of choosing the proper flower essence to prescribe. This is done by having the person being tested hold a flower-essence vial in one hand, and with the other arm outstretched, downward pressure is made on the arm. The arm will increase in strength when the **best** essence is held. It is a popular form of divination.

Dr. Bach—an English homeopathic physician, a psychic, a believer in subtle energies—started the use of flower remedies. He developed thirty-eight different flower essences, which are still available after eighty years. Since the death of Dr. Bach in 1936, many other flower essences have been added to the treatment protocol. At least five hundred different essences are available for treatment of a variety of maladies.

How are these flower essences discovered for use in a specific ailment? Richard Gerber in his book *Vibrational Medicine* (p. 512) explains:

> The information guiding their usage, like the information on previous Pegasus Products, comes from *channeled* sources.[10]

Flower essences are directed mainly at treatment of emotional imbalances and personality dysfunctions.

> Unlike conventional drug therapies which impact solely at the level of physical cellular pathology, the energetic patterns contained within the flower essence work at the level of the emotional, mental, and spiritual vehicles.[11]

> Bach correctly perceived that the illness-personality link was an out-growth of dysfunctional energetic patterns within the subtle bodies. He felt that illness was a reflection of disharmony between

---

[9] Pfeifer, Samuel M.D., *Healing at Any Price*, Word (UK) Ltd. Milton Keynes, England, (1980), p. 124–125. Reported in Ankerberg, op. cit., p. 259.

[10] Gerber, Richard, M.D., *Vibrational Medicine, the # 1 Handbook of Subtle-Energy Therapies,* Bear and company, One Park Street, Rochester, VT, (2001), p. 512.

[11] *Ibid.*, p. 247.

the physical personality and the Higher Self or soul.... Bach links this relationship of the physical personality to the Higher Self (Godhood of man) via a re-incarnational philosophy.[12]

ESSENTIAL OILS AND AROMATHERAPY

Another part of herbology that has grown very popular is **aromatherapy**. It too has its ancient origin in Ayurveda medicine. Its use is an attempt to heal through use of fragrances of botanical origin. The fragrances are extracted from plants by removing oils called essential oils. Oils are obtained from plants by *compression* or by various *distillation* methods. *Life force, universal energy*, is believed to be contained within the oils and fragrance. By the application of the fragrance internally or externally, this life force is believed to be transferred to an individual. The scientifically non-demonstrable concept of electromagnetic *frequency* or *vibration* of a plant is proclaimed to be within the fragrance and is said to be of a frequency faster than light, affecting the "higher consciousness" of an individual so as to be useful for healing emotional and mental faculties. The fragrance is considered to be the "personality" or "spirit" of the plant. It is believed to balance *subtle energy* flow (universal energy of high frequency). Aromas are used in Ayurveda to calm aggravated doshas (vata, pitta, kapha), three forces taught in Ayurveda that govern biological processes. Topical application with oil or creams containing the fragrance is said to affect the organ or organs in close proximity to where the application was made, imparting increased flow of energy. The fragrances are also used in baths and are administered by inhalation.[13]

The chemistry of the fragrances is complex, consisting of alcohols, esters, ketones, aldehydes, and terpenes. They do not dissolve in water, only in oil, ether, or alcohol. Aromatic oils are used in three classes of consumer goods: food, toiletries, and medicines.

- *Foods*: natural flavorings, such as oil of lemon, lime, and orange;
- *Cosmetics*: perfumes, toothpaste, etc.;
- *Medicine*: flavoring of medicinals, as therapeutics of their own right, such as oil of wintergreen, clove oil, peppermint oil, and eucalyptus oil used in steam inhalations and ointments for topical applications.[14]

---

[12] *Ibid.*, p. 244.

[13] Tisserand, Op. cit., p. 8.

[14] *Ibid.*, p. 13.

I can hear your thoughts!

> First, you tell me in the first paragraph above that use of essential oils and the fragrances they contain is spiritistic, then you list many common scents and fragrances used in foods, cosmetics and medicinals. Are you trying to tell me that their use is spiritistic also? You just lost me! Bye.

No! no! no! There is a difference—a distinct difference. Yet this is a very difficult subject to make clear and of which to have a correct understanding. I am not sure I can give an answer applicable in all situations discerning which use is proper and which is not. I will try to give principles; and each person will have to use caution, wisdom, and prayer to make that choice.

Let us look first at the principles of use for these scents, flavorings, and therapeutic substances that are not considered a part of *aromatherapy*. The reason for their use is to utilize their *biochemical properties*. The chemicals in an aroma such as eucalyptus oil are soothing to an irritated throat and bronchus and are used for respiratory infections. We are not using it because of some vibration of high frequency or spirit connection. Oil of peppermint is useful for simple gastrointestinal distresses because of its biochemical properties. Most anesthetics are gases used because of their effect on the central nervous system to allow painful procedures to be done without experiencing pain. Using these substances would not come under the definition of aromatherapy as the term is understood by holistic medicine practitioners. The above mentioned examples and many other substances have been safely used for ages totally apart from any religious spiritistic connotation.

Let us go back and look again at principles proclaimed in the use of aromatherapy by holistic healers. The following quotation is taken from the text *The Art of Aromatherapy* by Robert Tisserand, a frequently quoted author on the subject of aromatherapy:

> Aromatherapy belongs to the realm of natural therapeutics. As such it is based on certain principles which are shared by acupuncture, herbal medicine, homeopathy, etc. These principles are complementary, and are based on man's interpretation of nature from his understanding of life. . . . Surely the universe was created and is sustained on one set of principles, so there can only be one truth. . . . The main principles of our therapy are: *life force, yin-yang,* and *organic foods.*[15]

---

[15] *Ibid.*, p. 45.

Life force: synonyms are chi, prana, mana, logos, orenda, the innate, animal magnetism, odic force, bioplasma, monism, Self, Higher Self, Divine Self, purer consciousness, creative principle, essence, supreme ultimate, etc. I refer the reader back to chapter 5 on universal energy.

Tisserand continues, elaborating on life force, by telling us it is the same all-pervading force that is continually bringing about a state of health and harmony in the body. He tells us that it is the only power that can produce health for us. What the author does here is to describe the sustaining power of the Creator God but separates God from His power and makes the power "god itself." It is part of the pagan's counterfeit story of creation in contrast to the true creation by the Son of God, Jesus Christ, in harmony with the Holy Spirit and God the Father.

Yin-yang: *Yin* and *yang* are words taken from the Chinese and used since there are no English words for direct translation. They are intrinsic to the Chinese story of creation, a story that removes a personal Being as the Creator and applies credit to a *force*, or as now referred to as an energy. This is seen in the following quote:

> The physical universe was created when Oneness became duality, and we can see this duality, this yin and yang, everywhere in the universe, in every atom, every action, and in every function of the human body. Yin and yang are manifest everywhere, except at the very centre of being, the perfect point of balance, at that infinite moment when the future becomes the past." . . . "Every single function of a living organism manifests these two forces." . . . To know which oils are predominantly yin or yang gives a basic guide to their application in sickness.[16]

Organic foods: When we think of people choosing to purchase and/or eat only "organic" food, our understanding is that this involves a desire to avoid as much as possible contaminants in food such as the chemicals used in insect control, etc. It is also thought that organic foods will have a better balance of the constituents of which they are made when not pushed in growth by various added minerals. The reason for choosing organic by many is all of the above, but also for some people, there is a pagan religious belief involved. They believe that any interference with the growth of the plant will alter its *life force*. The fragrances—essences of a plant—are considered organic and work in harmony to organize the body and its chemistry. They recognize the *life force* as the only power that can

---

[16] *Ibid.*, p. 49.

produce health. Aromas are a constituent of plants and are considered to be a concentration of *life force*.

I wish to share with the reader a few more comments made from a text on aroma therapy:

Essential oils contain this mystery of life; they have powerful inexplicable energies too. . . . Plants are the interface between cosmic energies and the earth, upon which we depend.[17]

> From a brain biochemistry point of view, the pursuit of spirituality through aroma makes a great deal of sense, as the mechanics of smell are but one short biological step away from consciousness, including higher consciousness (godhood). Thinking of it in terms of light, essential oils are captured light, passed from the heavens, by plants, to us. From a vibrational, electromagnetic, and energetic point of view essential oils are in harmony with life.[18]

I wish to share one more comment from this text of *Aroma Therapy for the Soul*:

> Twenty years ago in aromatherapy, there was an unwritten rule that we would not be open about the spiritual side of the essential oils we worked with. We talked about their anti-infectious qualities and their beautifying effects on the skin, or about any number of benefits to body and mind. The positive spiritual changes were recognized, but silently. It seemed far too bold to suggest light and wisdom of the universe flowed through them, their fragrance like messengers from heaven, aromatic angels that come and touch us with the positivity and love of the deity.
>
> With an etheric quality, essential oils activate the receptors of love, compassion, and empathy. They are an informational network, carrying messages and crossing boundaries, operating on many different levels. Through them, we can contact the wisdom of nature, the power of light, the energy of the universe and the love in our hearts.[19]

---

[17] Worwood, op. cit., p. xviii.
[18] *Ibid.*, p. xix.
[19] *Ibid.*, p. xix.

This comment opens to us the deceptiveness of the holistic movement. These healers capture the minds of people by the teachings that holistic healing therapies are actually effective on the biochemistry and physiological functioning of our bodies, that their actions can be explained by the sciences of physics and chemistry. This is a charade. That which gives power to these holistic methods is the act of giving our "will" to that power. The physical methods of therapy are meaningless; it is the acceptance of the method and its perceived power that then allows Satan to exercise his power over us.

Ayurvedic medicine and the Hindu religion of which Ayurveda is a component were established more than 3,500 years in the past. Aromatherapy is an integral part of Ayurveda and Hinduism. The aromas are used to pacify aggravated doshas. *Doshas* (rajas-tamas), the dualism of "prana," is the equivalent word in Sanskrit language to *yin-yang* in Chinese. Aromatherapy is used to balance doshas.[20]

A question arises, how and by what means are these different aromas selected for use in treatment of various disorders? An answer comes from the book *Vibrational Medicine: The Handbook of Subtle-Energy Therapies*. Here, Dr. Gerber, the author, is speaking of flower essences, but his words apply to aromas as well. Note the following quote:

> A number of flower-essence practitioners are learning to combine the knowledge and techniques of acupuncture, herbal medicine, and homeopathy with their use of flower essences, some practitioners use flower essences potentized as high homeopathic dilutions in order to release a higher energy and stronger life-force pattern to the patient. . . . He is now producing a new class of vibrational tinctures that are made from the captured light of stars and planets. Most flower essences and gem elixirs are produced utilizing the light of our local star, the sun, to imprint the various life-energy patterns into the storage medium of water (and alcohol). However, unlike conventional vibrational essences, these *intuitively* created star elixirs carry the energy and informational patterns of various stars and planets that can be ingested for particular vibrational and healing benefits. The information guiding their usage, like the information on previous Pegasus Products, comes from *channeled sources* (by spirits through mediums).[21] (emphasis added)

---

[20] Gerson, Scott M.D., *Ayurveda, The Ancient Indian healing Art*, Element Books Limited (1997), p. 104.

[21] Gerber, op. cit., pp. 511, 512.

Clearly, there are two purposes in use of aromas that come to us in oils or a tincture. One uses them to utilize their *biochemical properties* in foods, cosmetics, and medicinals; the other use seeks to use them so as to *partake of their spiritual power*. I think that after considering all of the information presented in this chapter, few Christians are going to choose to use aromas in order to gain a higher spiritual experience. We would not desire to have contact with spirits in our quest to secure healing. However, it is not uncommon for sincere devout Christians to seek out flower essences, essential oils, and aromas to find healing for some discomfort and/or ailment. Often the purchase of these substances is done from a shop carrying all sorts of New Age merchandise. By entering into aromatherapy, do I place myself in a position to be deceived even if I am aware of Satan's counterfeit and my desire is to only use the biochemical properties of the essential oil or aroma? Important question!

How can I know that I am not choosing the power of spirits when I partake of aromatherapy? If I am a person who seeks to be a consultant or therapist in "natural healing" and wants to be sure of avoiding entanglement in a method that is a counterfeit and is one of Satan's deceptions, how can I recognize and avoid such? People tell me that when they purchase the essential oil containing a certain aroma that they in no way believe in or accept the spiritistic background associated with aromatherapy. They just want to get the *good* out of it and do not accept it as being spirit discovered and/or empowered for its effectiveness. They use it because *it works*, and they want no part in the rest of its trappings. They say they are strictly partaking of its biochemical properties to treat their malady.

How do we know if an essence, essential oil, or its aroma really is able to do what we take it for? Has it been tested on thousands of people for those same symptoms, tested against a placebo? Has the aroma been tested by being exposed to the patient without his or her awareness and it gave the same relief even when one was not aware of receiving it? Does it do the same for most everyone with the same symptoms? Does it create the same response in animals when it is feasible to so test? Does it give immediate results when we are exposed to it, or does it take time and repeated application for it to begin to give relief? These are a few of the questions we need to ask when considering as to whether the relief we receive from its use is really physiologic or an influence from a spirit.

Am I spiritually safe to go to the New Age store to buy or to try out the different essences from the many varieties of aromas to find the one that heals me? Has someone chosen the aroma for my therapy by use of the pendulum, the sway test, or muscle testing? I believe that there are spirits and that they have power, but I am not going to have anything to do with them. I just want to get the substance that is helpful for me, and I reject any spirit connection. That should prevent any spirit influence over me

I ask: is that possible? Let us consider the first great deception in the Garden. Adam and Eve were told to avoid going near the Tree of Knowledge of Good and Evil as that was the only place Satan could tempt them, which was *his ground*. If they stayed away from there, Satan would have no influence on them. When Eve found herself near the tree, she reasoned that she was capable of recognizing and resisting the foe God had warned of. She had no concept that the voice speaking to her was from Satan. Her protection vanished as she began to parley with the serpent. We too have been warned to stay off Satan's ground as our protection will be diminished.

Where and what is Satan's ground? It was my understanding that he is able to roam the whole earth. Yes, that is true; but there are places we may visit or frequent, attitudes we harbor, mistrust of God's leading, looking outside of His plan for aid, etc., that causes our guardian angel to separate from us. At that point, the warnings for our protection that God has given may well fade from our memories, leaving us on our own to face the tempter. And we are no match—no match at all.

As we near the close of this chapter, I wish to quote a paragraph from a book that contains an excellent review of the source and power behind aromatherapy:

> But in almost all these systems which claim to utilize herbs, plants, and their etheric energies for diagnosis, healing, psychic development, altered states of consciousness, etc., the herbs and plants themselves possess no mystical power. As in crystal healing and similar methods, they are merely implements behind which spirit powers can work. They are no different than dowsing rods, crystals, radionic devices, Tarot cards, I Ching sticks, rune dice, or the Ouija board. No power resides in any of these implements themselves; they merely become a focal point behind which the spirits secure their goals.[22]

Can Christians safely partake a healing method that Satan invented for his use and for 3,500 years has been an integral part of pagan religions as a component of his counterfeit healing system, then give it a new face of proclaimed scientific properties, and incorporate it into our healing system by saying, "I do not take of the belief system. I just take the good from it"?

---

[22] Ankerberg, op. cit., p. 261.

The answer for myself is no! The reader will make his or her own decision.

Postscript

The writing of this chapter had been concluded, and I was planning to send it to the editor for a professional touchup. I received e-mail correspondence from an individual unknown to me, asking me to defend my position of naming the alternative therapeutic discipline of "essential oils-aromatherapy" as being spiritistically deceptive. This individual was a spokesperson for a large company that grew various herbs and plants from which they extracted *essential oils* and in turn marketed them. She had displeasure with me because my book *Spiritualistic Deceptions in Health and Healing* had a few paragraphs that referred to essential oils and aromatherapy. She felt that my stand on this subject was detrimental to the "mission" of teaching people of the benefits of essential oils as medicinals for health.

I will share with you some of our correspondence as it did bring up a few issues I had not included in this chapter. I believe it to be important to write a brief of our interchange of correspondence. Points she used to justify the use of essential oils-aromatherapy were presented to me in a way that I had not previously heard from individuals attempting to justify their use of aromatherapy. Covering some of these teachings and beliefs may be of value to others.

It is not unusual for proponents of and especially marketers of various holistic therapeutic disciplines and/or products to attempt to tie in their use as being "biblical." So did my correspondent. I was informed that the Bible referred to essential oils 188 times. Frankincense and myrrh were aromatic oils and were given as gifts to the infant Jesus. (Actually, they are resins, not oils.)

Twelve different aromatic oils are mentioned in the scriptures, with references to different uses for oils, cooking oils, oil for lamps, anointing, incense, etc. I checked all those verses. Out of 188 references to oil, there was one mention of its being used as a medicinal, and that was the parable of the man who was beaten and robbed on his way to Jericho. The scriptures tell us that the Good Samaritan who took care of him placed oil on his wounds. It did not state which type of oil. Many medical therapeutic practices have been standard over time, yet that does not establish that they were effective.

In the website given to me to check out, I found a very interesting article on essential oils. It's titled *Twelve Oils of Ancient Scripture*. The author Judy DeRuvo elaborated on each of the twelve. Listed in the next paragraph is a brief of the proclaimed uses and effects of using these aromatic oils. It is interesting that in the first sentence on the first oil, *aloe/sandalwood* she refers to India; and thereafter, the explanations are tied into Ayurveda (Hindu) vocabulary and principles. I will list some of her "quips" below, referring to the actions of these twelve oils she listed as being in Biblical scripture.

> Enhancement to meditation; allows mind to move into the deepest states of meditation; connects with the great cosmic prayer; affects chakra energy; links the kundalini energy at the base chakra with the crown chakra; aligns all the chakras and subtle bodies; keeps you grounded, close to your divine essence; empowers the will; supports the sacral chakra; helps release emotional toxins lodged in the subtle bodies; aligns the heart chakra of the mental body to the physical; cypress has frequencies that are in transition between the physical and spiritual (etheric) plane; clears blockage in energy flow; cypress oil disconnects spleen energy attachments.; spiritual and karmic implications; operates beyond the auric field; frankincense helps each of us to connect to that part of us which is eternal and divine; promoting clairvoyance; it opens the 3rd eye for connection; sheds light on life's purpose and on the inner self; it clears the aura and energy fields; it transmutes dense thought forms.[23]

The many paragraphs that contain these remarks also contain Bible verses, attempting to blend them with the above Hindu terms and concepts.

My first response to give an answer to the question as to how I could include essential oils in my book on exposing spiritualistic deceptive practices in the medical field was to send this book's chapter on "Mystical Herbology" to the individual contesting my writings. The response back was that my chapter is only "RHETORIC writing." It did not line up with scripture.

Another teaching that seems common in *aromatherapy lore* is that at the time of the great black plague in the fourteenth century, physicians put certain essential oils in a face mask in such a way that air breathed through a cloth soaked in essential oils, which would protect from the

---

[23] http://www.experience-essential-oils.com/twelve-oils-of-ancient-scripture.html

infectious plague. This practice did occur, but it was to offset the stench of death. Medical history books record this practice. There are no comments in the history books that it was protective from infection by destroying bacteria. The cause of the plague was then totally unknown. Bacteria were not discovered until the nineteenth century, five hundred years after the plagues. I have a copy of an ancient drawing of this practice of a physician using a nosepiece soaked in perfume.

In the above dialogue, two books were recommended in support of essential oils and aromatherapy being based in Judeo-Christian scripture: *The Chemistry of Essential Oils Made Simple: God's Love Manifest in Molecules* and *Healing Oils of the Bible* by David Stewart, PhD. Recently, I received an e-mail request to give my opinion on these two books by an individual who has dabbled in essential oils and has a serious question as to where is the border between the mystical aspect of use of essential oils and aromatherapy and a non-mystical use. This question is not new and has been difficult to answer.

I have just finished reviewing the book on chemistry of essential oils. The author David Stewart has had significant education in physics and chemistry and lays out the chemical structures of many aromatic molecules and gives a synopsis of organic chemistry in an attempt to make clear to students of essential oils their molecular structure. He shares that he also is a Methodist minister. Stewart expresses his belief in a Creator God, one that made man in the image of God. I did not find a sentence establishing for certain his belief in a six-day creation, yet I gathered that such is his belief. There are direct comments made, however, that reveal a belief akin to pantheism (*panentheism*) concept of God's creation—i.e., a spark of divinity in man and all creation. His discourse on the action of essential oils' influence on the chemistry and physiology of man definitely includes the concept of plants and their oils containing a *divine* attribute.

> When molecules of essential oils are inhaled, swallowed, applied to the skin, or internalized into your body in any way, they resonate with your bodily tissues at the frequencies intrinsic to their molecular spectrum as well as their resultant harmonic and beat frequencies. This increases your own natural electromagnetic vibrations and restores coherence to your electric fields to produce healing and maintain wellness.[24]

---

[24] Stewart, David, Ph.D., *The Chemistry of Essential Oils: God's Love Manifest in Molecules*, Care Publication, Marble Hill, MO, (2005), p. 181.

Science does not recognize such "harmonic and beat frequencies." Such expressions are found only in the writing of New Age–neo-pagan literature. Essential oils also are said to respond to prayer/words and negative-positive thoughts, demonstrated by their changing frequencies. Even the "intent" of the therapists or patient will guide the molecules of essential oils to the location in the body where they are to restore health.[25] Molecules of essential oils are purported to contain "subtle electromagnetic properties," which allow them to communicate directly with "cellular intelligence," similar to homeopathy remedies.[26] Stewart presents support for these concepts by referring to the book *Vibrational Medicine* by Richard Gerber, MD.

In the book, *Vibrational Medicine*, mentioned above, you will read a comment made by its author Dr. Gerber, wherein he states that much of the information in that book came from *channeling of spirits*. Some other books that David Stewart recommends are from authors with similar beliefs. As I read further in Dr. Stewart's writings, it seemed to me he has attempted to blend pantheistic concepts with Christianity and applied them to the scientific world. He does not document by references to scientific studies in presenting his concepts and conclusions *Healing Oils of the Bible*, another book by David Stewart, follows a similar pattern of thought as the first book. I share with you my analysis of that text:

In response to requests for me to write an appraisal of the book, *Healing Oils of the Bible* by David Stewart Ph.D., it is necessary to again understand the author's *world view* as expressed throughout the text of his book. Vocabulary used by authors of different world views may be similar but with significantly different meanings. This is especially true of religious terms.

David Stewart, is a Methodist minister who has had advanced education in biology, chemistry and physics. He freely expresses belief in creation by a God of the universe, *by the breath of His mouth* as recorded in the Bible. However he blends the Biblical account with a *"panentheistic"* concept—*God in everything—divinity in all;* that even plants have *divinity within* of which they can impart. He attempts to blend Eastern view of *Reality* with Biblical world view and they do not mix.

In the Introduction of the book, a statement is made that plants and their essential oils contain an "essence," have "Life force," "divine intelligence," and "vibrational energy." Words that at first view might not

---

[25] Ibid., p. 183.
[26] Ibid., p. 229.

be recognized for what the author is saying. The correct understanding of his use of these terms is ascertained more clearly as one reads through the book. They have definitely been used in the setting of a *pantheistic* world view.

Stewart's intrigue continues as he explains that plants were brought into existence by the Thought and Word of God. No argument, however, he then tells us that the plants are also *responsive* to our thoughts and will respond accordingly.[27] Essential oils are said to have:

Theological applications:

1. purification from sin[28]
2. spiritual up lifting[29]
3. possess divine intelligence[30]
4. Impossible for God to lie therefore essential oils are *truth*[31]
5. demons are repulsed by essential oils' molecular high vibrational energies[32]

Psychological responses:

6. enhance spiritual state in worship[33]
7. bring emotional releases[34]
8. essential oils can release, unblock emotional congestion stored in various tissues other than brain[35]
9. open up subconscious mind to release deep seated emotional trauma[36]
10. elevate spiritual consciousness[37]

---

[27] Stewart, David, Ph.D., Healing Oils of the Bible, Care Publications, (2014) 7th Edition, p. xvii.

[28] *Ibid.*, p. xvi.

[29] *Ibid.*, p. 34.

[30] *Ibid.*, xvii, p. 19, 20.

[31] *Ibid.*, p. 47.

[32] *Ibid.*, p. 89.

[33] *Ibid.*, p. xvi.

[34] *Ibid.*, p. xvi, 79.

[35] *Ibid.*, p. 79.

[36] *Ibid.*

[37] *Ibid.*,

11. balance electrical energies within the body giving courage, confidence, and self-esteem[38]

Paranormal influence:

12. cause growth up to one inch in height of person[39]
13. rapid correction of scoliosis and or kyphosis[40]
14. able to repulse demons[41]
15. able to be directed by thought or word to the part of body desired[42]
16. possess divine intelligence[43]
17. use of oil by priests in ceremonial cleansing of a leper purported to be "reflexology" practice in Bible days[44]
18. able to determine disease causing bacteria, virus, or parasite, from non-disease causing and eradicate the pathogenic (disease causing) ones[45]

Dr. Stewart blends science with Eastern religious concepts to the degree it is hard to know which he is relating to. He gives zero references to back up any conclusions he makes. Never did I find any reference to scientific studies to support his hypothesis and conclusions. He did mention that science at times has to use supposition and that he is free to do the same. The difference here is science gathers all the evidence that it is able to secure which came about by rigorous testing and evaluation and then makes a judgment call, willing to change with new evidence. I do not find such trend in his text.

Is use of essential oils medically dangerous? Not likely. However, there needs to be an accurate diagnosis made before treatment with any method. To not treat a serious illness with a known beneficial treatment method presents a danger, especially when we seek out medically untrained to give us care. The most danger of all, however, is the participation in a proclaimed healing technique that has its roots in the Eastern dogma of reality. This association over time blurs our concept of origins and the mind

---

[38] *Ibid.*
[39] *Ibid.*, p. 80.
[40] *Ibid.*, p. 79.
[41] *Ibid.*, p. 89.
[42] *Ibid.*, p. 93.
[43] *Ibid.*, p. 19.
[44] *Ibid.*, p. 51.
[45] *Ibid.*, p. 74.

more easily accepts the explanations given for healing by Eastern thought. We get caught in the web of false theory and give Satan homage and think we are honoring the Creator God. I believe it leads us into Satan's trap.

Also the chemicals shown to have biological beneficial effects in animal and man as outlined in the book can be found in a variety of foods. It is not necessary to extract them by distillation to have access to such; they are referred to as *phytochemicals*.

I close this chapter with a short quote from David Stewart and then you decide if use of essential oils is biblical:

> Oil molecules are both receivers and transmitters of thought. They can receive and respond to our thoughts and, in turn, broadcast messages back to us and to our bodies. In fact, the best way to learn about essential oils is to talk to them and let them teach you as you use them. Sleep with them and pray with them and they will reveal their secrets to you.[46]

---

[46] Stewart, op. cit., *Chemistry of Essential Oils*, p. 733.

14

CRYSTAL HEALING, TALISMANS, AMULETS

God added luster to His creation when he made thousands of different types of precious stones and gems. Even before the creation of this world, the Bible tells of God's creation of decorative stone:

> You were in Eden, the Garden of God: Every precious stone was thy covering: the sardius, topaz, and diamond, beryl, onyx, and jasper, Sapphire, turquoise and emerald, with gold. The workmanship of your timbrels and pipes was prepared for you on the day that you were created. (Ezekiel 28:13, 14)

At the time of Exodus from Egypt and building of the sanctuary in the wilderness, explicit instructions were given by God concerning the garments of the high priest Aaron and his breast plate. First, two onyx stones were to have engraved on each the names of six tribes of Israel, then set in ornaments of gold, placed on an ephod worn on the shoulders. A breast plate was crafted with twelve gemstones, four rows of three stones:

Row 1: sardius, topaz, carbuncle
Row 2: emerald, sapphire, diamond
Row 3: ligure, agate, amethyst
Row 4: beryl, onyx, jasper

On each stone was engraved the name of a tribe.

The names of gemstones were often used to emphasize a description of some scene or event. Job spoke of precious stones to make scripture the emphasis between material and spiritual riches:

> It cannot be valued in the gold of Ophir, in precious onyx, or sapphire. Neither gold or crystal can equal it. Nor can it be exchanged for jewelry of fine gold. No mention shall be made of coral or quartz, for the price of wisdom is above rubies. The topaz of Ethiopia cannot equal it. Nor can it be valued in pure gold. (Job 28:16–19)

The prophets Ezekiel and John were both shown scenes in heaven and the throne of God, with the names of precious stones used in their descriptions of it.

> And I looked and, behold, a whirlwind was coming out of the north, a great cloud with raging fire engulfing itself; and brightness was all around it and radiating out of its midst like the color of amber, out of the midst of the fire. . . . The Appearance of the wheels and their workings was like the color of beryl, . . . the likeness of the firmament above the heads of the living creature was like the color of an awesome crystal, stretched out over their heads. (Ezek. 1:4, 16, 22)

The Apostle John's vision of the New Jerusalem coming down from heaven to earth also described a variety of gemstones:

> Having the glory of God: and her light was like unto a stone most precious, even like a jasper stone, clear as crystal; . . . And the building of the wall of it was of jasper: and the city was pure gold, like unto clear glass. And the foundations of the wall of the city were garnished with all manner of precious stones. The first foundation was jasper; the second, sapphire; the third, a chalcedony; the fourth an emerald; The fifth, sardonyx; the sixth sardius; the seventh, chrysolite; the eighth, beryl; the ninth, topaz; the tenth a chrysoprasus; the eleventh, a jacinth; the twelfth an amethyst. And the twelve gates were twelve pearls: every several gate was of one pearl: and the street of the city was pure gold, as it were transparent glass. (Rev. 21:11, 18, 19, 20 KJV)

God truly loves beauty in all His creation. His adversary, the devil, takes God's creative beauty of gemstones and applies it to his use in deceiving mankind. Let us now turn our attention to a masterful deception in health and healing by Satan in crystals and gemstones.

Simon Lilly, in *The Complete Illustrated Guide to Crystal Healing* (p. 190), states that the oldest written recordings of the use of precious stones for healing come from a variety of writings recorded in India. Their use was closely associated with beliefs and practices of astrology. Gemstones were believed to absorb and transmit energy radiating from the planets and to facilitate balancing of negative and positive energy in man. If the position of the planets were not satisfactory according to a person's birth chart, then crystals and gems were supposed to be able to improve the relationship of energies coming from the planets to man. The teachings from India spread across the world and left their influence in most civilizations.

Even civilizations that had little contact with, or influence from, India or other advanced civilizations developed some type of use of precious stones in the practice of health and healing. This concept is clear when one reads the history of shamans, medicine men of the Americas, witch doctors of Africa, native healers of Australia, and elsewhere. Michael Harner, present-day shaman and instructor of shamans, shares with us some of the history of shaman use of crystals and gemstones. In his book *The Way of the Shaman*, he quotes Jerome Myer Levi:

> The wide spread employment of quartz crystals in shamanism spans thousands of years. In California, for example, quartz crystals have been found in archaeological sites and prehistoric burials dating as far back as 8000 years.[1]

Harner summarizes this history of the shaman's use and belief in crystals with the following statement:

> Western science has obviously advanced to the point that it recognizes the quartz crystal as a power object, something the shamans have known for thousands of years.[2]

---

[1] Levi, Jerome Meyer, "*Wii'ipay*: The Living Rocks—Ethnographic Notes on Crystal Magic among Some California Yumans." *Journal of California Anthropology* 5 (1): (1978), p. 42. Reported in Harner, Michael, *The Way of the Shaman*, Harper Collins Publishers, New York, NY, (1990), p. 109.

[2] Harner, Michael, *The Way of the Shaman*, HarperCollins Publishers, New York, NY, (1990), p. 112.

Alternative & Mystical Healing Therapies

Stone has been an integral part of man's history—in building structures, in use as tools, in ornamentation, and in healing through shaman (witch doctors). Quartz crystal is the favored stone for healing by a shaman. The shaman is closely connected to the spirit world and its gods. In Australia and Southeast Asia, the supreme god is Baiame, the power believed to be behind healers and magicians who use quartz crystals. The indigenous people of Australia associate quartz crystals with the Rainbow Serpent, a fertility god.

> Here are the associations with rainbows, water, rain, clouds, and heaven that link to quartz as belonging to the upper world of the *spirits* and ancestors.[3]

The quartz crystal is considered by the shaman as solidified light. To be initiated into the shaman's domain, it is necessary to be filled with solidified light of quartz. The apprentices will have quartz crystals put into their bodies by rubbing ground quartz into their skin and will drink water in which crystals have been placed, ostensibly enabling them to see *spirits*. The initiate is taken to a grave where the dead come and give him magical stones. Afterward, a snake appears as an ally and ushers him deep into the earth where he meets more snakes. From there, he goes to the supreme being (Baiame) and receives crystals for his own healing.

In Malaysia shamans believe that spirits in the air cut quartz crystals out of the sky in order to use them in healing. Similar stories of crystals and spirits are common with the ancient healing practices. North American natives were closely allied with quartz crystals for healing and higher spiritual power. The crystals are kept in leather pouches and consulted frequently by the shaman in order to better understand and work with the world of spirits. Rattles used in dance and healing ceremonies to summon helpful spirits are often filled with pieces of quartz.

In the Southwestern United States, Indian tribes valued turquoise as a stone possessing power. In Central America as well, the turquoise stones were thought to connect heaven and earth to give protection and strength via the *spirit* world. The various natives of the world all had their witch doctors; *shaman* is a name coming from the witch doctors of Siberia.

Crystal and gemstone healing has the longest history in the Ayurvedic system of healing. The explanation for their power and healing is tied in with astrology, as is all of Ayurveda. Health is maintained as the body

---

[3] Lilly, Simon, *The Complete Illustrated Guide to Crystal Healing*, Element Books Inc., Boston, MA, (2000), p. 184.

remains in balance with its energies' three divisions or doshas: pitta, vata, and kapha (similar to yin and yang). Imbalance equals illness, and powdered gemstones given in water mixed with honey or cream are prescribed to balance doshas.[4]

The shaman of all cultures treated their crystal with special reverence by keeping it in a special container separate from the other objects in his medicine bag. He avoided talking about it lest it lose power. The crystal was viewed as a "spirit helper," and a special partnership might be entered between the shaman and his crystal; it was considered as "living," or a "live stone." The Yuman tribe shamans of California felt they must feed their crystals, hence the placement in tobacco water.[5]

In the last thirty-five years, we have seen a public explosion of practices and beliefs that were for centuries kept in the quiet. Neo-paganism/Western occultism has ushered into our midst the nature worship of ancient paganism from the pagan societies of the East, African animism, and American Native practices under the title of "holistic medicine." Harner expresses it this way:

> The burgeoning field of holistic medicine shows a tremendous amount of experimentation involving the reinvention of many techniques long practiced in shamanism, such as visualization, altered state of consciousness, aspects of psychoanalysis, hypnotherapy, meditation, positive attitude, stress-reduction, and mental and emotional expression of personal will for health and healing. In a sense, shamanism is being reinvented in the West precisely because it is needed.[6]

Crystal work is a component of both ancient and modern shamanism. In Native American healing, the shaman will utilize the crystal as a method for both diagnosis and treatment; the crystal is believed to be a vehicle through which the healing spirits work.[7]

What is so special about crystal that has brought it so much attention? First, let us look at its chemical and physical properties. Nearly all the rocks on the crust of the earth are crystalline with most being formed of oxygen and silicon. Aluminum, iron, calcium, sodium, potassium, and magnesium combined with oxygen comprise the rest. Every crystal consists of a single

---

[4] *Ibid.*, pp. 184–191.

[5] Harner, op. cit. p. 109.

[6] *Ibid.*, p. 136.

[7] *Ibid.*, pp. 108–112.

chemical molecular compound; one molecule is repeated throughout, forming a geometric internal structure. A crystal is defined by its internal structure. It is made up of atoms that have bonded together, creating molecules forming regular repeating patterns. These patterns, arranged in precise geometry, create a crystal's solid form with flat faces. The internal repeating molecule forms a crystal lattice. A lattice would be similar to stacking boxes of the same size and shape in the exact same position in relationship to all other boxes, and so filling a room or warehouse.

When electricity is delivered to a crystal, it expands in regular pulses. A quartz crystal, when compressed, will emit a measureable voltage, called the piezoelectric effect. Crystals are used in most electric instruments. For example, watches are dependent on crystals for their accurate timing. A crystal's internal geometric form determines its physical properties and supposedly "its healing."

Seven geometric forms of lattices are found among crystal formations: cubic, tetragonal, hexagonal, trigonal, orthorhombic, monoclinic, and triclinic. This would be analogous to having seven shapes of boxes, with each group of shaped boxes filling a separate room and stacked in a repetitive manner, leaving no free space. It is this internal *lattice* formation that determines the type of crystal and its physical properties.

When a quartz crystal lattice is distorted by heat, pressure, light, or friction, electrons flow, creating electricity. Electricity delivered to a quartz crystal creates expansion of the crystal in regular pulses. This physical property makes it possible with a perfect crystal to create timepieces that are exactly accurate. Thus, most watches today have a quartz crystal with a battery connected to it, causing impulses in absolute regularity, enabling the watch to show time.

Crystals have many properties. One is the ability to transform and transmit light. Glass fiber optics (crystals) transmit communication by light. Small quartz crystals have the ability to possess vast amounts of memory. The first laser was formed by using a ruby gemstone. Light usually diffuse in nature was concentrated on the ruby, which then emitted a single beam of light, carrying intense energy. Most electrical kitchen appliances will have a crystal involved in their functions. Solar cells are dependent upon crystals. The electronic industry also is dependent upon crystals for the function of computers and similar instruments. The understanding and ability to manufacture perfect crystal has revolutionized our electronics world.

I have mentioned only a little of the understanding of crystal formation and the physics involved; we now turn to the subject of the use of gems and crystals for healing. Shaman and similar healers did not have the knowledge of a crystal's physical properties as we have now; however, they did believe that precious stones had the ability to transmit, transform, and amplify energy. They believed that a *"universal energy" "life force,"* underlying the powers of the universe, was transmitted by the planets to earth. This life force power was accepted as that which replenished, transformed, and renewed all things in the universe. The so-called universal energy is described as being composed of a light layer and a dense layer. The dense layer transformed itself into material substance, encompassing all material things of the universe, including earth and all life on earth. The lighter forms of the *universal life force* formed the elements of the spirit world.[8] Author Henry Mason explains further:

> So, the universe is energy. That energy is the universe, and the source of everything manifested in our universe: the stars, our sun in particular, our planet, our lives, and our selves. We are part and parcel of the universe. We are dense, self-aware energy beings. We are part of the Universal Life Force, and we live on a planet that is a part of the Universal Life Force. We came from the same place. We are made of the same elements, coalesced from the same energy.[9]

You may have noticed that no mention of a Creator God is made in this description of the universe. Satan's counterfeit story of creation is what is depicted above. God's power of creation and of sustaining creation is "hijacked" and the personality of the Creator is taken out. The power is divided into spiritual and material, and again divided into positive and negative energy. As explained in a previous chapter, it is also divided into seven different electromagnetic frequencies. The first level, the slowest frequency, is said to be the material physical substance of the universe: planets, earth, man. The remaining six increasing levels of energy frequency comprise the spiritual division of the so-called universal energy. Richard Gerber, MD, in his book *Vibrational Medicine*, makes the following comment about the proclaimed higher levels of energy:

> To most individuals, the higher dimensional energies are in the realm of invisibility. To a fortunate few with *clairvoyant* perception, the beauty of these invisible realms can be perceived

---

[8] Mason, Henry M., *The Seven Secrets of Crystal Talismans*, Llewellyn Worldwide, St. Paul, MN, p. 11

[9] Ibid.

with great ease. The only thing that seems to limit human potential is its definition of itself. As technology makes visible what was previously seen only by clairvoyants, the invisible becomes visible.[10]

The false creation story continues: life force energy comes to earth from three sources, namely, the sun, the moon from its reflection of the sun, and the perceived molten mass from the center of the earth. The claim is made that this is pure science and not religion. I disagree; it is religion from ancient Babylon. Author Henry Mason continues:

> In a like manner, the sun projects tremendous spiritual energy to the earth. Virtually all cultures with recorded history have a sun god or goddess or the equivalent that embodied their understanding of that *spiritual strength and power*. He is Tonatiuh to the Aztecs, Horus to the ancient Egyptians, Apollo to the Romans, Tsohanoai to the Navaho, and Freyr to some Norse. She is Sol in Norse mythology, and Sunna to the Germans. But whatever the name and whatever the culture, we instinctively understand the sun as the source of *spiritual* strength.
>
> Like the sun, the moon is also a source of spiritual strength to Earth. The moon has been worshiped, like the sun, since recorded time. While in some cultures the moon was a god, in many it takes the feminine form. For example, to the Chinese she is Shin Moo, to the Celts she is Morgana. Again, different names in different cultures, but a universal recognition that the moon is a power in the affairs of men and women, and one that should be respected and honored.[11]
>
> The earth also absorbs the Universal Life Force from the sun and moon, uses it, and transmits it to the wind, the waves, and the life-giving atmosphere we need. In a like manner, it absorbs the spiritual energy of the Universal Life Force from the sun and moon, uses it to nourish itself, and transmits that *spiritual*

---

[10] Gerber, Richard, *Vibrational Medicine the Number One Hand Book Subtle Energy* Therapies, Bear and Company, One Park Street, Rochester, Vermont, (2001), p. 325.

[11] Mason, op. cit., pp. 12, 13.

energy through its elements and compounds into the plants and animals that absorb it to sustain life."[12]

The apostle Paul discusses this subject of worshiping the created instead of the Creator:

> The wrath of God is being revealed from heaven against all the godlessness and wickedness of men who suppress the truth by their wickedness, since what may be known about God is plain to them, because God has made it plain to them. For since the creation of the world God's invisible qualities—his eternal power and divine nature—have been clearly seen, being understood from what has been made, so that men are without excuse. For although they claimed to be wise, they became fools and exchanged the glory of the immortal God for images made to look like mortal man and birds and animals and reptiles." (Rom. 1:18–23 KJV)

A *Talisman* can be a *gemstone*, a *crystal* worn about the body in the belief that this object can aid us in our life; it is considered to act as a charm. This "aid" comes from the stone, supposedly, by amplifying our own powers, by focusing our feelings, thoughts, actions, and habits, thus benefitting us in reaching our goals. Secondly, it is taught that a talisman is a source of energy and power in and of itself due to its mineral nature and its ability to amplify our own power by channeling in more universal life force from the *sun*, *moon*, and *earth*. The mineral crystals have seven fundamental structural arrangements in their molecular lattice, and each type will have a specific type of influence on a person. Example: a triclinic crystal system produces a talisman that is believed to have *barrier* properties. A barrier talisman supposedly is protective against illness and injury. The monoclinic crystal system is considered to produce a talisman that is *protective* physically and spiritually. It then is called an amulet.

Not only the molecular structure and lattice type, but the color and even the shape of the gem are considered to influence its effect. Talismans and amulets are used to maintain the optimum function of the physical and spiritual attributes of man.

We now turn to the use of crystals in illness and disease. The discipline of crystal healing is totally dependent upon the hypothesis of *universal energy* and its believed negative and positive characteristics. This teaching

---

[12] *Ibid.*, p. 13.

is out of *astrology*. Subtle energy system concepts, such as electrical polarity, meridians, pressure points, chakras, aura, and subtle bodies, are used to assess and correct what are perceived as energy imbalances.

Crystal healers view the human body in totally different ways than orthodox scientists and doctors. Completely different languages and terms are used respectively in each system.[13]

A most important aspect of crystal healing is for the healer to be *grounded* and *centered* prior a healing session.

Grounding means total focus. All energy believed to be passing through the body will remain in balance, but if any excess energy flows, it will *go into the earth* where it is safely dissipated. Grounding is accomplished by the use of gems, usually dark colored; the best place to set them is near the throat and coccyx. Grounding can be done by Hindu-type meditation, guided imagery, and visualization (using the imagination to create a view of the change desired) and by tree meditation (visualizing a tree and its roots with the tree representing the healer and the roots the "ground" connection with mother earth).

Centering happens when all physical, mental, and emotional energies are integrated and balanced. Centering can be done by imagery and visualization such as drawing the *earth energy* up through your body by deep breathing focus, sight focus, or voice focus, or by sounding "om" or "aum," or by "tapping in." Tapping in is done by tapping lightly with the fingertips on the chest below the clavicle on either side. It is said to bring into balance all the *meridians* of the body (meridians are energy flow channels of Chinese traditional medicine and not recognized to exist by science).[14]

When grounded and centered, the healer will then proceed to the therapeutic act of using the crystals and gemstones. The following are examples of ways that the healing sessions are to be conducted. By these descriptions, we recognize the absurdity of crystal therapy and spiritually dangerous to partake of the practices.

- Place stones in positions upon or about the body, where disease or distress is felt to be present, in arrangement so as to depict the Seal of Solomon or Star of David, thus symbolizing a connection between heaven and earth.
- To recharge your body and spirit, do the following: place a crystal over a pulse point such as the wrist; when done in the sunlight, it will supposedly increase the therapeutic benefit.

---

[13] Lilly, op. cit., p. 34.

[14] *Ibid.*, pp 45–47.

- Healing by use of crystals and breathing techniques could be as follows: Inhale to bring energy into your aura; hold your breath several seconds as you focus your thoughts on the crystal held in your hand. With a forceful effort, expel your breath out, thus causing the energy within the crystal to be expelled through the top of the crystal as it is pointed toward the area of the body in need of healing. This effort must be repeated several times to be effective.
- One technique for self-healing is as follows: place a crystal over a *chakra* area of the body. While inhaling, place both hands on top of the stone being used and draw energy through it into the chakra. Hold the breath for 5–6 seconds, concentrating energy in that location, then exhale forcefully while throwing your hands out to each side of your body, thus dispersing negative energy. As you inhale bring the hands back to the same location on the body, then repeat.[15]

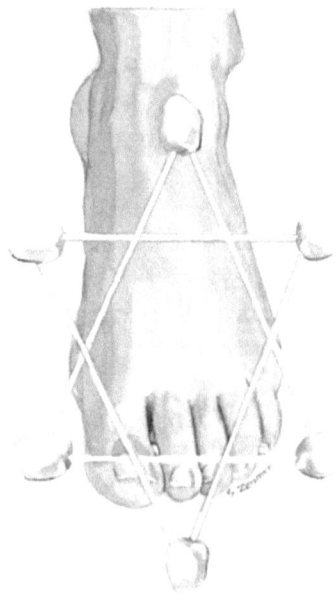

Figure 34. Crystals in formation of Solomon's Seal

---

[15] *Ibid.*, pp. 52, 53.

Water is believed by crystal healers to be able to hold a memory of an energy pattern of some object placed within it. The following practices are based upon this concept. Take a crystal and grind it into a very fine powder, place in a bowl of spring water for several hours, transfer the water into a dark glass jar, and refrigerate. Or one may place the ground stone in a bowl of tap water and expose it to sunlight for several hours; this creates an "*essence*" of sun energy, universal energy. Next, withdraw the water from the bowl and place it into a jar with 50 percent brandy; this becomes a "mother tincture." In turn, place a few drops of the mother tincture into another small bottle of 50 percent brandy. It is then ready to be consumed by drops as a medicinal, or placed in bathwater, in steam inhalation, etc. Both solutions of regular spring water or the essence water can be used similarly.

The particular crystal that is selected for therapy may be chosen not only because of its lattice structure but also because of its color. The color of the gem is contingent upon the crystal formation and its atomic structure, which, in turn, bends the rays of sunlight. Some colors depend upon the basic mineral while others are colored by impurities. When all colors are absorbed in the stone, it is then black; when all light is reflected, the stone is white.

Different colors are believed, by crystal healers, to affect different aspects of health. Each color represents a specific wavelength of light and may be referred to as "vibration" of energy, of creativity, of balance, etc. Different colors are said to affect the body in different ways. Examples: *orange* is supposed to influence physical rigidity, restricted feelings, digestive disorders, lack of focus, lack of vitality, inability to let go of past memories, etc.; green is equated with abnormal growths, sense of claustrophobia, being trapped, unfulfilled, restricted, dominated, a need to be in control or to be controlled, invasive illness, etc.

Problems occurred in the past because of the use of ground gems, as not all gems are safe. Minerals have been used since ancient times as source of colored pigments. Their colors do not fade because of sunlight but may change with extensive time because of oxidation. Some of these colored pigments are toxic and are no longer used. Red was from mercuric oxide and arsenic oxide—toxic. Orange is also from toxic minerals, yellow from arsenic and sulfur, etc.

Another practice in crystal healing involves "*chakra balancing.*" The Indian Ayurveda system of healing believes that there is a network of subtle energy channels that run through the body. This network is said to be composed of a central channel along the spine and which is made up of seven centers of energy called chakras. The seven chakras are proclaimed to be linked to the

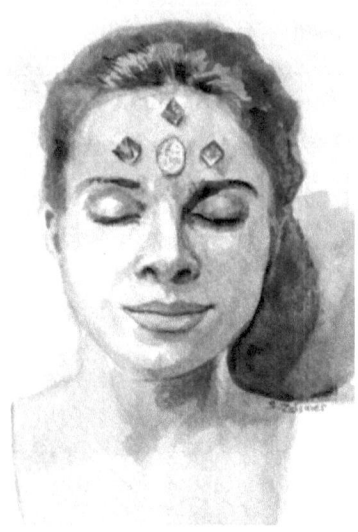

Figure 35. Crystals on forehead chakra

seven colors of the rainbow, with each chakra being of one of the seven colors. The chakra system is also believed to be influenced by a set of associated symbols, sound, color, shape, animal and god forms, as well as the senses.

The goal of chakra crystal balancing and healing is to empower each chakra to its optimal function as well as to the system as a whole. The most fundamental chakra balancing act is Hindu-type mediation, but the crystal healer supplements that act with use of his crystals. Choice of crystals for healing is determined by the problems the individual may have, or it may be just to maintain health. Once the chakra felt to be most associated with a health situation is determined, then it is necessary to select more specifically the optimum crystal needed to place over the chakra as therapy. Selection of a color and mineral type of stone to match the chakra is done by visualization, intuition (divine inspiration), applied kinesiology (divination by muscle testing), color meditation by visualization, or dowsing with a pendulum.

WAND HEALING

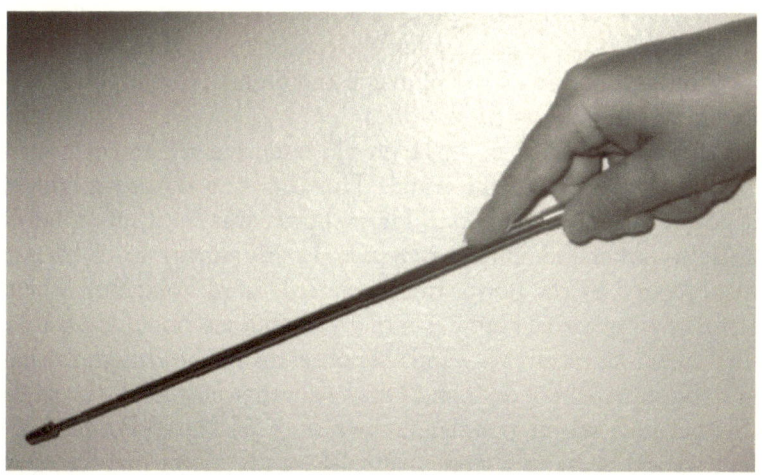

Figure 36. Wand

Wand is a word that we do not often hear in the health and healing arena, yet it is still being used and promoted as if it was of great value. At a large religious assembly in June 2010, I was sitting at a table, signing copies of the book *Spiritualistic Deceptions of Health and Healing*. The book exposes spiritualism in certain health and healing methods. I was approached by an individual who with enthusiasm presented to me his healing *wand* as an instrument that would remove pain by use of *life force energy*. A wand is an object usually a thin rod or stick ranging from a few inches in length to several feet long. A dictionary definition explains it as a "staff of a diviner, a fairy, or a magician."

This wand I was shown was the size of a ballpoint pen, platinum in color, and was said to be filled with crystals. Its magic was promoted as a "reliever of pain." Point it at pain anywhere on the body, and the pain was said to vanish. I asked if it worked on chronic low back pain; the answer was slow in coming, but the advocate of the wand had to admit defeat for this malady yet was claiming great success for headaches, small joint pains, soreness, and minor discomforts. This person was truly sincere in his belief of the wand; in fact, he was a distributor of such. He shared with me that some members of his church were concerned about his use of this healing wand therapy and had even suggested to him that he might be partaking of occultic power. He told me this in a manner and tone that led me to believe that he felt those who had warned him about the wand really did not understand the value and true scientific power he felt was truly within his wand.

A dictionary definition explains a wand as a "staff of a diviner, a fairy, or a magician." It has been a tool of the magician for thousands of years; its use is often found in stories of magic and fantasy. Great power is often attributed to the wand in these stories.

In the popular Harry Potter novel, extensive references are found pertaining to the use of the wand. Through it, a wizard might effect great power for good or for evil. Harry Potter was born into a family of wizards; his father and mother were such. In this fantasy novel, his parents were obliterated by the power from a wizard, Lord Voldemort, the most powerful of all wizards. Harry eventually attends a school for wizards and witches where he receives a wand. He observes his headmaster using his wand to blast through a door and knocks another powerful wizard flat.

In the most recent popular fantasy story of Harry Potter, he, as a student wizard, goes to a store that sells wands. After inspecting many different ones for size and feel, he chooses the one best for him. As he raises this wand in the air and quickly presses the tip toward the floor, sparks and light flash from the distal end of the wand, and Harry receives a feeling of exhilaration.

There is a claim made by some that the use of the wand is biblical! How can anyone make that claim? There is the story of Moses and Aaron using their shepherd staffs as a magic wand and with great power. The story starts in the fourth chapter of Exodus as Moses was talking to God at the burning bush. God told him He would give to Moses **a sign** he could use to impress Pharaoh that he, Moses, was sent to Pharaoh by the God of the Hebrews. At the bush encounter in the desert in Mount Horeb/Sinai, God told Moses to cast his staff to the ground; it became a moving snake, and Moses ran from it. He was told by God to pick it up by the tail, and it became a staff again.

The story continues as Aaron cast down his staff at the feet of Pharaoh, and it became a snake. Pharaoh's magicians were able to do the same, but Aaron's rod—snake—swallowed up the magicians' snakes.

The staff of Aaron was used to bring on several of the ten plagues that God placed upon the Egyptians so they would understand that the God of the Hebrews was the God of the universe. Aaron's staff was used to strike the Nile River to turn it to blood, stretched over the river to cause it to bring forth frogs, and struck on the ground and covered the nation with gnats. Moses stretched out his rod to bring on the plague of locusts, pointed it skyward causing a great hailstorm, and used it to bring darkness over the land. When Moses came to the Red Sea and Pharaoh was behind them with his army, Moses stretched his staff over the sea, and it parted (Ex. 14:16). After crossing to the other side, Moses held up his staff and pointed toward the passageway between the walls of water, and God allowed the water to come together, covering the Egyptians. As they journeyed in the dry desert and water had vanished, God directed Moses to strike a rock with his staff. The rock split open, and water gushed out (Ex. 17:6).

At a later time, when Israel was traveling in the desert and water was not obtainable, God asked Moses to speak to a rock to cause it to give forth water (Num. 20:10–12). But Moses in his anger with the people for their complaining said, "Hear now ye rebels; must **we** fetch you water out of this rock?" Moses struck the rock two times with his rod, and the rock gave forth water in abundance.

> Then the Lord spoke unto Moses and Aaron, "Because you did not believe Me, to hallow Me in the eyes of the children of Israel, therefore ye shall not bring this congregation into the land which I have given them." (vs. 12)

The rock from which flowed water at Mt. Horeb and the water that flowed from the rock as they journeyed represented the living water of grace which flows from Christ, the Son of God. When Moses was told to speak to the rock, it represented our privilege to ask of God for the water of life, to be given in abundance. Moses assumed that *he and Aaron* had the power to bring forth the water with his staff. For this error, he and Aaron were not permitted to enter Canaan. It was God directing Moses and through the use of his staff that God's power was made manifest; there was no innate power from Moses or the staff.

When a person takes up the *magic wand*, he is assuming he has power within himself to project power through the rod to accomplish some feat. There might be some response, but if so, it is not power of one's own self; it is the power of Satan working through the person and the wand.

Divination is a common component of crystal work and healing practices. It is often done by the use of a crystal pendulum or may be done by muscle testing called applied kinesiology. Healing may be performed using a pendulum made of crystal.

Geomancy, an ancient practice of "casting stones" then reading the resulting patterns as the stones came to rest, was practiced in many civilizations on many continents. The stone may be cast on a cloth with areas of the cloth demarcated to mean certain things and the stones also pre-chosen to represent various meanings. As the stones come to rest, the diviner will interpret the fall of the stones.[16]

Scrying is crystal ball gazing. It is a way to access the unconscious, or subconscious, mind.

> A crystal, or some other polished surface, is used to amplify or act as a screen for knowledge held in symbolic form within the mind." "The mind dives down into itself, leaving the familiar clear coordinates of time and space experienced as an individual wave, and centers the deep ocean of consciousness where collective and universal currents are to be found.[16]

The warning God gave the nation of Israel just before they were to enter the Promised Land, as recorded in Deuteronomy 18:9–12, should be a warning to us as well and help us choose to have nothing to do with crystal healing or any aspect of the crystal, gemstone, precious stone false premise.

> When you are come into the land which the Lord your God is giving you, you shall not learn to follow the abomination of those nations. There shall not be found among you any one that makes his son or his daughter to pass through the fire, or one that practices witchcraft (divination), or a soothsayer, or one who interprets omens, or a sorcerer, or one who conjures spells, or a medium, or a spiritist, or one who calls up the dead. For all who do these things are an abomination unto the Lord: and because of these abominations the Lord thy God drives them out from before you. (Deut. 18:9–12)

Absent healing with crystals is done, with permission, for those who may be long distances from the healer. This permission can be obtained by dowsing, intuition, or meditation if the individual has not previously given permission. A "witness" will be used—that is, a picture or lock of hair, a signature, drop of blood, or something the person has handled. The "witness" is said to carry the energy pattern of the individual desiring healing.

The Complete Illustrated Guide to Crystal Healing tells us no one understands how long-distance healing works but that it works. As with all crystal healing acts, it is important to have been "grounded" and "centered" (in a meditative state) before attempting the art of distant healing using a pendulum over the "witness." Also, simply placing chosen gems on a mirror that lies next to a "witness" may work.

---

[16] *Ibid.*, p. 176.

Alternative & Mystical Healing Therapies

Belief in *astrology* and its signs and symbols is very popular. Ancient Indian healing tradition, Ayurveda, developed a complex system of the relationship of the planets to stones and their use in health and healing. Today Eastern and Western theories of astrological crystal relationships have merged so that there are stones for each month, each planet, and each zodiac sign. Wearing of copper is believed to reduce the effects of planetary forces on health. Dowsing for a stone to use in dealing with astrological influences is also a common practice.

The quartz crystal has entered the mind—control field of therapy as well. Marcel Vogel, senior scientist with IBM for twenty-seven years, concludes that the natural energies of a healer can be amplified and directed to heal another's mind problems. His quote is below:

> The crystal is a neutral object whose inner structure exhibits a state of perfection and balance. When it's cut to the proper form and perfection, the crystal emits a vibration which extends and amplifies the powers of the user's mind. Like a laser, it radiates energy in a coherent, highly concentrated form, and this energy may be transmitted into objects or people at will.
>
> Although the crystal may be used for "mind to mind" communication, its higher purpose . . . is in the service of humanity for the removal of pain and suffering. With proper training, a healer can release negative thought forms which have taken shape as disease patterns in a patient's physical body.
>
> As psychics have often pointed out, when a person becomes emotionally distressed, a weakness forms in his subtle energy body and disease may soon follow. With a properly cut crystal, however, a healer can, like a surgeon cutting away a tumor, release negative patterns in the energy body, allowing the physical body to return to a state of wholeness.[17]

John Ankerberg and John Weldon present an in-depth discussion of the use of crystals in their book *Can You Trust Your Doctor?* Therein, we learn that the real power from crystals is derived from the spirit world and many who become involved in crystals for health move on to channeling

---

[17] Miller, R., *The Science of the Mind*, The Healing Magic of Crystals: an Interview with Marcel Vogel, August 1984: Reported in Gerber, op. cit., pp. 338, 9.

with spirit guides. Crystal healers claim that the crystals are mere devices for attracting the spirits, who then supply the real power. Even when the crystals are not used, the occult power remains.[18]

> According to the nature of the illness, the crystal will become hot or cold as it is passed over the person's aura. The crystal is absorbing the bad energy out of the body, according to these teachings. It is important to remember that "the crystals are your teachers. Hold one in your hand. Be open to its power. It will teach you."[19]

Is there danger in consulting cultist physicians? Isaiah 8:19–20 makes it very plain:

> And when they shall say unto you, "Seek those who are mediums, and wizards (diviners) who whisper and mutter," should not a people seek their God? Should they seek the dead on behalf of the living?" To the law and to the testimony! If they do not speak according to this word, it is because there is not light in them.

This system of deception that Satan has devised starts very innocently. When our interest is developed, we are led on to more involved practices. This, in turn, can lead to developing psychic powers and communicating with spirit entities, animal entities, etc. This *channeling* allows for demonic possession of our minds and souls. The end result is loss of eternal life. Clearly, the whole practice of crystal healing and crystal divination is a form of "spiritualism."

---

[18] Ankeberg, John, Weldon, John, *Can You Trust Your Doctor?*, Wolgemuth and Hyatt, Brentwood, TN, (1991), p. 243, 249.

[19] Newhouse, Sandy, Amoeda, John, *Native American Healing*, [Holistic Health Handbook, "A Tool for Attaining Wholeness of Body, Mind and Spirit" Berkeley California Press, Berkeley, CA, (1978), p. 67. Reported in Gerber, op. cit., p. 243.

15

HOMEOPATHY

SAMUEL HAHNEMANN MD

Samuel Hahnemann MD (1755–1843) was a German physician who was appalled at the results of conventional medical care and refused to prescribe the drugs and bleeding treatments used by physicians of his day.

> Hahnemann attacked the extreme medical practices of the day, advocating instead, good public hygiene, improved housing conditions, better nutrition, fresh air, and exercise.[1]

He believed that if a healthy person was given enough of a substance to produce symptoms similar to the symptoms of a particular illness, then by diluting that substance to minute doses and ingesting, the body would be stimulated to heal itself of the illness. This "presumed" phenomenon he called *homeopathy*.

Homeopathy is a discipline of therapy for illness that Hahnemann initiated and which subsequently became popular in his day. The use of this therapy has continued ever since. It is a method of treatment utilizing an extremely diluted preparation of a "mother tincture" of a plant, mineral, or animal substance. It began in Germany and spread throughout Europe, being brought to the United States in the early 1800s.

---

[1] Lockie, Andrew, MB, ChB, MRCGP, MF Hom. Dip obst RCOG, *Natural Health Encyclopedia of Homeopathy*, Dorling Kindersley, London, New York, 2000), p. 14

It became very popular and was commonly practiced until the ascendancy of scientific medicine. After the turn of the century and in the early part of the twentieth century, there were twenty-two medical schools following this type of discipline in the United States. There were more than one hundred hospitals and over one thousand pharmacies devoted to homeopathic medicine.[2] It was commonly practiced in the United States since people were able to purchase a home kit of homeopathy remedies and treat themselves. I have in my library a home medical text dated 1918, which has instructions and guidelines for homeopathy treatments for home use. However, by the mid-1900s, the use of homeopathy had almost died out in the United States. Yet in the last forty years, there has been a rapid resurgence of the practice among various practitioners.

Hahnemann once took a large dose of Peruvian bark (quinine) while he was healthy and said that he developed symptoms similar to malaria. He thereafter initiated a theory that if very small doses of quinine were administered, standard doses would not be necessary for treatment of malaria. To understand how Hahnemann arrived at this conclusion, we need to understand his concept of disease.

In his text *Organon*, paragraph 11, he defines the bodily condition we call disease. First, he states that all disease manifests *subjective* and *objective* symptoms. This situation, in turn, is caused by *vital energy* being in an "untuned spirit-like *dynamis*"—unbalanced universal energy status. He reasoned that if disease was a result of spirit-like energy being "out of tune," then it could only be corrected by "retuning" through the action of another spirit. He further reasoned that if the "spirit" of animal, plant, or mineral, when given in large doses, would create similar symptoms as the disease under consideration, then this same spirit taken in a very minute quantity would correct the unturned-unbalanced spirit causing the disease, thereby, effecting a cure.

Symptoms are the key to understanding his reasoning. When disease was present, symptoms were present. To eliminate the symptoms would, he believed, cure the malady. These correcting spirits were found by trial and error. A mineral or plant substance would be taken by a healthy individual in sufficient quantity (dose) to bring on symptoms. If those symptoms were similar to symptoms peculiar to a disease, then this substance under test would be considered the "remedy" for that particular disease. This whole concept was built upon belief in the *spirit dynamis* of vital energy—life force. Every plant, mineral, or animal was considered to have its specific spirit dynamis.

---

[2] Ankerberg, H. John, Weldon, John, *Can You Trust Your Doctor?* Wolgemuth & Hyatt, Brentwood TN., (1991), p. 264

Alternative & Mystical Healing Therapies

The cause and correction of disease was considered to be by action of "spirit." Biochemical, infectious agents, lack of or insufficient nutrients, toxic substance ingested causing biochemical interaction, etc., were not understood and had no part in the thinking of Hahnemann. Today, individuals accepting homeopathic therapy as being legitimate therapy are thinking in the terms of correcting a disorder by a biochemical adjustment or interaction; however, there is no scientific evidence to substantiate the remedying claims of homeopathic substances.

It is very important to understand Hahnemann's *world view* in order to comprehend the rationale of his conclusions regarding disease, its cause, and treatment. Understanding his belief in man's origin will help to clarify why he formed certain conclusions.

> First Hahnemann was a follower of the powerful spiritist and medium Emanuel Swedenborg. Those familiar with the occultic philosophy and theology of Swedenborg, such as his blending of the world of nature and the occult, can recognize the parallels in Hahnemann's thinking. Andrew Weil received his M.D. from Harvard Medical School, is a research associate in Ethno pharmacology at Harvard, and is somewhat sympathetic with aspects of new age medicine. He observes that Hahnemann was "steeped in the mysticism of Emanuel Swedenborg." [3]
>
> Hahnemann was also a Freemason, and as the authors have demonstrated elsewhere, the study of Freemasonry presents an excellent opportunity for delving into mysticism and the occult.[4]
>
> Hahnemann was also an admirer of the occultists Paracelsus and Mesmer.[5]

He was a believer in the concept of animal magnetism, which is the same power behind psychic healing. In his *Organon* (textbook on

---

[3] Weil, Andrew; *Health and Healing: Understanding Conventional and Alternative Medicine,* Houghton Mifflin, Boston, MA, (1983), p.14. Reported in Ankerberg, John, Weldon, John; *Can You Trust Your Doctor? p. 315*

[4] Ankerberg, John, Weldon, John; *Can you Trust Your Doctor?* Wolgemuth & Hyatt, Brentwood TN., (1991), [sold to Word] p. 316.

[5] Gumpert, Martin; *Hahnemann*: *The Adventurous Career of a Medical Rebel,* L.B. Fisher, (1945), New York, NY, p. 25. Reported in Ankerberg, John, Weldon, John; *Can You Trust Your Doctor?* P. 316

homeopathy), Hahnemann confessed similarities between the practice of homeopathy and mesmerism. He wrote:

> I find it yet necessary to allude here to animal magnetism, as it is termed, or rather Mesmerism. . . . It is a marvelous, priceless gift of God . . . by means of which the strong will of a well intentioned person upon a sick one by contact and even without this and even at some distance, can bring the vital energy of the healthy mesmerizer endowed with this power into another person dynamically. . . . The above mentioned methods of practicing Mesmerism depend upon an influx of more or less vital force into the patient.[6]

Hahnemann was also influenced by animism and Eastern religion. In discussing Hahnemann's writings and that of other leading homeopaths, Dr. H. J. Bopp, in his book *Homeopathy*, comments:

> As a matter of fact the vocabulary is esoteric and the ideas are impregnated with oriental philosophies like Hinduism. The predominant strain of pantheism would place God everywhere, in each man, each animal, plant, flower, cell, even in homoeopathic medicine.[7]

Dr. Samuel D. Pfeifer, in his book *Healing at Any Price*, mentions the influence of Eastern thinking upon Hahnemann by quoting a biographer who reveals that

> he is strongly attracted to the East. Confucius is his ideal.[8]

Dr. Pfeifer continues:

> On Confucius, Hahnemann himself writes in a letter:
>
> This is where you can read divine wisdom, without (*e.g.,* Christian) miracle–myths and superstition. I regard it as an

---

[6] Hahnemann, Samuel; *Organon of Medicine*, 6th edition, reprint, B Jain Publishing, New Delhi, India, (1978), pp. 309, 311

[7] Bopp, H.J.; *Homoeopathy*, Down, North Ireland, Word of Life Publishing, (1984), p. 9. Reported in Ankerberg, John, Weldon, John; *Can you Trust Your Doctor?* p. 317

important sign of our times that Confucius is now available for us to read. Soon I will embrace him in the kingdom of blissful spirits, the benefactor of humanity, who has shown us the straight path to wisdom and to God, already six hundred sixty years before [650 B.C.] the archenthusiast.[8,9] (*Jesus Christ, Divine Son of God*).

His reverence for Eastern thought was the fundamental philosophy behind the preparation of homoeopathic remedies. Hahnemann claimed inspiration, as seen in a letter he wrote to the town clerk of Kothen in 1828. He said he had been

guided by the invisible powers of the Almighty, listening, observing, tuning in to His instruction, paying most earnest heed and religious attention to this inspiration.[10]

Hahnemann believed in universal energy or "vital force" as some called it. He believed that the power, or effects, of his minutely diluted remedies resulted from the working of "vital force." Hahnemann's *vital force*, which is believed to *rule* the *physical body*, is similar to the soul, or the *etheric* and *astral bodies* of many occult disciplines.[11,12]

What does this mean? In the chapter on universal energy, we learned about vital force and the dividing of universal energy into seven frequencies or levels. Level one is said to be our material world and our physical bodies. The belief is that the level of energy above this first level is in a plane with "frequencies faster than light" and that the *etheric body* is an electromagnetic template of our physical body. The *astral body* is said to be an even higher level of frequency from which we can have *out-of-body* experiences and astral travel.

From the above paragraph, we understand the belief that the vital force in the remedies of homeopathy is purported to be actually influencing and treating the higher levels or bodies of energy rather than just the physical body. This is truly *mysticism*.

---

[8] Pfeifer, Samuel M.D., *Healing at Any Price*, Word Limited, Milton Keynes, England, (1988), p. 68.

[9] Bopp, op. cit., p. 3; Ankerberg, op. cit., p. 318.

[10] Pfeifer, op. Cit., pp. 68–69.

[11] *Ibid.*

[12] Kent, James Tyler, *Lectures on Homoeopathic Philosophy*; Reported in Ankerberg, op. cit., p. 326.

Because homoeopathists operate in the realm of the "invisible" and not in that of the visible and material, many of them admit to the belief that homeopathic medicines really work upon the etheric or astral bodies.

> This is where disease begins and spreads outward into the physical body presenting as *symptoms*.[13]
>
> This is why a number of occultic religions such as Hinduism and anthroposophy employ homeopathy. Its philosophy fits well with their occultic views of man and health.[14]

The power that is transmitted directly in psychic healing through the laying on of the healer's hand, or from a distance, is no different than the power to heal that occurs in the homoeopathic remedy. Homoeopathic practitioners claim that a cosmic *vital force* is transferred from the homeopathic *medicine* into the patient. But the same effect is supposedly accomplished by radionic devices (see section "Radionics" in chapter on divination), which employ spiritistic power.[15] Using these devices, it is said, makes the use of homoeopathic remedies unnecessary.

LAWS OF HOMEOPATHY

This system is built on the theory that

(1) most diseases are caused by an infectious disorder called the *psora* (itch) (see glossary);
(2) life is a spiritual force (vitalism) that directs the body's healing;
(3) remedies can be discerned by noting the symptoms that substances produce in overdose (proving) and applying them to conditions with similar symptoms in highly diluted doses (laws of similia); and

---

[13] Ankerberg, op. cit., p. 326.
[14] Weldon, John; Levitt, Zola; *Psychic Healing An Exposé of an Occult Phenomenon*, Moody Press, 1982, pp. 53–65.
[15] *Position Paper of National Council Against Health Fraud*, Feb 1994; p. 5. http://www.ncahf.org/pp/homeop.html

(4) remedies become more effective with greater dilution (law of infinitesimals) and become more potent when containers are tapped on the heel of the hand or a leather pad (potentizing).[16, 17]

Proving is a term used to describe the process used by homeopathic practitioners to select new substances for inclusion in the list of therapeutic remedies. A substance will be tested by taking it in high doses, then recording the symptoms it creates. In testing, a substance may be taken daily in high doses for as long as a month, and any type of sensation or supposed change is recorded during this time.

> Consider the alleged 'symptoms' of chamomilla as given by Hahnemann in his *Materia Medica Pura* [1846, Vol. 2, pp. 7–20]: "Vertigo ... Dull ... aching pain in the head ... Violent desire for coffee ... Grumbling and creeping in the upper teeth... Great aversion to the wind ... Burning pain in the hand ... Quarrelsome, vexatious dreams ... heat and redness of the right cheek."[18]

One author, writing about Hahnemann, said he (Hahnemann) documented thirteen pages of symptoms from taking chamomile. If such is the case when healthy people take this substance, how can we expect it to cure sick people?[19]

A very interesting comment about "proving" of the remedies is made by Ankerberg in *Can You Trust Your Doctor?* (p. 273). We are told that the remedies that are listed in the homoeopathic *Materia Medicas,* when tested or proved over the past 150 years by nonhomoeopaths, have never given the responses found by homoeopaths.

CHOOSING THE PROPER REMEDY

In a pharmacy with inventory of more than two thousand homeopathic remedies, how do I select the proper substance that is closest to my symptoms? This is the decision the homoeopathic doctor has to make

---

[16] *Ibid.,* pp. 3–4.

[17] Stalker, Douglas, Glymour, eds.; *Examining Holistic Medicine,* Buffalo, NY, Prometheus books, 1985, p. 32, Sobel, David S., ed.; *Ways of Health: Wholistic Approaches to Ancient and Contemporary Medicine,* Harcourt Brace Jovanich, New York, NY, 1979 pp. 295–297 Reported in Ankerberg, op. cit., p. 274.

[18] Ankeberg, *Can you Trust Your Doctor?,* op. cit., pp. 275–276.

[19] Bopp, op. cit., p. 5.

when prescribing for a patient. Homeopathy teaches that it is important to get the exact medicinal for the specific illness and the patient's constitution. The following procedures may be used to choose a specific substance for therapy:

1. Astrological signs or other modes of astrology may be used to determine the proper diagnosis and therapy.[20]
2. Dr. Bopp writes about the use of the pendulum in choosing the proper remedy for homeopathic treatment. Dr. A. Voegeli, a famous homoeopathic doctor, has confirmed that a very high percentage of homeopaths work with the pendulum.[21] Dr. Pfeifer also notes the use of pendulums by homeopaths because "it is easier to take a shortcut with the radionic pendulum."[22]
3. John Weldon, author of *Psychic Healing: An Exposé of an Occult Phenomenon*, reports that many homoeopaths today have spirit guides with research on homeopathy being done in séances. There are groups whose (homoeopathic) research is carried out during séances, through mediums who seek information from spirits.[23]

Dr. Bopp tells in his book *Homeopathy* about a woman who worked in a homoeopathic laboratory in France. She personally related the story of an interview she had on applying for a job in a specific homoeopath laboratory. She was asked about which astrological sign she was born under and whether or not she was a medium. She told the sign and answered yes to the question about being a medium. She was then informed that new treatments to be produced by the laboratory were researched in séances.[24]

As "conventional" doctors of the past used large doses of toxic drugs, "eclectic" physicians discontinued the use of mercury and the heavy toxic substances and tended to be better at diagnosing but prescribed small doses for every symptom. The homeopathic physician, though ridiculing conventional doctors, continued to use toxic drugs in his treatments. He simply used extremely weak dilutions. The following are examples of drugs used in homeopathy: "Nux vomica (strychnine), sulphur, lobelia (nicotine), phosphorus, ipecac, hydrochloric acid, alcohol, lead, arsenic, colchicine,

---

[20] *Ibid.*, p. 8.
[21] Pfeifer, op. cit., pp. 79–80.
[22] Ankerberg, John; Weldon, John; op. cit., pp. 328–329.
[23] Bopp, op. cit., p. 8.
[24] Marcy, E.E. and Hunt, F.W.; *The Homoeopathic Theory and Practice of Medicine*, Vol. I, pp. vii-xxxii; Reported in Hardinge op. cit., p. 82.

jalap, senna, mercury, aconite, belladonna (atropine), podophyllum, camphor, veratrum, staphysagria, opium, quinine, cantharides, croton oil, phosphoric acid, tartar emetic, iodine, and numerous other agents."[25] The solution made by repeated dilution often surpasses the point of having any molecules of the original substance left, yet the homeopathic doctor claims these extreme dilutions are the most potent of the preparations. How can this be? Let us consider the process of dilution.

When each dilution takes place, the solution is shaken vigorously by hitting the hand that holds the dilution on a hard surface so as to thump the solution. This is called succession. It is claimed that this process causes the remedy to be more *potent*. This is believed to be the critical part in preparation of the remedies. Notice the following comments by leading homeopaths Dana Ullman and Stephen Cunnings:

> Homoeopaths have found that the medicines do not work if they are simply diluted repeatedly without vigorous shaking or if they are just diluted in vast amounts of liquid. Nor do the medicines work if they are only vigorously shaken. It is the *combined* process of dilution and vigorous shaking that makes the medicine effective.[26]

How can the medicine get stronger and stronger with increasing dilution? The homeopathic practitioner says that the solution (water) receives an *imprint* or *signature* from the original substance (mother tincture), and this is passed along, thereby increasing the potency. Chemists and physicists find no scientific evidence to support this theory.[27]

There have been homoeopaths who claimed that homoeopathic remedies act similar to vaccinations, a theory that was quickly and unwisely accepted by some adherents of homeopathy. When a vaccination is administered, the immune system manufactures protective proteins and stimulates specific white blood cells to respond to the organism or allergen contained in the vaccination. A memory is created within the immune system, which allows it to respond powerfully to this specific organism or allergen should it be encountered at another time.

---

[25] Ullman, Dana; Cummings, Stephen; *The Science of Homoeopathy*, New Realities, [journal] Summer of (1985) p. 20. Reported in Ankeberg, op. cit., p. 330

[26] *NCAHF Position Paper on Homoeopathy*, (1994), http://www.ncahf.org/

[27] *Ibid.*, p. 5.

The proponents of homeopathy claim that the small homoeopathic dose will trigger an immune response. This is not true. The quantity of active ingredients in the homoeopathic remedy usually is too small to trigger an immune response. A vaccination will have far greater concentration of an organism or allergen. The response of the body from an immunization can be measured chemically. The high-dilution homeopathic remedies do not produce measurable responses. Vaccines are used as prevention, not as a cure. Homoeopathic remedies have no relationship to immunization science.

PREPARATION OF HOMEOPATHIC REMEDIES

Materials for use in remedies are finely ground or dissolved in water. They are then mixed with a solvent, and the mixture is allowed to soak. The fluid containing the original substance is then filtered or strained. The filtered solution—the *mother tincture*—is placed in a dark jar for keeping.

One drop of the mother tincture can be diluted one of two ways: using either a nine-part solvent or a ninety-nine parts solvent, and then shaken vigorously. The solution banged down firmly on a hard surface after each dilution, a process devised by Hahnemann. The "thumping" after the dilution is believed to transfer the "spirit" from the remedy substance into the solvent. Homeopathy teaches that the *essence* (spirit—remedy) can be carried by water even after all molecules of the original substance are diluted out of the solution. Once the mixture has reached the required strength and potency, a few drops of it are added to lactose tablets, pills, granules, or powder so as to impregnate the carrier with the remedy. It is then stored in dark glass bottles.

Dilutions are most often made by using one part of the mother tincture and nine parts solvent (1-X). With each additional dilution, the labeling would be 2-X, 3-X, etc. When dilutions go beyond 24-X, there may not be one molecule left of the original remedy substance in the solution. Homeopaths do not depend on molecules of the original substance to effect healing. They are looking to the *signature/energy—imprint/spirit—* of the original substance to be passed on and magnified by dilution. This signature or imprint said to be in the solution has not been scientifically demonstrated.

Given below are examples of common "remedies" as listed in *Natural Health, Encyclopedia of Homeopathy* by Dr. Andrew Lockie (2000):

Mercury: found in cinnabar ore from Spain, Italy, US, Peru, China
Rx for symptoms of:

  a. Foul smelling discharge
  b. Reserved, suspicious state of mind
  c. Insecurity
  d. Copious perspiration that does not relieve condition
  e. Person feels worse at night

Hellborus: Southern Europe—extremely poisonous
Rx for symptoms of:

  a. Mental dullness
  b. Chilliness
  c. Tendency to drop things
  d. Person feels worse between 4 pm and 8 pm

Aconite: Europe, Central Asia—deadly poisonous, handling root can cause poisoning
Rx for symptoms of:

  a. Symptoms triggered by shock or cold wind
  b. Panic attack and fear of death
  c. Acute infection with sudden onset

Nux Vomica: (strychnine) (poison nut tree) India, Burma, Thailand, China, Australia
Rx for symptoms of:

  a. Irritability
  b. Over-critical nature
  c. Tendency to be highly driven and ambitious
  d. Chilliness
  e. Desire for rich foods

Carcinosin: Cancer cells usually from breast
Rx for symptoms of:

  a. Workaholic, of passionate nature
  b. Conditions that are affected by being at the beach
  c. Desire for travel

d. Desire for butter or chocolate
   e. Sleeping difficulty

Remember, there are more than two thousand remedies in the homeopathy pharmacy! In review, homeopathy came from the concept of one man's beliefs that were not scientifically verified. However, it had a great advantage over the common medical care of his day. He did not advocate the use of harmful drugs in large doses. He promoted not only good personal hygiene but also good hygienic conditions for the home and its surroundings. Diet, fresh air, and exercise were also part of his regimen. The remedies (substances given in minute doses) were given credit for the improvements in health without any scientific evidence to verify that they had anything to do with improvement.

HAS HOMEOPATHY BEEN VERIFIED?

Studies have been done to test the value of these remedies, but there is no clear proof that they have any effect on the body in minute doses. Larger (more concentrated) doses have shown some effect on the system. This effect may not always be good. Some remedies available may contain regular modern drugs added to them, so they will have an effect on human physiology.

There has been a strong effort on the part of believers in alternative therapeutic modalities to scientifically explain the perceived effects of such methods as acupuncture, homeopathic, therapeutic touch, Rolfing, osteopathic, chiropractic, hypnosis, and many other therapy techniques. James Oschman, in his book *Energy Medicine: The Scientific Basis*, makes a strong argument for the scientific explanation. He presents the recent advances in the understanding of electromagnetic physiology in biology. Some researchers who are adherents of the concept of *vitalism* have reported advances in laboratory research of electromagnetic discharges of body, organs, cells, and molecules. Other researchers are unable to reproduce these same laboratory results. The gap is still wide between hypothesis and true scientific proof of cause and effect. Many believers in alternative medicine, or energy medicine, tend to proclaim that energy medicine is now proven to be scientific. They have ignored this gap of proof in a presumptuous manner.

Controlled studies of homoeopathic remedies, when done by the homoeopaths, tend to show positive results. However, most other studies do not support these positive results. Studies should be repeated by objective investigators, with independent analyses of the homoeopathic formulations employed, to ensure that they have not been adulterated with active medications.

A recent meta-analysis of 107 controlled homeopath trials appearing in 96 published reports also found "the evidence of clinical trials is positive but not sufficient to draw definitive conclusions because most trials are of low methodological quality and because of the unknown role of publication bias." The reports also concluded that there is a legitimate case for further evaluation of homeopathy "but only by means of well performed trials" (Kleijnen, 1991).[28]

In the British medical journal *Lancet*, August 27, 2005, a large study made by the University of Berne in Switzerland reported the results of a meta-analysis of 110 trials, each of homeopathy and conventional medicine. No convincing evidence was found that the homeopathic approach to illness was any different from using a placebo. Conventional medicine did significantly better.

April 19, 2010, *Med J Aust*. 192(8):458–60 carried an article "Homeopathy: What Does the 'Best' Evidence Tell Us?" The author Edzard Ernst of Peninsula Medical School, University of Exeter, Exeter, United Kingdom, summarized his study of homeopathy. He had searched the Cochrane Database of Systematic Reviews (most reliable information source) in 2010 for studies on homeopathy.

> The reviews covered the following conditions: cancer, attention-deficit defect, hyperactivity disorder, asthma, dementia, influenza and induction of labour. DATA SYNTHESIS: The findings of the reviews were discussed narratively (the reviews; clinical and statistical heterogeneity precluded meta-analysis). **CONCLUSION**: The finding of currently available Cochrane reviews of studies of homeopathy does not show that homoeopathic medicines have effects beyond placebo. (http:www.ncbi.nlm.nih.gov/pubmed/20402610)

WORLD HEALTH CONDEMNS HOMEOPATHIC Rx

Homeopathy is not a cure, says World Health Organization:

> Homoeopathic remedies often contain few or no active ingredients. People with conditions such as HIV, TB and

---

[28] *NCAHF Position Paper on Homeopathy, pp. 3,4 (1994)*, http://www.ncahf.org/

malaria should not rely on homeopathic treatments, the World Health Organization has warned. It was responding to calls from young researchers who fear the promotion of homeopathy in the developing world could put people's lives at risk.[29]

The group Voice of Young Science Network has written to health ministers to set out the WHO view. Objective evidence that homeopathy is effective on these infections does not exist, says Dr. Nick Beeching, Royal Liverpool University Hospital, by letter on June 2010 to WHO. The doctors from the UK and Africa said:

> We are calling on the WHO to condemn the promotion of homeopathy for treating TB, infant diarrhea, influenza, malaria and HIV. Homeopathy does not protect people from, or treat, these diseases. Those of us working with the most rural and impoverished people of the world already struggle to deliver the medical help that is needed. When homeopathy stands in place of effective treatment, lives are lost.[30]

Dr. Robert Hagan, a researcher in bimolecular science at the University of St. Andrews and also a member of *Voice of Young Science Network*, which is a part of *Sense About Science* that promotes evidence-based medical care said:

> We need governments around the world to recognize the dangers of promoting homeopathy for life-threatening illnesses. We hope that by raising awareness of the WHO's position on homeopathy we will be supporting those people who are taking a stand against these potentially disastrous practices.[31]

Dr. Mario Raviglione, director of the Stop TB department at the WHO, said:

> Our evidence-based WHO TB treatment/management guidelines, as well as the International Standards of Tuberculosis Care do not recommend use of homeopathy.[32]

---

[29] http://ww.news.bbc.co.uk/2/hi/8211925.stm
[30] *Ibid*
[31] *Ibid.*
[32] *Ibid.*

Physicians also complained that homeopathy was being promoted as a treatment of children with diarrhea. A representative of the WHO department of child and adolescent health and development said:

> We have found no evidence to date that homeopathy would bring any benefit. Homeopathy does not focus on the treatment and prevention of dehydration—in total contradiction with the scientific basis and our recommendations for the management of diarrhea.[33]

Dr. Nick Beeching, a specialist in infectious diseases at the Royal Liverpool University Hospital, said:

> Infections such as malaria, HIV and tuberculosis all have a high mortality rate but can usually be controlled or cured by a variety of proven treatments, for which there is ample experience and scientific trial data. "There is no objective evidence that homeopathy has any effect on these infections, and I think it is irresponsible for a healthcare worker to promote the use of homeopathy in place of proven treatment for any life-threatening illness."[34]

In June 2010, delegates to the British Medical Association's conference were expected to support seven motions opposing the use of public money to pay for remedies they claimed have no place in modern medicine and health care. Hundreds of delegates called for a ban on funding homeopathic remedies by the National Health Service. The British Medical Society's position comes as a result of an absence of evidence that use of homoeopathic remedies are more effective than placebo.

In March 2015, a report by the Australian government's National Health and Medical Research Council, after an exhaustive study on homeopathy, was released. This was a report on a review of 176 scientific studies on homeopathic treatment. The conclusion: **It does not work. It is no better than a placebo.**

In the first half of the twentieth century, the twenty-two homeopathy medical schools in the United States closed or converted to regular medical schools. With the advance of scientific evaluation in medical care, the old harmful way of using dangerous drugs slowly changed. The homeopathic

---

[33] *Ibid.*

[34] *Ibid.*

doctor was no longer having better results than the MD. The public turned to *science-driven* medicine. There is now a resurgence of homeopathy among New Age adherents and some others that consider it to be more "natural." Its return in America is not based on science, but is the end result of the belief in *vitalism*. A man's belief in his origin has great influence in his choice of healing methods.

I refer again to James L. Oschman, a biology scientist, who, in his book *Energy Medicine: The Scientific Basis*, speaks of his belief in alternative medicine therapies and of having felt the electrical charges enter his body as applied by *energy therapists*. He expresses his belief that these electrical charges are explained by electromagnetism. He writes that the electromagnetism of one person can restore balance to the electromagnetism of another. He tells of laboratory testing of healers using therapeutic touch and other methods with tools for measuring electromagnetic charges. He admits to the problem of the reproducibility of these experiments by other investigators.

We have received wise counsel regarding the type of medical care we choose, following God's "will" versus gain and life itself. I wish to share with you the words of a Christian physician who has written on this subject:

> There are to be sure some honorable and conscientious ones seeking to utilize homeopathy detached from its obscure practices. Yet, the occult influence, by nature hidden, disguised, often dissimulated behind para scientific theory, does not disappear and does not happen to be rendered harmless by the mere fact of a superficial approach contenting itself simply with denying its existence. *Homeopathy is dangerous*. It is quite contrary to the teaching of the word of God. It willingly favors healing through substances made dynamic, that is to say, *charged with occult forces*. Homoeopathic treatment is the fruit of a philosophy and religion that are at the same time Hinduistic, pantheistic and esoteric.[35]

When God led Israel from Egypt to Canaan, He gave them health laws and statutes. Israel was the only nation in the history of the world that had a medical and health system that was based on prevention. The

---

[35] Bopp. Op. cit., p. 9; Reported in Ankeberg, *Can You Trust Your Doctor?* p. 336

Mosaic health code is medically and scientifically reliable, based on sound physiology and proven principles of hygiene.[36]

> If you diligently heed the voice of the LORD your God and do what is right in His sight, give ear to His commandments and keep all His statutes, I will put none of the diseases on you which I have brought on the Egyptians. For I am the LORD who heals you. (Ex. 15:26)

---

[36] Hubbard, Reuben A., *Historical Perspectives of Health,* Printed by the Department of Health Education School of Health Loma Linda University, Loma Linda, CA, (1975), pp. 23–38.

16

DIVINATION AS A DIAGNOSTIC TOOL

A young American woman had been living in a Southeast Asian country. She developed an earache and sought medical care at a modern hospital in an Asian city. One complaint led to another, and an abdominal ultrasound (exam of the abdomen by use of sound waves) was ordered, then an abdominal CT scan (machine that makes computer-generated pictures of the insides of the abdomen). A diagnosis was made of a cancerous fatty tumor surrounding the right kidney that had spread to other areas of the abdomen. The woman was devastated with this diagnosis. The attending physicians desired to proceed with surgery, but she elected to return to America.

Her American doctor ordered a PET-CT scan (a $5,000+ test, which is better able than the CT scan to determine if cancer is present). The test indicated active tissue in the abdomen that could be cancer. A laparoscopic surgical procedure (looking in the abdomen by optics) was scheduled to be done. A blood test prior to this procedure revealed severe anemia (low number of red blood cells), which made it unsafe to proceed with surgery. Additional blood studies and another ultrasound were ordered in a further attempt to define the disorder. A repeat ultrasound exam of the abdomen did not add any new information. At this point, the expenses had reached nearly $10,000, and the doctors were still not able to determine the exact diagnosis.

Study results to this time could not differentiate between a malignancy and endometriosis, a non-malignant disorder. A laparoscopic procedure was done, which revealed tumors spread in various areas inside the abdomen. Biopsy of the tumors established the diagnosis of ovarian cancer. Extensive surgery to remove as much cancer as possible was performed. Following surgery, treatment would be needed for many months in an attempt to control the disease.

So goes the story for many people seeking definite answers to medical problems in an age of very sophisticated diagnostic equipment and highly trained physicians. Thousands of dollars can be spent, yet the question still remains as to the exact diagnosis, which is so important in order that the proper treatment can be given, in the best sequence, to receive the best results.

Why not seek out some "alternative"-style practitioner with a Homo-Vibra Ray or the Mora machine or the Rife machine or some similar-type instrument to make the diagnosis and treat at the same time with little expense? These machines are said to be able to read energy-wave frequencies or vibrational energy of the cells of the body. (Such energy frequencies and/or vibrations from cells cannot be demonstrated by physical science.) However, this is a belief of some alternative medicine practitioners. By tuning in to those frequencies, the machine is said to compare them to the assumed normal frequency. Then, by the operator spinning a few dials, frequencies are said to be sent back into the body to correct the body's cell frequencies, thereby correcting disease and restoring health.

Another choice is to find a holistic medical doctor who can pass his hands over the abdomen or hold a pendulum above the abdomen in order to localize tumors. Questions can be asked of the pendulum, as it is held above the spot where it has located a tumor, as to whether or not the tumor is a cancer. The pendulum can spin clockwise if a positive answer is given or counterclockwise if it is negative. Any question under the sun can be asked, and a yes-or-no answer can be obtained. The pendulum can be asked what type of therapy would be best. Should the answer be homeopathy, the pendulum can pick out the proper remedy.

This "alternative" method is quick, non-invasive, and inexpensive compared to the above-described conventional medical tests and treatment. Is the machine and/or the hands-on technique accurate? Can they be trusted? Why are scientifically trained physicians not using these techniques? Is it because more money can be made doing many tests? Let us proceed in a search for answers to these questions.

Let me give a definition at this point for the word *alternative therapy*: therapy that is not shown to be *evidence based* (evidence-based means there is an accepted body of peer-reviewed, statistically significant evidence that raises probability of effectiveness to a scientifically convincing level) by quality scientific testing. When an *alternative* method of treatment is shown to be *evidence based*, it then becomes *scientific medicine*.

The following paragraph tells of incidences involving Christian church members and church institutional workers, as was reported in a special report:

- A nurse corrected chronic constipation by repeated application of her hands to her abdomen during the day, to correct *electrical currents*.
- A mother swings a pendulum over her son afflicted with cancer to determine the herbs he needs for healing.
- A young person was tied to a tree so his back was against "its window" to effect healing; the window had been located on the tree by use of the pendulum.
- Women shopping for groceries use a pendulum to select the best products.
- Books on iridology, a method for diagnosing disease through the iris of the eye, were on sale in a college-operated supermarket. Another popular volume on the same shelf was *Magnetic Therapy: Healing in Your Own Hands*, by Abbot George Burke. The author refers with approval to the studies of Dr. Franz Mesmer (from whom the term "mesmerism-hypnotism" derives) and traces his research through pagan thought to Isis, a famous goddess of ancient Egypt.

The nation of Israel was admonished by God just as they were about to enter the Promised Land:

> When you come into the land which the Lord thy God is giving you, you shall not learn to follow the abominations of those nations. There shall not be found among you any one who makes his son or his daughter to pass through the fire, or one that practices witchcraft (divination KJV), or a soothsayer, or one who interprets omens, or a sorcerer, or one who conjures spells, or a medium, or a spiritist, or one who calls up the dead. For all who do these things are an abomination to the Lord, and because of these abominations the Lord your God drives them out from before you.[1]

Caution was also given in regard to false prophets and their proclamations:

---

[1] Deuteronomy 18:9–14.

They have envisioned futility and false *divination*, saying. "Thus says the Lord!" But the Lord has not sent them; yet they hope that the word may be confirmed. "Have you not seen a futile vision, and have you not spoken false divination? You say, 'The Lord says, but I have not spoken.' Therefore thus says the Lord God: "Because you have spoken nonsense and envisioned lies, therefore I am indeed against you," says the Lord God. "My hand will be against the prophets who envision futility and who divine lies: they shall not be in the assembly of My people, nor be written in the record of the house of Israel, nor shall they enter into the land of Israel. Then you shall know that I am the Lord God."[2]

In studying the history of divination, it soon becomes obvious that every civilization used various forms of divination in an attempt to obtain knowledge not obtainable by the usual means. It is of ancient origin. Reading of omens is recognized as a very early divining practice. A child born with an abnormality might well be looked upon as revealing something of the future. Reading the stars and using the zodiac were common. Tarot cards, palm reading, crystal balls, and séances all contributed to the use of divination in daily life.

Dictionary definitions of divination are the following:

> The act or practice of trying to foretell the future or explore the unknown by occult means.[3]

From the *Catholic Encyclopedia*:

> Divination is a form of occultism wherein the person uses objects such as tea leaves, a crystal ball, tarot cards, Ouija board, or any superstitiously interpreted object as the means of attempting to gain or elicit knowledge or information that is beyond ordinary human intelligence. The attempts to contact the dead through a séance, for example, are spiritistic divinations that have been contested by parapsychological testing and proved false. Likewise astrology, witchcraft, zodiac readings or horoscopes are forms of divination. Although it is natural for human beings

---

[2] Ezekiel 13:6–10.

[3] *Webster's New World Dictionary, 3rd College Edition,* Published by Webster's New World dictionaries A Division of Simon & Shuster, Inc., (1988).

to attempt to 'lift the curtain' and see beyond the present, the tendency should be controlled lest it distract from the unfolded and true vision of God contained in His revelation to mankind.[4]

The Bible records the use of divination, but it does not always say what method was used. Does the Bible promote the use of divination by stories? Joseph had his cup placed in the sack of grain belonging to his brother Benjamin. He called it his "divining cup." Joseph's servant said to the brothers:

> Isn't this the cup my master drinks from and also uses for divination? This is a wicked thing you have done. (Gen. 44:5 KJV)

When his brothers were brought to Joseph, he said to them:

> What is this you have done? Don't you know that a man like me can find things out by divination? (Gen. 44:15 KJV)

This verse does not tell us Joseph used divination, but he wanted his brothers to believe he did and could discover their secrets.

Over four hundred years later, God told the descendants of Joseph and his brothers that He was going to give them a land that others possessed because those people were practicing divination along with other acts of which God did not approve. Their degree of iniquity had come to its full. But Israel did not heed God's command to abstain from divination, for we read that the divining rod was in use in Hosea's day.

> My people ask counsel from their wooden idols, And their staff informs them. (Hosea 4:12)

King Ahaziah of Israel sent messengers to Ekron, a city of the Philistines, to inquire of Baalzebub, the god of Ekron, as to whether or not the king of Israel, Ahaziah, would recover from his injuries of falling through the lattice. When Elijah was sent of God to intercept those servants of the king, he asked them this question:

> Is it because there is no God in Israel that you are going off to consult Baal-Zebub, the god of Ekron? (2 Kings 1:3 NIV)

---

[4] *The Catholic Encyclopedia,* Thomas Nelson Inc. Publishers, Nashville, NY, (1976), p. 168.

The servants returned to the king who then sent fifty soldiers to bring Elijah to him. When the soldiers came near Elijah, God sent fire down from heaven and consumed the captain and the fifty soldiers. The king sent another fifty, and again fire consumed them. The captain of the next fifty asked Elijah for mercy, whereupon God told Elijah to go with him to the king with a message from God. Elijah told the king that he would not get up from his bed because he inquired of Baalzebub rather than inquiring of the God of Israel (2 Kings 1).

King Nebuchadnezzar, while traveling with his army, came to a division in the road. He could proceed to Egypt, or he could travel toward Jerusalem. He did not know which way to go first, so he had an animal killed and "read the liver" as a method of divination.

> For the King of Babylon stands at the parting of the road, at the fork of the two roads, to use divination: he shakes the arrows, he consults the images, he looks at the liver. (Ezek. 21:21 NKJ)

The use of various methods of divining has been presented including the rod, cup, arrows, and the liver. There are scores of other methods. Divination by astrology to establish medical diagnosis has also been a common practice. Is divining used in medical practice today? In the scientific method of medical care, divining is not used. It is used, however, by some of the "alternative" and "holistic" practitioners. This fact is to be found in the writings of those alternative disciplines.

Ankerberg and Weldon, in their book *Can You Trust Your Doctor?*, lists the names of several alternative healing disciplines that in their own literature state that some practitioners may use divination. These disciplines are psychic healing, reflexology, herbal medicine, naturopathy, dowsing, iridology, color therapy, chiropractic, homeopathy, astrologic medicine, and therapeutic touch. The pendulum is the most common method of divination.[5]

PENDULUMS

The practice of divining using a rod, wand, or pendulum is ancient. No exact history is available to pinpoint the start, but some drawings found in China show evidence of this practice as far back as 1400 BC. In the Bible (Deut. 18:9–14), which is dated around 1450 BC, strong words of warning

---

[5] Ankerberg, John; Weldon, John; *Can You Trust Your Doctor?*, Wolgemuth and Hyatt, Brentwood, TN, (1991), pp. 100–101.

were given to the people of Israel concerning divining as they were about to enter Canaan. Divination was recorded in the Bible as having been used five hundred years prior to the writing of Deuteronomy 18. This passage does not state the method of divining that was practiced. In the Bible, it is recorded that *divining by a staff* was practiced in Israel around 750 BC (Hosea 4:12).

Divining with a rod can be considered the same act as using a pendulum. When was it first used in medical diagnosis? We do not know, but early in history, the rod became connected with health and healing as evidenced by the following examples. Greek mythology shows ties to serpent power and the use of a "rod" when Apollo handed over to Hermes (Mercury) a magic wand. Homer, in his *Odyssey*, tells how this rod could send men's souls to Hades or return them; it had power to bring winds and storms. Another name for the rod was *caduceus* and was depicted as entwined with snakes. The rod was passed on to Aesculapius, the Greek god of healing, and has since become the symbol of medicine.

The pendulum is one of the most frequently used methods of divination. It may be used in psychology to assess personality disorders, to make diagnosis in medical conditions, to choose treatments or medicinals, to find oil in the ground, to locate different metals in the earth, and most frequent of all, to find water underground.

Around 1900, a Catholic priest, Alexis Mermet, who was a dowser for underground water and metals, concluded that dowsing should be amenable in medical diagnosis for humans and animals as well. He wrote the book *How I Proceed in the Discovery of Near or Distant Water, Metals, Hidden Objects, and Illnesses*. He makes the following statement:

> I invented the method of "pendular diagnosis."[6]

It is unlikely that Mermet was really the first to use the pendulum in medical diagnosis, but at least, he thought so.

A question was asked, why does a pendulum appear to react to a metallic substance or an underground water vein as well as to a simple act of thought—an action of the mind? In 1806, a bright young German scientist, Johann Wilhelm Ritter, took up this question. While experimenting with a variety of pendulums on various metals, he noticed that the pendulum would swing in a specific pattern for each type of object over which it was suspended. He demonstrated that the swinging or rotating of the

---

[6] Bird, Christofer; *The Divining Hand*; New Age Press, Black Mountain, NC, (1979) p. 289.

pendulum, when held at the top versus the bottom of an object, would give different directions of motion in the pendulum. He did this on the human body and mapped out different anatomical areas showing how the pendulum would spin in one direction, but at other places, it would reverse its direction of spinning. Because this reaction reminded him of magnetic characteristics, he called this polarity.

Today, there are healers who teach that illness is a result of an organ's or the body's polarity becoming disturbed and out of balance. They also teach that in order to bring healing, it is useful to apply magnets about the body. There are "magnetic healers" who apply magnets to the body to balance the polarity. Then there are other healers who do not consider polarity but apply magnets in various places for almost any symptom common to man. They may not have a philosophy as to how it works, but they say it works, and that is good enough for them. The philosopher Friedrich Wilhelm Joseph von Schelling explained it as follows:

> There was a "force" in nature that could be revealed mechanically, chemically, electrically, magnetically, and also vitally.[7]

He concluded that when a pendulum is used by a "sensitive" operator, it was possible to detect the force described. He believed there was a polarity throughout the universe, which was the source of all substance. Ritter, a member of the Bavarian Academy of Sciences, in the early 1800s summarized it this way:

> What we have, then, are the celestial movements themselves here repeated in microcosm. Could it be that the whole organism of the universe is reflected in the human body?[8]

The book continues:

> What Ritter had stumbled upon at the start of the nineteenth century was the fact that a pendulum or dowsing rod could be used to extract pure information from the universe about any subject no matter how abstract or nebulous.[9]

---

[7] *Ibid.*, p. 126.
[8] *Ibid.*, p. 128.
[9] *Ibid.*, p. 129.

The dowsing instrument would respond to the questions or commands of the dowser as long as it could be answered by a yes or no.

Many people have had very little contact with dowsing, or pendulum exposure, and may only have heard of one or two styles. If their experience has been that they have witnessed or heard only of positive responses from this particular technique, they may be convinced that there is some physical explanation for its function. A knowledge of the various ways pendulums are used will undermine confidence in there being a true physical explanation for the information obtained by their use.

DIVINING FOR WATER

Christopher Bird, in his book *The Divining Hand* (p. 110), tells of a miner and diviner of metals who would dowse with his arm outstretched and fist clenched. His arm shook when near a vein of metal, and his whole body shook when he was directly over it. The miner was asked why he does not shake and vibrate when he is working in the mine and next to the vein all the time. He answered:

> If I do not "orient" my thoughts specifically to finding a vein of ore, I get no reaction when I cross over a vein or work near one.

A very common practice is to "witch" for water before a well is drilled or dug. Witching is most often done by using a forked tree branch. Many well drillers will not drill until someone has witched for water. There is a very strong belief in this practice, even within the Christian church. To suggest to people that the power in this act is of the occult and not of science is to ignite an argument. Those who have accepted dowsing as being scientific do not easily change their minds. It is believed that there is some physical force connecting the tree branch, the person doing the witching, and the water in the ground. The explanation as to why some people can do it and others cannot is proclaimed to be because of the differences in the electrical activity in our bodies.

These explanations are wishful thinking. The science of physics has not been able to demonstrate any of these claims. The more one studies the variety of ways of witching for water and divining for other objects or information, the easier it is to be persuaded that there is no scientific physical explanation for divining. For instance, some utility crews will use two copper wires bent at a right angle and held in each hand. One part of the wire held in the hand will be at ninety degrees to the ground, the other part bent at a ninety-degree angle so as to be horizontal to the ground.

When a water or gas pipe is located underground, the horizontal wires will swing and cross, not dip down as is done with the tree branch.

Witching may be done with a forked stick, a strait rod, wires bent at a ninety-degree angle, a plain stick held in the palms of outstretched arms, a coin resting in the palm of the hand, outstretched hands alone, or just the mind with no tools of the trade. The stick may point up or down, or it may vibrate or oscillate. The wires may turn inward, or they may turn outward; they may also turn opposite each other as they are held in the hand. A wire may oscillate up and down, sideways, or in other modes of gyrations. The hand may shake; a coin in the palm may turn over. The stick may turn round and round in the palm of an outstretched hand or be thrown clear out of the diviner's hands. When divining with no instrument, the taste of water may be the sign that water, or whatever is being dowsed, is beneath the dowser. The diviner chooses what method he wants to use, and before he divines, he decides the reaction that is to occur with his instrument.

Witching may be done from a map thousands of miles from the area of interest. It may be done for any substance: fluid, solid, mineral, or water. It can be done for any object on earth. It may even be done for an underground tunnel. Bird, in his book *The Divining Hand*, tells of the use of the divining rod by marines in Vietnam to find tunnels and even to locate the Viet Cong in the tunnel. Divining by map was used to locate prisoners of war and the location of Viet Cong prisons. Any question under the sun could be asked and would receive an answer as long as it involved a yes-or-no response.

In 2013, while attending a church social, three members cornered me and with vigor attempted to "straighten me out" concerning this subject of witching. One of them had a short time prior our conversation sent to a "diviner" in a distant city a copy of a surveyor's plot of his property. Prior sending, he and his wife had prayed over the copy, asking God to bless the work of the dowser so that upon drilling they would find water. A pendulum was held over the copy of land plot where it located the correct locus to drill; upon drilling, water was found. I was asked to give my response to this act. My answer: this was a clear act of divination. The response back was, well, since they had prayed over the copy before sending and water was found, it had to have been blessed by God. Is this presumption?

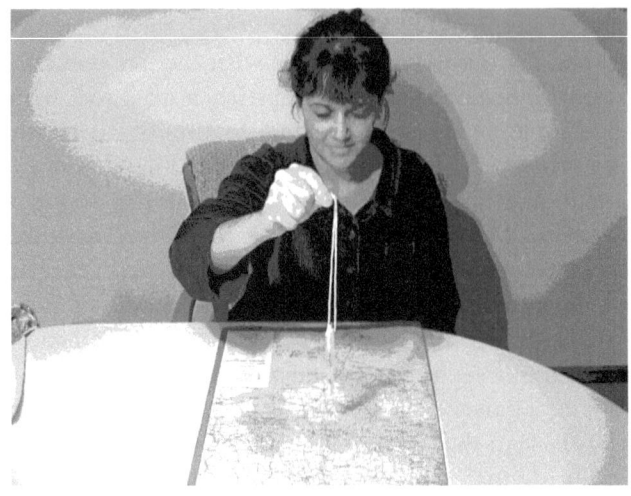

Figure 37. Map dowsing

A gentleman once came to my office for treatment of a very swollen and painful shoulder. After injection with medication, he was promptly healed. He later returned and told me I had ruined his "bobbing arm." I asked what a bobbing arm was. He stated that when the arm was very tender, he was able to more accurately sense the pull on the wire he would use in witching for water. Later, he came to my home to demonstrate to me his technique for witching.

He took a bucket and turned it upside down, using it for a stool. Sitting on the bucket, he took a strong stiff wire about a meter long and bent a coil on the end to hold a lightbulb. A bulb was placed in the coiled wire, and the wire was held on his knee, pointing out in front of his knee about twenty-five inches, with the light bulb on the end. He held a pencil in the other hand and placed a tablet on the free knee. The wire began to bend up and down, causing the lightbulb to rise and fall eight to ten inches. He would count the number of times it would flex till it stopped. When it stopped, the wire began to bend back and forth in horizontal moves. After ten to twelve moves this way, the wire would stop and begin to bend up and down again. He counted the up-and-down moves, and he also counted the horizontal moves, recording them. The up-and-down moves represented one foot for each bend, and the horizontal moves represented the volume of water at that depth. The distance was thus calculated to each level where water would be found and an estimate given for the volume at the different levels. I asked him why it was that in America each "bob" of the wire is counted as a foot and in Europe each "bob" of the wire is calculated as one meter. He had no answer.

Later, I found the answer to the question. A relative came to visit whom I learned belonged to a dowsing club of "water witches." I asked him the same question, and this is his answer:

> That is no problem, a person doing the *bobbing* just determines in his mind what measurements he is going to use before he starts.

Many who are involved in divination for metal or water continue their attempts to find some scientific association or answer so that dowsing will be accepted by the scientific world. However, there seems to be no common ground with science.

RADIONICS

Radionics, psychotronics, etc., involves the occult use of technology (various devices). It does not really deal in heretofore undiscovered areas of undetected energy but rather is *dependent on the psychic ability of the operator, referred to as* radiesthesia. For example, radionics is divination (not always recognized or admitted) and the same as using a rod or pendulum. Radionics is divination aided by a mechanical apparatus: Abrams's box, black box, or any one of the numerous machines used for such work.

Some years ago I had a family come to my office in great distress. They had secured the services of a "medical practitioner" who had sent a saliva specimen of their little girl to a lab that used a radionic machine. The family was told that the machine made the diagnosis of acute leukemia. They were shaken and frightened. They asked for my help in determining if this was so. The child had no symptoms that would have caused a physician to suspect such an illness. A blood count was ordered and done at a hospital laboratory. It was normal with no hint of leukemia. Their medical practitioner had given them the diagnosis of leukemia because the machine had diagnosed leukemia. The family did not understand what clinical and lab findings go with leukemia, and my assurance that the child did not have the disease was not enough to relieve their fears. I sent them to a pediatrician who had advanced training in leukemia. He agreed with me, but their doubts lingered. It took many months of normal life before they were free of the fear caused by this wrong diagnosis.

What concept of science did this medical practitioner have that caused him to believe the diagnosis made by the machine? This introduces a belief that is common in the non-scientific world of health and healing, that of *vibrational medicine*. The radionic machine is said to be able to detect *vibrations* or *frequencies* from the saliva. If any disharmony is in the salivary vibrations, the machine can analyze in such a manner as to detect and diagnose the abnormality. Where does the idea originate that saliva has vibrations, or frequencies? How does vibration from saliva relate to an individual and make it possible for a machine to make a diagnosis of leukemia?

We have to return to the basic pagan belief that every existing thing has a common origin from a non-describable energy (*vitalism*) that is present throughout the universe. This energy is said to be manifest in every *living* substance (some authors, writing on this subject, include *inanimate* substances) and that there is an *aura* of radiating energy that emanates and surrounds those substances. This radiating energy is believed to have a specific vibrational or electromagnetic frequency. If the particular frequency is off normal, it indicates an imbalance of energy. Electronic machines have been made that are supposed to detect the vibrational imbalance, ascertain the reason for the imbalance, and make a diagnosis. It is simply another form of divination. It is not true science. *Vibrational medicine* is simply a synonym for *energy medicine*.

A commonly used radionic machine is the EAV machine, or electro acupuncture according to Voll (Reinhold Voll). Voll was a German physician engaged in acupuncture, starting in the 1950s. EAV technique is a form of radionics, with the concept of measuring by use of an electronic machine, hypothesized electric impulses from specific acupuncture points, which, in turn, are said to have originated from an organ having "meridian connections" to that specific point. The machine is supposed to reveal low, normal, or high electronic vibrations from the organ. Low-amplitude electronic vibration reveals a weak organ; a high signal reveals "inflammation."

Then, if you find an organ that has a low energy, for example, you insert a medicine contained in a vial into that electrical circuit, which also consists of the patient and the machine. If the medicine vibrates at the same frequency as the weak signal being tested, synchronizes, harmonizes literally, electronically, with the low signal from the weak organ, the amplitude or strength of the signal will get higher as the two frequencies will superimpose and add together. Then you know that what is in the vial is the right medicine for that organ, for that patient. The person doing the testing must be *highly sensitive*—that is, have high occult powers.

The American Cancer Society, exposing nonscientific alternative medical treatments, lists the following synonyms regarding terms used by

Alternative & Mystical Healing Therapies

proponents of various alternative treatment methods: electromagnetism, bioelectricity, magnetic field therapy, bioelectromagnetics, bioenergy therapy, bioresonance tumor therapy, energy medicine, black boxes, electronic devices, electrical devices, zapping machine, Rife machine, cell com system.

These terms refer to names given by alternative healers to the energy they say comes from the body, which machines are said to be able to detect, diagnose, and use to treat for different medical disorders.

It is claimed by radionic practitioners that when electromagnetic frequencies, or energy fields, proclaimed to be within the body are unbalanced, disease and illness occur. The belief is that these imbalances disrupt the body's chemical makeup. By applying electromagnetic energy from outside the body, either by the hands of a *healer* or by electronic devices, practitioners claim they can correct the electrical imbalances in the body.

There are a variety of radionic machines for sale on the Internet. You may find a practitioner that uses one, but most physicians will not do so. What are these machines? How do they work? Why don't most medical doctors use them? Let me present my answer.

The machines are simply "galvanometers" that measure the electrical resistance of a person's skin. The machine will usually have two electrodes, one the patient will hold or someway be attached to the patient. The other electrode in the form of a pointed wand—probe—will be held by the operator of the machine and apply to "acupuncture points" on the body. The machine has a dial with a needle or has a screen that shows some type of graph, which will change in response to flow of electricity through the machine. The machine sends a current through an electrode held by the patient: the other electrode (probe) held on the skin by the operator receives the electricity flowing through the body and carries it back into the machine, which has a gauge. The needle on the gauge moves according to the strength of electrical flow, which is determined by (1) amplitude of electricity generated by the machine and (2) the quality of contact on the skin of the two electrodes. If the probe is pushed hard, making better skin contact, the electrical flow increases; if a poor contact on the skin is made, then there's less electrical flow. That's it! Nothing more!

A galvanometer is the same electrical tool as the "volt meter" most men have in their toolboxes. I took my volt meter, turned it on so it emitted a low-amplitude electric current, and then grasped an electrode in each hand. No swing of the needle. Then I moistened the fingers holding the electrodes, and the needle moved. I squeezed harder and the needle moved farther. I took one probe and touched a spot on my body and no motion of the needle. I moistened the skin, and now the needle moved; and the harder I pushed the probe, the greater the swing of the needle in the dial.

An acupuncture point is considered by its proponents to connect to and reveal the status of energy balance of an organ, endocrine gland, immune system, or some other body response such as allergy, etc. The results of the test really depend upon the operator, not some hypothetical energy balance. This type of testing is often promoted as being able to detect any and every type of disease even before it manifests in the body. Machine testing is also proclaimed to be able to detect vitamin and mineral deficiencies or excesses, to check substances for allergic response, to select appropriate homeopathic medicinal remedies and even to treat. Real science! NO! This is fraud or divination or both!

Let's look at some names applied to these radionic instruments: electro acupuncture according to Voll (EAV), electrodermal screening (EDS), bioelectric functions diagnosis (BFD), bioresonance therapy (BRT), bioenergy regulatory technique (BER), biocybernetic medicine (BM), computerized electrodermal screening (CEDS), electrodermal testing (EDT), limbic stress assessment (LSA), meridian energy analysis (MEA), or point testing. Additional names one may encounter are Dermatron, Vegatest, Accupath 1000, Asyra, Avatar, BICOM, Bio-Tron, Biomeridian, Computron, Drmatron, DiagnoMetre, Eclosion, e-Lybra 8, ELAST, Interro, Interactive Query System (IQS0), I-Tronic, Kindling, LISTEN System, Mora, Matrix Physiques System, Meridian energy Analysis Device (MEAD), MSAS, Oberon, Omega, Acubase, Omega Vision, Orion System Phazx, Prognos, Prophyle, Punctos III, Syncrometer, Vantage, Victor-Vitalpunkt diagnose, Vitel 618 and ZYTO, zapping machine, Royal Rife machine, Cell com system.[10]

What are the claims about the machines' capabilities? Let us look at an advertisement connected with the **Mora machine**. The machine is used as a health detective for its practitioner supposedly delivering information that he/she believes is a true picture of bodily functions at all levels. It is offered as able to test for chemical imbalances, food intolerances and allergies, nutritional deficiencies, and is able to select appropriate homeopathy remedies. It is a painless form of electro acupuncture as no needles are inserted.

> Originally created for use by holistic skin therapists who continue to use it to treat disorders such as eczema, psoriasis

---

[10] http://www.experiencefestival.com/alternative_health_dictionary (dictionary now removed from Internet)

and acne, it is now widely used to detect most disorders that manifest themselves physically, no matter what the cause.

The Mora machine itself picks up electromagnetic waves from the body and then manipulates those that have gone out of kilter by increasing or decreasing their amplitude before sending them back to the body to effect a cure. Where the detective work comes into force is in finding which nutritional or mineral deficiencies are responsible and which ones and what doses or cocktail mix of them will correct them.[11]

Bioresonance frequency therapy is vibrational technique of *recording a person's voice* and submitting it to machine analysis. It is claimed to check for nutritional imbalances, stress, and illness. The acoustical vocal recording is claimed to provide information so that specific frequencies can be ascertained and returned, which are said to resonate and support the body. With this technique, it is not necessary to make a diagnosis as the frequencies imparted back to the body go to the core of the energy imbalance problem.

Practitioners claim that these above mentioned methods can treat ulcers, headaches, burns, chronic pain, nerve disorders, spinal cord injuries, diabetes, gum infections, asthma, bronchitis, arthritis, cerebral palsy, heart disease, and cancer. There is no scientific evidence to support any of the claims made for these devices.

VIBRATIONAL MEDICINE

I suggest that the reader do an Internet search for the term *vibrational medicine* and read some of the nine hundred thousand websites available under this heading. The heading on one entry I found is as follows: "VIBRATIONAL MEDICINE, ENERGY MEDICINE, AND VIBRATIONAL RESONANCE." As I looked through more than three hundred websites, I soon realized that the term *vibrational medicine* is used in referring to any or all of the subjects I present in this book. The following definitions are from the *Alternative Health Dictionary*:

> Vibrational medicine (energetic medicine, energetics medicine, energy medicine, subtle-energy medicine, vibrational healing, vibrational therapies): "Healing philosophy" whose main

---

[11] http://www.mora-akademie.org/mora-mglichkeiten.html?&L=1 (if web site does not open try "mora machine")

"tenet" is that humans are "dynamic energy systems" ("body/mind/spirit" complexes) and reflect "evolutionary patterns" of "soul growth." Its postulates include the following. (a) Health and illness originate in subtle energy systems, (b) These systems coordinate the "life-force" and the "physical body." (c) Emotions, spirituality, and nutritional and environmental factors affect the "subtle energy systems." Vibrational medicine embraces acupuncture, aromatherapy, Bach flower therapy, chakra rebalancing, channeling, color breathing, color therapy, crystal healing, absent healing, Electroacupuncture According to Voll (EAV), etheric touch, flower essence therapy, homeopathy, Kirlian photography, laserpuncture, the laying on of hands, meridian therapy, mesmerism, moxibustion, orthomolecular medicine, Past-life Regression, Polarity Therapy, psychic healing, psychic surgery, radionics, the Simonton method, sonopuncture, Toning, Transcendental Meditation, and Therapeutic Touch. The expressions "energy healing," "energy work," and "energetic healing work" appear synonymous with "vibrational medicine."[12]

These vibrations, frequencies, and auras that all objects are said to possess are not demonstrable by science despite the use of extremely sensitive instrumentation. This concept is found only in the writings of theosophy (pagan theology), occult writings, believers in *vitalism*, energy medicine, and New Age writings. True science is often quoted with an attempt to blend it into the vital force concept so that it looks like true science, but the connection is just not there. Yes, sometimes the machine or pendulum makes a correct diagnosis; but mostly, it is incorrect. If it is not true science, how can it be correct anytime? How does divination give correct answers at any time or with any method? A power does direct divination—the power of demons or fallen angels. Because a machine gives a correct diagnosis at times does not prove it works by the laws of science. Because a method of treatment may seem to bring healing does not prove the method is following God's laws of physics.

It is worth noting the conclusions of the Theosophical Research Center in its publication *The Mystery of Healing* (p. 63):

> It is now admitted by those who use the various types of diagnostic machines associated with radiesthesia that for successful work it is necessary to have present a human operator of a special type

---

[12] http://www.experiencefestival.com/alternat health dictionary - v (reference is now removed from Internet)

(*i.e.*, one with occult abilities). It is also well known that some operators are more proficient than others, while in the case of certain people, the machine will not work at all.[13]

In psychometry, an object that a person has handled such as a glass, book, or anything else can be taken and *dowsed* (using pendulum or radionic machine) to answer questions or to determine the proclaimed energy imbalance in the person, thus giving answers as to how to treat for illness. A doll may be used to represent a person and the pendulum held over it to identify the location of illness.

OUIJA BOARD

The forms of divination used for medical reasons presented in the preceding pages are performed on, or for, someone. They are not designed to be used by oneself. The Ouija board allows a person to divine for himself. If there are questions concerning health relating to diagnosis or treatment, these questions can be asked so as to receive a yes-or-no answer. The Ouija board can spell out words and give numbers.

The Ouija board is flat with the words *yes* to one side (left or right) and *no* to the other. The letters of the alphabet are also on the face of the board, along with numbers zero through nine. There is a small heart-shaped board on which to place one's hands. When questions are asked of the Ouija board, the small heart-shaped board will slide on the surface of the Ouija board and point with its tip to yes or no or to various letters and/or numbers so as to spell out words or numbers, thereby answering the question asked of the board.

The Ouija board is frequently used in parties or at other gatherings of people. This is a method of divination that began in Europe in the late 1700s or early 1800s. Baron von Reichenbach, a student of Mesmer, is credited by Garrison in *History of Medicine* (p. 369) with initiating it. However, almost all techniques have an ancient history of use.

This method of divination, like crystals, seems to be a fast-track for contact with the spirits. Where there has been use of the board, it is not unusual to hear of strange physical phenomena occurring in the home or location of use. This may manifest by objects moving around the house, doors opening and closing with no one present, and many other physical

---

[13] Wilson, Weldon; *Occult Shock and Psychic Forces*, Master Books, San Diego, CA, (1980), p. 198.

manifestations. A person repeatedly using the Ouija board is subject to demon possession.

The answers coming from divination are accurate and true many times, but at other times they lie. The devil uses these answers to his advantage; an accurate answer may be given in order to gain our interest and confidence. We can be sure that in the long run, his, Satan's, interest is in our destruction. The highest level and most deceptive divination is when man is led to believe he is communicating with the dead.

> For the living know that they shall die, but the dead know not anything. (Eccles. 9:5 KJV)

Isaiah 8:19, 20 states it very plain:

> And when they say to you, "Seek those who are mediums and wizards (diviners), who whisper and mutter," should not a people seek their God? Should they seek the dead on behalf of the living? To the law and to the testimony! if they do not speak according to this word, it is because there is no light in them.

Satan's systems of deception start very innocently; then when our interest is developed, we are led on to more involved practices. These in turn can lead to developing psychic powers and communication with spirit entities, animal entities, etc. Channeling allows for demonic possession of our minds and souls. The end result is loss of eternal life.

When so many different instruments and methods can be used to obtain answers to questions and to receive information that is requested, it becomes obvious that the instruments are only a ploy. The real reason is the connection between the mind of the one seeking information and the *intelligence* that gives the answers, namely, Satan or his angels. This same situation is seen in the practice of the different martial arts derived from qi gong (manipulation of vital energy) or use of a crystal to direct channeling of energy and spirits.

CONCLUSIONS ON DIVINATION

In the use of the pendulum, what can it do that scientific instruments cannot do? The pendulum can work from maps or dolls, and from long distances; it can find a vein of water or metal, making it possible to cover a considerable area in a rapid manner. It can diagnose and select the remedy.

One can ask the pendulum questions and receive a yes-or-no answer. These are things scientific instrumentation cannot do.

It is interesting to note that the dowser's ability may be blunted or turned off by his own doubts or by the presence of someone who is a strong disbeliever.

> The rod must be held with indifference, for if the mind is occupied by doubts, reasoning, or other operation that engages the animal spirits, it will divert their powers from being exerted in this process, in which their instrumentality is absolutely necessary: from whence it is that the rod constantly answers in the hands of peasants, women and children, who hold it simply without puzzling their minds with doubts and reasoning. Whatever may be thought of this observation it is a very just one, and of great consequence in the practice of the rod.[14]

It is obvious that the power and intelligence involved is not operating under the rules of our physical laws, which do not vary and do not depend upon a *sensitive* person to demonstrate or utilize them. Ben Hester, in his book *Dowsing: An Exposé of Hidden Occult Forces*, shares with us his and his two friends' eight-year foray into searching for answers to the power behind these practices. He started as an avid believer that the power in dowsing could be explained and was seated in the science of physics that is yet unknown. His friends held the opposite opinion. They joined their talents, energy, and time to pursue an exhaustive study and examination of the subject.

They examined a large volume of the writing and history of dowsing. What stood out was that those writers believing in the subject of dowsing tended to exclude negative remarks, and this same trait of presenting only biased views seemed to prevail in books against the practice. There is a five-hundred-year history of writings in many languages telling of dowsing accomplishments but also books showing the failures of the practice. Throughout this period, the explanation for the power that often did perform some outstanding feat of delivering knowledge could never be arrived at, or agreed upon, even by the dowsers themselves. Hester makes the following comment:

> I had a nearly closed mind in favor of dowsing as a not-yet-understood physical phenomenon. The discovery of

---

[14] Hitching, Francis; *Earth Magic*, Morrow, NY, (1977), p. 196.

contradictions in the information from field interviews and written material on dowsing was the beginning.

Once my eyes were opened to the fact of the truly supernatural aspect of dowsing and the fact that it had never been satisfactorily explained in the five hundred years of written material—even to the community of dowsers—my own questioning began.[15]

The answers found by Hester and his friends to the question of what power is involved in dowsing were "found to be shocking."[16]

When all the theories were compared, all the opinions evaluated, and all the contradictions considered, the ancient biblical condemnation of *divination* began to make sense. In fact the biblical description of dowsing, the death penalty imposed for practicing it, and the exposing of its power source is the only reasonable consideration to be found. It is the only explanation avoided in all dowsing literature.[17]

The past two hundred years have seen contention between dowsers and science. Those involved in divination want so much to be able to show that their work is scientific, yet the proof has been elusive. It is an accepted truth that dowsing organizations admit and write that they have no explanation for the feats that they perform. The dowser sees it as a power that has yet to be discovered but is in the physical world, or as some extra talent given to an individual as is music or other artistic ability.

The pagan and nature worshiper sees divination as an extension of his mind, which has merely been expanded by a simple procedure. He believes that the intelligence of the universe rests within his mind and is only waiting to be released. The field of science that tests and observes for consistent results tends to see divination as trickery and chance and to deny that a special power is involved.

There is a third explanation to be considered as the Bible-believing Christian reads the Bible and he is told of the power of Satan and his angels. The Christian sees two conflicting powers: the devil and his angels and Christ, the divine Son of God, and His angels. The power of Satan

---

[15] Hester, Ben; *Dowsing an Exposé of Hidden Occult Forces*, Leaves of Autumn Books, Payson, AZ, (1982), p. ix–x.

[16] *Ibid.*, on exterior of back cover of book.

[17] *Ibid.*

does not always do evil; many times it will do good and marvelous acts to gain men's loyalty. Eventually, man will suffer the consequences for choosing to follow and utilize the directions and power of Satan, but it may not be until the judgment day. By accepting his power, we, in essence, choose him as our lord.

I believe the power and intelligence acting in divination to be of Satan. This power has intelligence to be able to answer yes or no to any question in the universe. It does not matter one twit as to the instrument used in the divination in obtaining the knowledge desired and sought. It has to do with giving the "will" of the diviner to this power. When the divining instrument "bobs," indicating one-foot distance in America but a meter in Europe, and this measurement is actually set by the mind of the dowser, there can be no other answer. When dowsing can be done over an individual or from a saliva sample, a hair, or an object the individual has handled, from a thousand-miles distant, there can be no other answer.

The Bible tells of the response of the Ephesians when they were converted and considered their interest in witchcraft prior to conversion. They made a bold move:

> Also, many of those who had practiced magic, brought their books together and burned them in the sight of all. And they counted up the value of them and it totaled fifty thousand pieces of silver. (Acts 19:19)

After conversion and conviction of the Holy Spirit, habits and practices changed, and they promptly laid bare the mysteries of their witchcraft. They chose to burn their books rather than sell so as not to involve others in witchcraft. Those treatises on divination contained rules and directions for communication with evil spirits. They were regulations for the worship of Satan, directions for obtaining his help and information from him. By retaining the books, the disciples would have exposed themselves to temptation; by selling them, they would have placed temptation in the way of others. They had renounced the realm of darkness and wished to destroy its power over them.

17

THOSE WHO PRACTICE MAGIC ARTS

In Greek mythology, Odysseus learns that his men have just been turned into swine when given a *potion* by Circe. Hermes gives Odysseus a protective herb, and when Circe offers him the *potion*, he drinks it without harm.

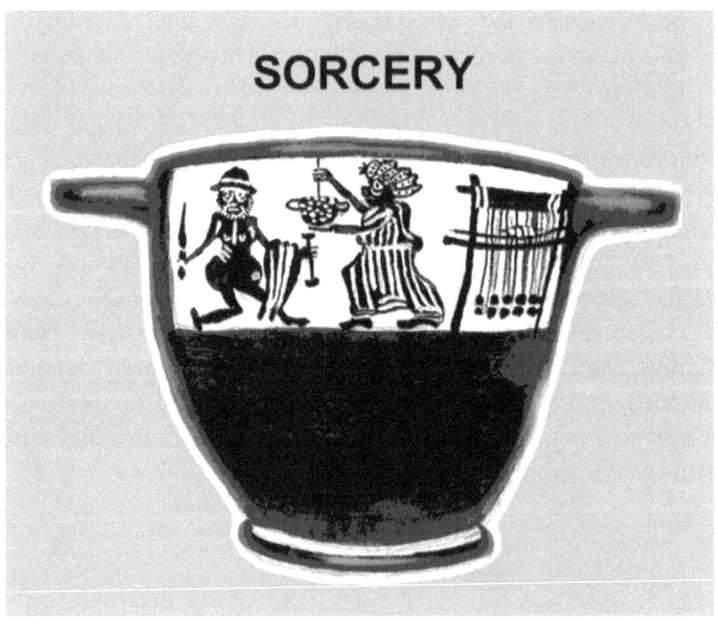

Figure 38. Sorcery cup

Alternative & Mystical Healing Therapies

In ancient times, the use of herbs, special concoctions for creating magic, and a variety of incantations were used to create mind-changing experiences. Plants with psychedelic properties are often used in Wicca (witchcraft), Satanism, occult magic, and shamanistic cultures to produce altered states of consciousness and to facilitate contact with the spirit world.[1] Today, many substances are commonly used to affect the mind; even though they are not taken for a psychic experience or to facilitate contact with the spirits, they actually do alter the mind to a varying extent. Mind-altering substances include tobacco, alcohol, marijuana, different narcotics, amphetamines (speed), cocaine, peyote, and other various plants such as certain mushrooms; even some prescription pharmaceuticals might be included in this list. Worldwide, there is "enchantment with the use of drugs." Should we also include caffeine?

The King James Bible tells us what will be the end of those practicing *"sorcery."* The New International Version of the Bible translates the same word from the original Greek as *"those who practice magic arts."* They do not obtain eternal life and translation to heaven.

> Blessed are they that do His commandments, that they may have the right to the tree of life, and may enter in through the gates into the city. But outside are dogs, and *sorcerers* (*those who practice magic arts*, NIV) and whoremongers and murderers and idolaters and whosoever loveth and maketh a lie. (Rev. 22:14, 15)

What is their eventual end?

> Sorcerers and idolaters and all liars, shall have their part in the lake which burneth with fire and brimstone, which is the second death. (Rev. 21:8)

Why does God destroy the sorcerers (those who practice magic arts)?

> For by their sorceries were all nations deceived. (Rev. 18:23–24)

> Neither repented they of their murders, nor of their sorceries, nor of their fornication, nor of their thefts. (Rev. 9:21)

---

[1] Ankerberg, John; Weldon, John; *Can You Trust Your Doctor?*, Wolgemuth & Hyatt, Brentwood, TN, (1991), p. 257.

What is *sorcery*, and who is a *sorcerer*? In the book of Revelation in the King James Version of the Bible, the word *sorcerer* has been translated from the Greek words *pharmakeia*, *pharmakeus*, and *pharmakos*; all, according to *Young's Analytical Analysis*, have the meaning of "enchantment with drugs," "charm," and/or "remedy." *Webster's New World Dictionary Third Edition* lists *witchcraft*, *magic*, and *enchantments* as synonyms for *sorcery*. It is defined as follows: (1) the supposed use of an evil supernatural power over people and their affairs: witchcraft, black magic." (Examples are: to cast a spell to cause harm to something or someone); 2) seemingly magical power, influence, or charm." This definition does not imply causing harm but influencing an event, situation, or person.

Young's Analytical Concordance of the Bible presents a broader definition of the word *sorcery* as it has been used in the King James Version. The Hebrew words *kashaph*, *kashap*, and *kashaphim*, meaning "wizard" or "witchcraft," are translated in the King James Bible as *sorcerer*, as is the Hebrew word *anan*, which refers to "observing the clouds," a form of divination. The Greek words *mageia* and *magos*, or *magic* in English, are likewise translated sorcerer. Witchcraft, one of the synonyms of sorcery, is given additional synonyms by the concordance: *divination*, *charm*, and *remedy*.

Webster's New World Dictionary further expands the meaning of *sorcerer* by defining *magic* as use of charms, spells, rituals to control and/or cause events or to govern forces such as occultism, baffling effects and or illusions—truly, the practice of magic arts. In this chapter, the word *sorcery* is used as defined by the synonyms and expanded definitions. I do not refer to black magic or a curse on something or someone. The sorcerers will, in all probability, have as their goal to be helpful and to do well for others, yet the end result of following their advice or leading will be our loss.

A sorcerer could be one associated with alchemy as the ancient alchemists concocted drugs and hallucinogens.[2] Manly Hall, in his book *The Secret Teachings of All Ages*, tells us that alchemy and astrology are the oldest sciences of the world. He tells us that mastery of these sciences would restore man from the curse of the forbidden fruit so that he could again enter the Garden of Eden.[3] Alchemy was considered a science of multiplication and a process of improving upon what already existed.

Not only was alchemy considered a science, it was a religion teaching that God is in everything, a universal intelligence, a universal spirit, found

---

[2] Steed, Earnest; *Two Be One*, Logos International, Plainsfield, NJ, (1978), p. 95.

[3] Hall, Manly P., *The Secret Teachings of All Ages*, Jeremy P. Tarcher/Penguin of Penguin Group Inc. New York, NY, (1928), p. 494.

in all matter.⁴ A common definition of an alchemist is one who tries to turn base metal into gold. Certainly, that was one goal, but it also was a ploy to divert the attention from the true nature of the alchemist—that of bringing about a transmutation of material substance. This, in turn, would bring about a change of his spirit from being mortal to immortal.

During the Middle Ages, alchemy was forbidden by the universal church, and one practicing it could be sentenced to death. The common definition of an alchemist was a person who tried to turn base metal into gold; but many alchemists, in truth, practiced an occultist pagan religion. They were ridiculed because people really thought they believed that substances could be turned into gold; however, they were able to practice their occultic religion unrecognized. Alchemists were found all over the world working not only with metals but experimenting with plants and subsequently finding many drugs and psychedelic substances. Hallucinogens and mind-altering substances were used at times to facilitate contact with the spirit world. One author's definition of alchemy is

> our work . . . is the conversion and change of one being into another being, one thing into another thing, weakness into strength, bodily into spiritual nature.⁵

The forerunner of a *chemist* was the alchemist. He not only looked for a way to transform one substance into another, but he also looked for some magical substance from mineral or herb that had the *secret of life, bringing immortality when consumed.*⁶

Earnest Steed, in his book *Two Be One*, makes the following statement:

> At the root of all alchemy was astrology with its macrocosm, microcosm, and transformation.⁷

Various secret societies—Cabalists, Masons, and Rosicrucians—adhered to the philosophy of alchemy down through the ages.⁸ *Morals and*

---

[4] Ibid., p. 498.

[5] Cirlot; *Dictionary of Symbols*, Philosophical Library, NY, (1962), p. 8 reported in *Two Be One* by Steed, p. 89.

[6] Steed, op. cit., p. 93.

[7] Ibid., p. 92.

[8] Pike, Albert, *Morals and Dogma of the Ancient Accepted Scottish Rite of Freemasonry*, LL.H. Jenkins, Inc., Edition Book Manufacturers, Richmond, VA, (1871), pp. 772–792.

Dogma of the Ancient Accepted Scottish Rite of Freemasonry by Albert Pike has twenty pages [772–792] on the philosophical doctrine of the alchemists.

THOTH'S SIGN

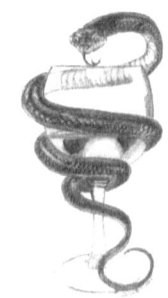

Figure 39. Thoth's sign

Manley Hall, a respected Masonic writer, tells us that alchemy was the secret art of the land of Khem (Ham), or Egypt.[9] Thoth (another name for Cush) was known as the moon god in Egypt. The same god, called Hermes in Greece, was also known as Mercury.[10] The Thoth sign is a flask with a snake coiled around it or a Y-shaped tree with the snake ascending it. This sign of a flask with the snake can be seen on signs at pharmacies in many countries.

The symbol of snakes entwining a rod, staff, or tree (a *caduceus*) is an ancient symbol associated with medicine and healing. Mesopotamians considered the intertwining of serpents as the god of healing. (A four-thousand-year-old beaker with a caduceus on its sides was found in Mesopotamia and is in the Louvre Museum in Paris. It is also shown in the book *Medicine: An Illustrated History* by Lyons and Petrucelli.) The Greek god of healing, Asclepius, had as its symbol *one* snake twined around a rod or staff (Thoth symbol).

---

[9] Hall, Manly P., *The Secret Teachings Of All Ages*, Tarcher/Penguin Books, 375 Hudson Street, New York, NY (1928), pp. 494–509.

[10] *Ibid.*, p. 494; Hislop, Alexander; *The Two Babylons*, Loizeaux Brothers, Neptune New Jersey, (1916), p. 25 and footnote, p. 26.

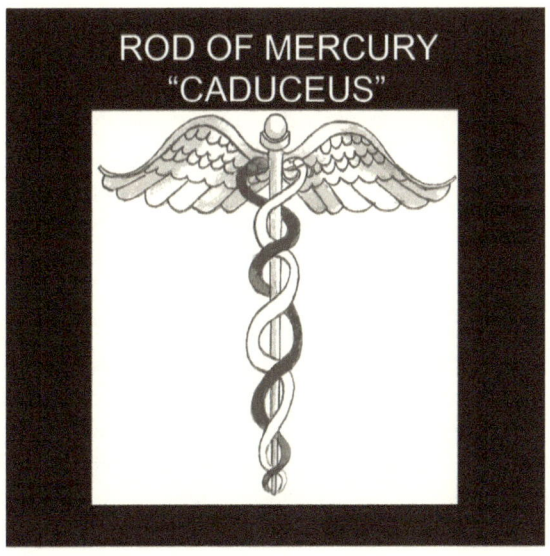

Figure 40. Caduceus

I had the privilege of visiting the ruins of an ancient Asclepius temple of healing in Pergamum, Turkey. The temple still had in its ruins this symbol of a snake climbing a flask and entwining itself around the base. This temple was associated with an ancient medical school, at which the physician Galen was a professor. His concept of disease and healing dominated the *mind-set* of medical science for more than 1,500 years.

The alchemist, the pseudo-scientist in China, also searched for the elixir of eternal life, which he felt was needed in order to harness the energy that created all things, including life. The Taoist alchemist thought he could find a "potion" that contained the secret to life. Over thousands of years, as the alchemist looked for that secret to life, he tested a vast array of substances. He did not comprehend the biochemical aspects of the substance he tested, so the testing of the potions was not always free of danger. In the book *Secrets of the Alchemist*, we are told of the ultimate goal of laboratory alchemy in China: produce the elixir of immortality and:

> according to Chinese records, a number of alchemists—and several emperors—succumbed to fatal doses of these mystical substances. Often the cause was mercury poisoning, since many

alchemical recipes called for ingredients of pure mercury or mercuric compounds.[11]

Pharmaceutical science of today is the study of the biochemical properties of a substance and its interaction with the biochemistry of a living subject. The ancient alchemist had no comprehension of either the biochemistry of a plant or understanding of living organisms. Since man sinned and was driven from the Garden of Eden and lost access to the tree of life, he has ever been looking for the *secret of life*. He attempted to find it through alchemy by blending substances, transforming a substance, or creating a potion that would hopefully give eternal life. The ancient pagan pantheistic beliefs teach that there is constant transformation and change. The pa kua (Chinese circle of harmony) is also a symbol of this concept.

The European alchemist sought to find and capture the *vital energy* that he thought gave life. It was very elusive. The Chinese alchemist looked for it in some herb or plant so as to make a potion that could then be administered. Perhaps this helps explain why the Chinese have so many herbs as medicinals—the constant quest to find one that would bestow eternal life.

Alcohol was called the water of life. It was cold but tasted hot; it was considered water and fire, elements that were regarded as creative.

> The words *whiskey* and *vodka* both mean, *water of life*, conveying the belief that opposites were blended to achieve life.[12]

Ancient medical treatment involved the use of a great many practices and substances in an attempt to relieve disease. It involved not only herbs and concoctions but also minerals, acts, dances, rituals of many types, and the many preparations the alchemists had made. *Hippocrates* (460–370 BC) *and Greek medicine* brought about a change to medical treatment and influenced the thinking of doctors for four hundred to five hundred years. He used very few of the usual treatment modalities and taught that disease was related to lifestyle. He believed in the cosmic forces, four humors (fluids) and the dualism concept; yet he felt that exercise and rest, nutrition, and excretion were the great influences for health or for disease.[13]

---

[11] Editors of Time-Life Books, Secrets of the Alchemists, Time-Life Books, Alexandria, VA, (1990), p. 110.

[12] Steed, op. cit. p. 93.

[13] Lyons, Albert S. M.D.; Petrucelli, H. M.D.; *Medicine an Illustrated History*, Harry N. Abrams, Inc. Publishers, NY, (1978), p. 195.

Alternative & Mystical Healing Therapies

After Hippocrates, the physician *Galen* (AD 129–200) changed the *mind-set* of medicine. Hippocrates's influence lasted 400 or more years, but Galen's influence lasted more than 1,500 years. Galen was at the Asclepius healing center and medical school in Pergamos of Asia Minor (Turkey). Hippocrates had brought in a breath of fresh air to medicine and looked at lifestyle as the greatest influence on disease. He advocated living in such a way as to lessen illness. Galen turned the mind of physicians the other way. He advocated the use of many drugs. *Theriac* was a mixture of more than seventy minerals and substances (eventually over two hundred) that Galen advocated. These herbs and substances were blended together for use as a universal antidote for illness, snake bites, or any type of disorder.[14] Theriac as a universal treatment concoction was used until the late 1800s in Europe. Today a similar popular medicinal is to be found in Russia. It is called mumio and contains approximately fifty different substances. Masonic writer Manley Palmer Hall states the following:

> Upon the authority of Hippocrates, Galen, and Avicenna, medieval astrologers and physicians developed an elaborate system of correspondences between the planets and herbs, chemicals, and mineral medicines. They administered them according to the rules of sympathy and antipathy, and judged the disease by the afflicting planet and its aspects.[15]

The intrigue to treat disease with some sort of mineral, herb, or concoction has been present throughout time and has continued to our present day. There are many proven valuable pharmaceutical therapies in use, but the need for their use often could be greatly reduced by following a different lifestyle of exercise and diet. Is it feasible that by depending upon a medicinal rather than lifestyle changes, thus eliminating or reducing the need for therapy, could fall under the definition of sorcery? Pharmaceuticals are heavily used in the mind therapy sciences, from anxiety to attention-deficit disorder, depression and psychosis. There are times when nothing short of a specific medicine will be of value in treatment; however, for many problems, there are other solutions. It is man's preoccupation with the belief that for every symptom and distress, there is a medicinal therapy that could be thought of as a deception or sorcery.

Wednesday, February 9, 2011, the *Oregonian*, a Portland, Oregon, newspaper carried and article titled "Take Two pills and Call Me in

---

[14] *Ibid.*, p. 259.
[15] Hall, Manley, *The Story of Healing*, Citadel Press, New York, (1928), p. 162.

2000 Years." Underwater archeologists had found a shipwreck (age: two-thousand-plus years) in the Mediterranean Sea forty years ago but just recently the Smithsonian Institute had analyzed pills found in a container in the ship. These were medicinal tablets. DNA revealed them to be a variety of herbs: celery, alfalfa, wild onion, radish, cabbage, wild carrot, yarrow, jack bean and hibiscus, willow, aster, common bean and nasturtium. This same article tells that *The Hippocratic Collection* is a series of ancient Greek texts attributed to Hippocrates, which refers to 380 medicinal herbs used for a variety of ailments. Records show that Greek physicians used 45 different herbs in the pharmaceutical approach to health and healing.

One of the leading causes of death is an adverse reaction from drugs even when given properly by the practitioner. When we combine the accidental wrong medicine, or overdose etc., we recognize there is a major problem with use of medicinal therapies. These problems not only occur from physicians but from patients as well. It would be a wise choice to seek ways of dealing with illness and disorders with as few medicines as possible.

There is a movement with some physicians across this country to blend conventional medicine with alternative and complementary methods; this blending is referred to as integrative medicine. There has been a rapid increase in the number of clinics adopting this *mix* of the scientific with the non-scientific. This blending is most deceptive for people who are unaware of the devil's sorceries.

> Andrew Weil M.D. has devoted the past 30 years to developing, teaching and educating others on the principles of integrative medicine. Weil is an internationally recognized expert on integrative medicine, medicinal herbs, and mind-body interactions. . . . He is a clinical professor of internal medicine and the founder and director of the Program of Integrative Medicine (PIM) at the College of Medicine, University of Arizona in Tucson, Arizona. Weil received both his medical degree and his undergraduate AB degree in biology (botany) from Harvard University.[16]

Dr. Weil is the author of many books. A review of the titles of these books reveals his interest in meditation, deep breathing, guided imagery, and sound and music therapy. He also has vast influence with the public. He trains other doctors in converting to the integrative method of practice.

---

[16]   *http://www.webmd.com/andrew-weil*

The following quotation will give some insight to the direction of his beliefs and teachings and their orientation. Dr. Weil wrote about his *fire walking*. He spoke of walking through forty feet of extremely hot coals and experienced no pain or burns or sensation of heat. He said that there was just a crunch as he stepped on the coals.

> This was in a large group with Tony Robins, where everyone got very charged dancing to African drums, chanting, and engaging in other rituals. On another occasion I got burned attempting a mere six-foot walk over cooler coals. On that occasion, there were no exciting rituals, no charismatic leader, and only a small group of not-very bonded individuals.[17]

Upon reading the above comment from Dr. Weil, I thought again of the verse in Deuteronomy 18:9–12:

> When thou art come into the land which the Lord thy God giveth thee, thou shalt not learn to do after the abominations of those nations. There shall not be found among you anyone that maketh his son or his daughter *to pass through the fire*, or that useth divination, or an observer of times, or an enchanter, or a witch. Or a charmer, or a consulter with familiar spirits, or a wizard, or a necromancer. *For all that do those things are an abomination unto the Lord;* and because of these abominations the Lord thy God doth drive them out from before you.

What is it that attracts and motivates people to fire-walk? What is to be gained from it? What prevents burns to the feet? It is an act performed in many places of the world. I lived for a short time in Phuket, Thailand, where once a year a festival was held for worshiping Satan. It was my understanding that fire walking was a part of this festival. I have been in *pagan provinces* of Russia where similar festivals are held. Revelation 13:13, 14 (NIV) gives an answer to the above question:

> And he performed great and miraculous signs, even causing fire to come down from heaven to earth in full view of men. *Because of the signs he was given power to do on behalf of the first beast, he deceived the inhabitants of the earth.*

---

[17] *www.drweil.com/u/QA/QA221693/*

Satan will use fire to cause men to believe he, man, is God. God sent fire from heaven to ignite the sacrifice of Abel, at Solomon's dedication of the temple, at the sacrifice Elijah offered on Mount Carmel. He sent fire to consume the soldiers of Ahaziah, king of Israel, when they went to arrest Elijah. In the days of Daniel, God preserved the three Hebrews in the fiery furnace. Just because God has allowed Satan to have power over fire, we need not be deceived if all miracles are tested by the scriptures.

By sending fire down from heaven at the end of time and protecting those who walk in fire, does not Satan hold himself out to be God? Does he not deceive by these miracles he performs? Should we not carefully consider the teachings of those people who are led by his power? They may be highly trained in the science of conventional medicine, yet the deception comes as they blend in Satan's method of healing with God's methods. Let the followers of Christ beware.

Another popular physician and author, Gabriel Cousens, MD, also leads the march toward integrative medicine. His orientation is revealed by his quotation found in chapter on Ayurveda in this book. Dr. Cousens has a popular following in regard to his dietary writings. He writes of foods being held over chakra areas of the body to establish which colored foods, when eaten, would most enhance the power of the chakras. His books strongly reflect Ayurvedic and Hindu concepts.

Another powerful influence enticing interest in New Age/new spirituality exists in the USA, Canada, and in areas of the world where the television show of Oprah Winfrey penetrates. She has featured many individuals on a repeated basis who, by their appearances on her show and their books promoted by Oprah, have given great exposure and the potential of acceptance of New Age/neo-pagan/new spirituality concepts by vast millions of people. Several of those individuals featured by Oprah were Marianne Williamson, famous for her *Course on Miracles*, which was channeled to her by a spirit; Gary Zukav and his book *Seat of a Soul* espouses the divinity of man; Oprah's endorsement of the book *The Secret* by Rhonda Byrne, which teaches that we are all *God*; Eckhart Tolle and his book published in 2008 titled *A New Earth: Awakening To Your Life's Purpose*, teaching a shift in consciousness with an indwelling of divinity referred to as "Christ"; promotion of the popular Dr. Mehmet Oz, a Muslim and Sufi (mystical order in Islam), intertwines the occult with his knowledge of nutrition and lifestyle; all recipients of powerful promotion by Oprah's show. Dr. Oz now has his own TV show wherein he mingles the good with the bad. His wife is a Reiki master, also a follower of the late world-renowned spiritualist Emanuel Swedenborg; Dr. Oz is a strong promoter of her spirit powered healing technique.

Alternative & Mystical Healing Therapies

Rick Warren—"America's pastor," author of *The Purpose-Driven Church* and *The Purpose-Driven Life*—recently launched on January 15, 2011, a fifty-two-week course from his Saddleback Church on wellness. This program is titled the Daniel Challenge and is a weekly program guided by Mehmet Oz, MD; Daniel Amen, MD; and Mark Hyman MD, all well-trained specialists and highly versed in health and nutrition but also heavily engaged in promoting New Age/neo-pagan concepts. They will be bringing up-to-date nutrition and healthful living information but will be blending in Eastern meditation techniques as an important component of health.

Rick Warren has far-reaching influence. His organization is extended to and has communication with more than 160 nation networks, and 400,000 ministers and priests have attended his teaching seminars.[18]

In the book of Acts 19, we are told that the God of heaven through the Holy Spirit empowered Paul; miracles were wrought. But there were seven sons of Sceva who tried to imitate the miracles of Paul, and the evil spirit fell upon them, and they were beaten and bruised and fled naked because they took the name of Jesus to use in their sorcery. They cannot mix; they cannot mix at all.

God's design for health and healing is not to be mixed with that of Satan's. Let us review the basics of what has been presented in this book. The devil desires to draw men's minds away from recognizing God the Creator. He devised a counterfeit story of creation based upon the blending of two opposing divisions of a supposed universal energy, which is considered god. This energy, when blended in the right proportions, brought about the creation of the universe (cosmos), earth, and man. This universal energy (god) is said to be in all substances of the universe, including man. Man need only to bring the god within himself to a higher level to obtain immortality and godhood.

Man's journey on earth, according to the pagan, is to escape from the cycle of reincarnation and to progress upward to become an ascended master or god himself. This may take many lifetimes. Many ways are promoted to shorten the journey to godhood, often called higher consciousness. Yoga meditation, yoga exercises, qi gong exercises, and psychedelic drugs used to connect with spirit entities are some of the ways believed to shorten the pathway to Nirvana or godhood. Another way to hasten this progression toward godhood is to be a follower of a guru. I invite the reader to pause and reflect upon the contrast between the theory and variety of modalities

---

[18] Smith, Warren, A Wonderful Deception, Lighthouse Trails Publishing, Silverton, OR, (2009), p. ix.

presented for healing by *energy or vibrational medicine* and that of being in harmony with the physical laws of God. Our Creator is to be upheld as the source of healing, and His physical and spiritual laws are to be followed.

There is a power in the universe, and it is the power of God. It is not inherent in the planets. It is not hidden away in the mind of man, waiting for some gimmick to release it. It is not accessed by pendulums or radionic machines or by mindless meditation. The power of God is accessed by prayer and Bible study and obedience to His physical and spiritual laws.

The Samaritans were deceived by Simon Magus; so do many Christians today give heed to Satan's sorceries. The ardent student of the scriptures will not be misled as the teachings of Satan are not in harmony.

> Take each verse of this chapter [Revelation 18], and read it carefully, especially the last two: 'And the light of a candle shall shine no more at all in thee; and the voice of the bridegroom and of the bride shall be heard no more at all in thee: for thy merchants were the great men of the earth; for by thy *sorceries (magic arts)* were all nations deceived. And in her was found the blood of prophets, and of saints, and of all that were slain upon the earth. (Rev. 18:23, 24)

Modern civilizations suppose that ancient heathen superstitions are not with us today, but the Word of God unmasks present practices that are the same as old-time practices of magic. Revelation 22:14, 15 shares with us a sobering consideration:

> Blessed are they that do his commandments, that they may have right to the tree of life, and may enter in through the gates into the city. For without are dogs, and **sorcerers**, and whoremongers, and murderers, and idolaters and whosoever loveth and maketh a lie.

18

Hypnosis

I once received a call from the hospital to come quickly to care for a lady who had been water skiing. She had fallen into the water and had been run over by a boat, sustaining severe injury to one leg. Upon reaching the emergency room, I saw the patient had several huge lacerations across her thigh inflicted by the propeller of the boat. She had lost much blood and looked pale. Bleeding had stopped, so there was time to give her blood and fluids intravenously before taking her to the operating room. The injuries were so large and destructive to her leg that I decided to ask a plastic surgeon to join me in caring for her in the operating room.

We were able to save the leg and expected proper healing and the return to normal use. Three days later, I scheduled a change of the bandages on the leg. By that time, the bandages had crusted and dried, sticking to the wounds. Changing the dressings was going to be painful.

The plastic surgeon arrived in her room before I did and proceeded to change the dressings. When I entered the room, the patient had her eyes closed; she was not showing any tension or any sign that she was in distress. When I spoke to her, the doctor said that she was sleeping but he would awaken her soon. He finished with the new dressings then told her that he was going to count backward from five, and when he got to zero, she would awake.

He counted, five, four, three, two—she began to move—one and zero. She awoke and was happy and smiling, as well as delighted that the dressings were changed and she knew nothing of the ordeal. It seemed wonderful. Who could object to such a pleasant method of dealing with injuries? I was surprised to learn that the surgeon used hypnosis. I had known him for several years and operated with him many times. I opposed hypnosis and never suggested it to my patients. I was embarrassed to have had this happen to one of my patients without first being able to share with her my concerns about its use.

Why should I object? Was it not wonderful to relieve someone from a painful procedure? Why would I oppose this humane approach? Was it not better than giving a pain medication an hour prior and then removing the bandages? She was wide awake and pain free and did not remember the procedure.

Some doctors in medical practice have used hypnosis for many years, and it is considered an acceptable method of treatment in the medical field. It has been used as an anesthetic in operative procedures, as well as in treatment of psychological ailments. Yet many physicians choose not to use it in their practices.

What is hypnosis? How does it work? Where does it come from? Why does not every doctor use it? These are important questions that deserve answers. Let us first look at a dictionary definition. Hypnosis is:

> An induced state of mind in which the subject is responsive to the suggestions of the hypnotist. This state may be to the degree of resembling sleep, called a hypnotic trance.[1]
>
> In hypnosis, the hypnotist talks directly to the unconscious of his subject and the cortex gets out of the way, sometimes so far out of the way that the subject cannot remember anything that happened during the hypnotic session.[2]
>
> Hypnosis is bypassing the critical faculty of the conscious mind in order to establish selective thinking within the subconscious mind. It is the ultimate means of heightening motivation by programming your subconscious mind to work in cooperation with your conscious desires. (Clinical Hypnosis Institute, http://www.ccnprogroup.com/id21.htm)

This suggests that there are degrees of hypnosis that are below the hypnotic trance. What of its origin? Was the encounter in the Garden between Eve and the serpent a form of hypnosis? Eve made a fatal mistake.

---

[1] *Mirriam Webster Advanced Dictionary.*
[2] Green, Elmer & Alyce, *Beyond Biofeedback*, fifth printing, Academy of Parapsychology and Medicine, Knoll Publishing Co., (1977) p. 164,5

Instead of leaving the proximity of the tree, she lingered and entered into dialogue with the voice apparently coming from the serpent. She was no match for the disguised foe.

> And he said to the woman, "Has God indeed said, 'You shall not eat of every tree of the garden'?" And the woman said unto the serpent, "We may eat of the fruit of the trees of the garden: But of the fruit of the tree which is in the midst of the garden, God hath said, 'Ye shall not eat of it, neither shall you touch it, lest you die.'" And the serpent said unto the woman, "You shall not surely die: For God knows that in the day ye eat of it, your eyes shall be opened, and you will be like God, knowing good and evil." (Gen. 3:1–4)

The apostle Paul wrote to the church at Corinth the following:

> But I fear, lest somehow as the serpent deceived Eve by his craftiness, so your minds may be corrupted from the simplicity which is in Christ. (2 Cor. 11:3)

Was the temptation of Christ by the devil in the Judean desert a form of hypnotism?

> Then Jesus was led up by the Spirit into the wilderness to be tempted by the devil. . . . Now when the tempter came to him he said, "*If* you be the Son of God, command that these stones become bread." . . . But He answered and said "It is written, Man shall not live by bread alone, but by every word that proceeds out of the mouth of God." . . . Then Jesus said to him, "Away with you, Satan! For it is written, 'You shall worship the Lord your God, and Him only you shall serve.'" (Matt. 4:1–10)

Let us consider comments made in the *New Age Encyclopedia*:

> What is now called hypnosis has existed in almost all societies in the past, though its nature was only rarely understood or appreciated. Hypnotic phenomena began to be studied in Europe in the sixteenth century, when these occurrences were attributed to magnetism, which was understood to be a subtle

influence exerted by every object in the universe on every other object.³

Medical history texts record hypnotic phenomena being studied by physicians, such as Paracelsus, in Europe in the midsixteenth century. Its power source was explained as a magnetic fluid that connected all substances in the universe and that which could not be seen, demonstrated, or measured. In the seventeenth century, it again appeared in the writings of several notorious physicians.⁴ The power of suggestion, or hypnosis, was used by these physicians to treat medical conditions.

In the eighteenth century, Emanuel Swedenborg (1688–1772) studied this "magnetism" credited to hypnotism and tied it in with his interest in the spiritual world. This, in turn, laid the grounds for spiritualism.⁵ Swedenborg and his ideas of spiritualism influenced the world of the occult for nearly two centuries.

If you were to consult an encyclopedia on the word *hypnosis*, you would most likely find that a physician, Franz Anton Mesmer, is referred to as the father of modern hypnosis. He is not truly the father of hypnosis, but he did make it so well-known that for nearly a century this phenomenon was known as mesmerism. Let us review Dr. Mesmer's history.

He graduated from medical school in Vienna in 1766. That same year, he published a book, *On the Influence of the Planets*, in which he proposed stroking diseased patients with magnets to effect a cure. In 1773, he claimed his first cure by the use of magnets. Mesmer was a believer in astrology and felt the body of man was a microcosm of the macrocosm (universe). He felt that man, earth, and the universe were tied together with a universal magnetic fluid. Mesmer continued his medical practice using magnets to cure disease.⁶

Mesmer heard of a Swabian priest, John Gassner, who was simply passing his hands across diseased bodies and effecting "cures":

> Mesmer observed Gassner and thought it was done by the power of the same magnetic fluid that he felt explained his activities with magnets. He then dispensed with the magnets and achieved equal results by use of his hands. Eventually he dispensed with the hand technique and used the mind only as

---

[3] *New Age Encyclopedia*, Gale Research, Detroit, MI, (1990), p. 28.
[4] *New Age Encyclopedia*, Gale Research, Detroit, MI, (1990), p. 28.
[5] *Ibid.*, p. 28.
[6] *Ibid.*, pp. 28, 58.

the modality of influencing animal magnetism (power believed to effect hypnotism).[7]

In 1784, a book written by French doctor and spiritualist Jean Philippe Francois Deleuze referred to this same phenomenon (hypnotism) as "animal magnetism." Deleuze seemed to want to separate the name "Mesmer" from the method.[8]

> For much of the nineteenth century, the term 'animal magnetism' also encompassed clairvoyance, empathy, mediumistic trances, and many other psychic abilities and psychological phenomena, the relationships between which were far from clear.[9]

Let us briefly review the influence of Dr. Mesmer and the different methods he used in his medical therapy. First, he started by passing magnets across the bodies of his patients. He would make large tubs and fill them with chemicals to produce an electrical charge; placed on the tubs were iron knobs. People would stand around the tubs, holding on to the iron knobs in order to receive *magnetic* therapy. His treatments progressed to simply passing of hands over the body.

Eventually, he used only the mind to accomplish the desired effect. The hypnotic state could be so deep that surgical procedures could be performed during the trance. To accomplish this involved not only an expert "mesmerist" but also a willing, submissive person. A British surgeon, James Esdaile (1805–1859), practiced in India and used the trance state for anesthesia during surgery. He performed 261 painless operations with mesmerism as the only anesthetic. When he returned to Scotland, he found that mesmerism used as an anesthetic did not work well there.[10]

The inducement of the hypnotic state by suggestion was used in many ways by the various practitioners who became skilled in its use.[11] The British Medical Society, in 1893, concluded that hypnosis was a true science even though they were not able to perfectly explain it. There could be no doubt that it was much more than a sham or fake act. Great influence

---

[7] *Ibid.*

[8] *Ibid.*, pp. 28–29, 58.

[9] *Ibid.*, p. 58.

[10] Garrison, Fielding H. M.D., *History of Medicine*, W.B. Saunders & Co., Philadelphia, PA, (1929), p. 428.

[11] *Ibid.*, p. 369; *New Age Encyclopedia*, p. 58.

and results did indeed occur with its use, and it appeared as though its action was only positive with little to no adverse side effects.

The American Medical Association was much slower in embracing this form of treatment. Physicians at large were not fully convinced of its value, though there was no denying that it had great power to affect a person. There was no real lasting effect on disease. It seemed to be more related to the treatment of the mind and so has not been widely used by all physicians. Hypnosis was given official sanction by the American Medical Association in 1958.

We are warned that it will be in the area of *science* that Satan will exert such deceptive practices in the last days. In the days of Paul and Timothy, there also existed false sciences, and Paul gives us warnings concerning them:

> O Timothy, keep that which is committed to thy trust, avoiding profane and vain babblings, and oppositions of science falsely so called. (1 Tim. 6:20 KJV).

Dr. Franz Joseph Gall (1757–1828) was an anatomy instructor. He was the first to show that different parts of the brain had specific functions.[12] He carried this too far, however, and felt that the character and personality could be recognized by observing the bumps and ridges on the skull. This idea he carried even further, suggesting that the mind, character, and personality could be altered by massage to the head or pressure applied to specific areas of the skull. This concept was named phrenology.

Phrenology was a pseudo-science and was adopted by those practicing mesmerism and other occult therapies. The spiritualist movement was attracted to phrenology and mesmerism. Psychology in the late 1800s and early 1900s commonly used mesmerism (hypnotism). Phrenology was popular with non-medical-trained practitioners in the late 1800s and early 1900s and then faded. In recent years, it has surfaced again along with the many other so-called alternative/complementary approaches to healing.

Mesmerism or hypnotism allowed one mind to be placed under the control of another mind. This is a method originated by Satan to further his control of man and separate man from his Creator—to place human philosophy where divine philosophy should be. In the long run, it is not restorative; it is a destructive influence on the mind.

---

[12] Garrison, op. cit., p. 539.

Michael Harner, the leading "shaman" of our time, an instructor of shamans, includes hypnotism as one of the techniques utilized by shamans through the ages in the following statement in his book *The Way of the Shaman* (p. 112):

> The burgeoning field of holistic medicine shows a tremendous amount of experimentation involving the reinvention of many techniques long practiced in shamanism, such as visualization, altered state of consciousness, aspects of psychoanalysis, *hypnotherapy*, meditation, positive attitude, stress-reduction, and mental and emotional expression of personal will for health and healing. In a sense, shamanism is being reinvented in the West precisely because it is needed. (emphasis added)

The business world is offered commercial mind-training courses by a variety of teachers. Some of these courses teach hypnotism even though the title of the course will not suggest so. Course titles such as "conditioning," "programming," "brain-wave training," "alpha training," etc., may actually be hypnosis. There can be consequential adverse effects to the student taking part in such a course. Elmer and Alyce Green (doctoral researchers in psychology), in their book *Beyond Biofeedback*, state that thousands of students in these courses will sooner or later experience serious mental changes such as neurosis or even psychosis. They warn that the greatest danger, however, is obtaining "psychic advisors" who are assistants in the course. The Greens warn that there is the possibility of mediumistic "possession" via the influence of the advisors.[13]

> Almost all of the popular commercial mind-training programs use a heavy dose of hypnotic programming. It may not be called hypnosis, and in fact it may be vehemently denied by instructors, but nevertheless many of the courses use hypnotic techniques that are "right out of the book." . . . The Attorney General of the State of Kansas sent us an instructors' manual from one of these four-day courses and asked for our evaluation. The hypnotic nature of the procedures was obvious. As an example, twelve times in the four-day course the instructor programmed his trainees with the following statements before

---

[13] Green, Elmer and Alyce, *Beyond Biofeedback*, Knoll Publishing Co., (1977), pp. 319–323.

> bringing them out of a state of suggestion achieved by hypnotic countdown: "You will continue to listen to my voice. You will continue to follow instructions at all levels of mind, including the outer conscious level. This is for your benefit, you desire it—and this is so." ... After a few days of programming during which the trainee is in a suggestive state much of the time, it is almost certain that behavioral and perceptual changes will occur. The changes may not last in every case, but for a period of time "graduates" do not seem the same to themselves and often seen different to friends.[14]

The point brought out by the Greens that there is great danger in allowing another individual to control or even strongly influence us in the science of *mind control* brings to mind the advice given long ago by practitioners who had abandoned the practice of hypnotism.

Elmer and Alyce Green wrote an article exposing the commercial mind-training courses and received not only some great stories of benefit but also stories of problems from receiving hypnosis. I will give one story and then copy their excerpts from the article.

> A woman wrote that after her husband had taken the course one of his "imaginary psychic advisers" unexpectedly began speaking to him without being asked. The adviser explained that he (the adviser) was God and that for spiritual reasons the wife also must take the course. When she refused to do this, "God" told him to get a divorce. She and her teenage sons were unable to influence her husband. He also developed some other peculiarities.[15]

In April 2011, I received a copy of an article that appeared in a Colorado town's newspaper, *Highlands Ranch Herald*, April 4, 2011. This article was lauding and promoting the value of using hypnotism in childbirth. I share with you some comments found in this article.

> HypnoBirthing, which is a registered trademark, has been found to significantly reduce stress and improve the well-being of newborns, and classes are now being offered at Westridge Recreation Center. Even the family education center at a

---

[14] *Ibid.*, p. 316,317
[15] *Ibid.*

Christian operated Littleton Hospital is planning on training nurses and physicians on how to assist mothers who use HypnoBirthing. . . . HynoBirthing classes teach expecting parents how to wipe away anxiety through positive thoughts and reassurance. Hypnosis CDs containing messages directed at *imaging* a healthy birth; *visualization* of good outcomes and pain-free childbirth are also part of the 2 ½ hour class sessions. (emphasis added)

Drs. Green, psychologists, continue their discussion of hypnotism by describing long-term effects of use of hypnotism in *Beyond Biofeedback* (pp. 320–321).

Facts that may relate to hypnobirthing training: Phenomena that are claimed by commercial mind training teachers and by many of their students, namely:

- A person can "go down" into his own "unconscious" and while in that deep "level" can program his own physiological and psychological processes so that various diseases in him that have not yielded to standard medical treatment can be brought under control.
- While at his deep "level" a person can learn to manipulate the physical, emotional, and mental natures of other persons, sick or healthy, and thereby modify their behavior.
- While at his "level" a person can learn to manipulate nature so that coincidences, "accidents," or lack of accidents, can come under his control. This is, essentially, a promise of psychokinetic powers.

They continue:

Now from a traditional psychological point of view, the above ideas are sheer nonsense, some would say 'sheer madness.' From that point of view, the tens of thousands who have taken mind-training courses and are convinced of the reality of some or all of the above claims have been programmed into a serious delusional system and can be expected sooner or later, if rationality is not reestablished, to develop, in consequence, some degree of neurosis or psychosis.

Reading this article on hypnobirthing brought to me a feeling of sadness as I remembered the many warnings given through the years by various Christian authors regarding Christians using hypnotism as individuals or of its practice being brought into Christian hospitals. Let us consider dealing with anxiety by claiming the promise given by Jesus:

> Come unto me, all you who labor and are heavy laden, and I will give you rest. Take my yoke upon you, and learn from me; for I am gentle and lowly in heart: and you will find rest for your souls. For my yoke is easy, and my burden is light. (Matt. 11:28–30)

> You will keep him in perfect peace, Whose mind is stayed on You, because he trusts in You. (Isa. 26:3)

A great danger occurs when we seek counseling from professional or lay counselors. The education and source of knowledge of so many of these individuals is from the cistern of modern psychology. The counselor may be a Christian, but if his education and mind are fixed in the philosophy of modern world's humanistic psychological principles, his very influence on you by accepting his advice has danger. The principles of counseling must come from the scriptures; our Creator is the Great Counselor.

> For unto us a child is born, unto us a son is given: And the government will be upon His shoulder. And his name will be called Wonderful, **Counsellor**, Mighty God, Everlasting Father, Prince of Peace. (Isa. 9:6)

There are people who feel they are wise enough to take parts of these false sciences and use them to their advantage, but the warning is given to have nothing to do with them. Even to investigate the theories can expose us to Satan's power. Our duty is to direct the mind of man to God, the true *Mind Therapist*.

> And do not be conformed to this world: but be transformed by the renewing of your mind, that you may prove what is that good, and acceptable, and perfect, will of God. (Rom. 12:2)

> Let this mind be in you, which was also in Christ Jesus. (Phil. 2:5)

19

BIOFEEDBACK

A common medical complaint with which doctors are challenged is headaches. When a patient complained of such to me, I would place my hand on the back of their neck and feel for tight muscles and tender points at the base of the skull where the neck muscles attach. When there was tenderness on the skull, I could be reasonably sure that that person had excess tension of the neck muscles, and the pain was a result of the chronic contraction of these muscles. The point on the skull where the muscles attach becomes sore and contributes to the headache. I would advise the patient to practice relaxing these muscles several times a day, massage the neck muscles, apply moist heat, and attempt to discover initiating stress factors that led to the tenseness.

In the 1960s, I read in medical journals of another method of treating people with stress headaches. This method was called biofeedback. Simply stated, it was a procedure where electrodes were attached to the muscles of the neck, which in turn would be attached to an oscilloscope indicating electrical nerve impulses stimulating the neck muscles. With conscious effort, an individual could learn to reduce the excess nerve impulses and tension in the muscles, and the headaches would cease. Biofeedback sounded harmless and possibly might work better than the method I used. The procedure was not done by physical therapists in my area, and so I never prescribed this treatment method.

Migraine headaches usually occur from a different physiological dysfunction than tension headaches. They occur on one side of the head and usually are preceded by symptoms of dimming vision on one side and strange sensations at various locations. Sometimes apparent weakness of certain muscles will be manifest. These symptoms occur, it is believed by physicians, as a result of artery constriction over one side of the brain; after a few minutes, the same vessels will dilate, resulting in pain. Many factors, including mental stress, can trigger such a headache. Present-day therapy involves using medicines to cause constriction of the dilated artery with varying degrees of relief. This type of headache may last from a few hours to days. It is often incapacitating, affecting the ability to attend school or work. Migraine headaches are notoriously difficult to treat.

Medical literature has featured articles telling of the use of "biofeedback" as treatment for migraine headaches. These articles reported that up to 80 percent of patients with migraines received great relief by using biofeedback treatments. It sounded like good, safe therapy, and I never had any adverse thoughts against such a method. Over time, it was shown that many other physical ailments, such as high blood pressure, some gastrointestinal disorders, asthma, neuromuscular disorders such as post-stroke rehabilitation, cerebral palsy, spinal cord injuries, anxiety states, Reynaud's phenomena, etc., have been helped with the use of biofeedback.

In the 1980s, I began to be aware of different types of medical treatments referred to as alternative or complementary medicine. I had concerns about those treatments as it appeared to me that hypnotism-spiritualism was probably the source of their power. When reading articles and books written by Christian authors explaining the nature of certain alternative therapies, I would notice that biofeedback was included in the list of treatment methods those books advised against.

In 1987, the Biblical Research Committee of a religious denomination presented a report on the *New Age Movement* and alternative medical therapies. In this paper is a section dealing with various medical treatment methods that were believed to be *spiritualistic* in nature. Three times the word *biofeedback* is mentioned as one such method. I found that this same labeling of biofeedback occurred in several other books written to expose spiritualism in alternative medicine methods. I was surprised and questioned this label against biofeedback. It occurred to me that I needed to do some in-depth study of biofeedback and to arrive at my own conclusion on this issue. I will share with you my discoveries.

Before proceeding with biofeedback investigation, I wish to establish the definition as to the word *biofeedback*. It is possible in this discussion for confusion to occur between the word *monitoring* and *biofeedback*. Monitoring refers to some mechanical or electrical device, such as an electroencephalogram, electrocardiogram, or electromyography, which reveals electrical biological functioning. Applying electrodes to neck muscles and to an oscilloscope, wearing any type of apparatus to reveal physiological functioning such as a blood pressure monitor, is using a monitor. When I use the word *biofeedback*, I am speaking specifically to a method that uses a combination of monitoring and adding a mental act to facilitate an altered state of consciousness. This is usually achieved by use of *muscle relaxation, deep breathing exercises*, use of a *mantra* or repetitive sentences/phrases, and *visualization*.

The special paper prepared by the Biblical Research Committee listed several sets of questions that need to be answered as a person studies medical treatment methods to determine if they are *spiritually* safe. The committee took these questions from Dr. Warren Peters's book, *Mystical Medicine*. They are excellent questions. No single question should determine the issue, but several questions, when answered, should give evidence of a spiritualistic relationship before you finalize judgment.

The first set of questions was: Where did the method come from? What is its source? Does it have mystical roots? With what other therapies is it often associated? What did the founder believe? What is the life story of the founder or founders?

A renowned German brain physiologist Oscar Vogt of the Berlin Institute, during the 1890s, was using hypnosis in guided sessions. Some of the people in the sessions learned to put themselves, for a self-determined time, into a state similar to the hypnotic state they achieved with the doctor's guidance.[1,2] Vogt found he could have these people, in their auto-hypnotic practices, treat and alleviate many different stress-like medical disorders with which they were afflicted. In the early 1900s, Johannes Schultz, a psychiatrist and neurologist in Berlin, continued the work that Vogt started. This state of self-hypnosis was called autohypnosis.

Schultz wanted to perfect autohypnosis because it would eliminate the tendency of the participant to develop dependence on the hypnotist. It was recognized that the state of self-hypnosis could be induced by (1) using certain basic verbal formulas repeated over and over by the individual desiring autohypnosis as repeating these phrases contributed to developing a state of pronounced, (2) *relaxation* of the muscular and vascular systems as did practicing, (3) *deep slow breathing*, and (4) *visualizing* colors, objects, and abstract concepts.

---

[1] Green, Elmer Ph.D., and Alyce M.A., *Beyond Biofeedback*, Knoll Publishing Co., (1989), p. 26.

[2] Hill, Ann, *A Visual Encyclopedia of Unconventional Medicine*, Crown Publishing Inc. NY, (1978), p. 190.

This is followed by meditating on one's own feelings or on the image of another person, and finally, at the deepest level, *one may interrogate and get* "answers from the unconscious" levels of one's own nature, as Schultz put it.[3]

Dr. Wolfgang Luthe had been a student of Schultz and continued the work after Schultz's death. Luthe called autohypnosis *autogenic training* in a book authored by Schultz and Luthe (1959). In the early 1960s, Dr. Joe Kamiya of San Francisco attached an electroencephalograph to college students' heads to see if they could, at will, change their brain-wave patterns. He found they could. He came up with the word *biofeedback*.

He studied the brain waves of Zen meditators and proposed that it might be possible to develop a "psychophysiology of consciousness."[4]

Dr. Kamiya presented a lecture at the Psychophysiological Research Society meeting in 1965, which was attended by one Elmer Green, PhD, a physicist and psychologist. It was the first time Dr. Green had heard of biofeedback. He was inspired to investigate this ability to self-control brain-wave patterns.[5]

There were many therapists who dabbled in the use of autogenic training, but one outstanding investigative group led the way to what we now call biofeedback. Dr. Green; Alyce Green, MA, a psychologist; and Dale Walters PhD, a colleague, were investigators at the Menninger Foundation, a psychiatric institute in Topeka, Kansas. In 1965, they began to explore the autogenic techniques in their research. Dr. Green developed electronic devices to monitor physiological changes while people were in autogenic training. They could see changes in the rate of nerve impulses, muscular tension and relaxation, temperature of the skin in specific locations, and brain-wave amplitude and rates.

From these studies of autohypnosis or biofeedback, brain-wave monitoring studies were done. By *muscle relaxation, deep slow breathing*, and use of *mantra* phrases along with *visualization*, a certain brain-wave rate called theta could be achieved. It is at this level of brain activity that the autohypnosis takes place. Dr. Green stated the following:

---

[3] Green, op. cit., p. 27.
[4] *Ibid.*, pp. 44, 118, 119.
[5] *Ibid.*

> In my view theta training is a form of accelerated meditation—and the benefits to students are incalculable. They range from better physical functioning, to improved emotional balance, to sharpened intellect, to true creativity—to the solution of insoluble problems in unpredictable ways, coming into mind as from another dimension.[6]

With the addition of electronic monitors, a person could see evidence of changes in his physiology as he practiced the *autohypnosis* or *autogenic training* or, as it is now called, biofeedback. The Greens' work and writing for scientific journals has made biofeedback well-known and has rapidly increased belief in, and use of, this technique.

At this point in our discussion of biofeedback, the difference should be made clear again between "monitoring" some physiologic function of the body and "biofeedback." Monitoring of blood pressure, skin temperature, brain wave, or heart by appropriate mechanisms is not biofeedback. Biofeedback is a procedure wherein monitoring various physiologic activities of the body is done, but the critical difference is the added emphasis of combined use of *muscle relaxation, deep slow breathing, visualization and repetition of a mantra word or phrase.* These practices together can bring about an altered state of consciousness, bringing the mind to a neutral or stilled state, opening it for spirit control.

Dr. Elmer and Alyce Green refer to biofeedback as Western yoga.[7] In their book *Beyond Biofeedback*, both Elmer and Alyce express their belief in the "energy concept" of the cosmos and its relationship to man. They have, from youth, studied and practiced the astrological concepts of the East. In their book preface (p. xix), they state:

> From our viewpoint, the development of full human potential starts most easily with mastery of *body* energies (through internal control of images, emotions, and volition), and the process can be extended to energies which influence the outside world.[8]

The book tells the story of their life, which is deeply entrenched in the Eastern teachings. I quote again from their book *Beyond Biofeedback*:

---

[6] *Ibid.*, preface xiv–xv.
[7] *Ibid.*, p. 16.
[8] *Ibid.*, Preface xix.

During those years Alyce and I read continuously in the fields of metaphysics, parapsychology, and theosophy, searching for and constructing a framework of ideas that would correspond with our own experiences and at the same time be reasonable in terms of a possible science in which mind and matter were not forever separate.[9]

The practice of using *mantras, muscle relaxation, rhythmic deep breathing,* and *visualization* to induce changes in brain-wave patterns and induce physiological function change is of concern. The use of mantras (repetitive phrases), relaxation, deep breathing, and visualization is an integral part of Eastern religions and has long since found its way into Christianity with the use of prayer beads and, more recently, in various styles of prayer, often referred to as contemplative prayer. Even Bible verses can be used as mantras. The Eastern religions use mantras to alter consciousness; actually, they eliminate thinking. Body and/or muscle relaxation practices are integral to hypnosis techniques. The Indian gurus have warned that rhythmic deep breathing is a time-honored method for entering altered states of consciousness and for developing psychic power. *Visualization* (forming a mind picture) is a method of attempting to change and manipulate the physical reality by mental pictures. Dave Hunt, in his book *Seduction of Christianity: Spiritual Discernment in the Last Days*, states:

> Shamanistic visualization is an attempt to create or manipulate the physical world by the practice of "mental alchemy." It is based upon the ancient sorcerer's belief that the entire universe is an illusion (called *maya* in Hinduism) created by the mind.[10]

One leading proponent of visualization, Adelaide Bry, says that it can be used to create whatever you want. Visualization, as practiced in this pagan philosophy, is an attempt to mimic God's power of creation: by the breath of His mouth" (Ps. 33:6).

The ancient roots of this type of thinking can be found in Greek mythology. Dave Hunt tells in *The Seduction of Christianity* that the Egyptian god Thoth (to the Greeks, Hermes) taught that the physical world could be transformed through *mental imagery*.[11] Also of bygone times

---

[9] *Ibid.*, p. 13.

[10] Hunt, David; McMahon T.A., *Seduction of Christianity, Spiritual Discernment in the Last Days*, Harvest House Publishing, Eugene, OR, (1985), p.138.

[11] *Ibid.*, p. 140.

has been the use of *visualization* in yoga to create reality with the mind and achieve union with the supreme Hindu god, Brahman. Also mentioned is the comment that visualization is a widely used technique in psychic healing.[12] It is a regular practice in training psychic healers. Do not confuse visualization (which is an attempt to bring something into reality or into materialization by the thought itself) with our creative ideas, plans, and mental activities that we use to work, design, and function by every day. That is not what is referred to by the word *visualization*.

Chapter 47 of Isaiah warns us of the end result of trusting in sorceries and enchantments. Evil and desolation and final destruction by fire will be our lot. The astrologers, stargazers, and sorcerers will not be able to save us. It is very clear that the most prominent investigators and authors on the subject of biofeedback are deep believers in, and practitioners of, Eastern mysticism.

Second set of questions: What company does this technique keep? Who uses it and what other therapies accompany its use? From the above information, we see that biofeedback developed out of hypnosis actually is hypnosis under a different name. In the book *The Illustrated Encyclopedia of Body-Mind Disciplines* by Nancy Allison, chapter 4 titled "Mind/Body Medicine" lists the names of therapeutic techniques that are associated. They are biofeedback training, guided imagery, hypnotherapy, interactive-guided imagery, and psycho-neuroimmunology.[13]

Chapter 4 of *The Illustrated Encyclopedia of Mind-Body* opens with the following paragraph:

> Mind/body medicine is a contemporary term used to describe a number of disciplines that study or approach, healing the physical body, transforming human behavior, by engaging the conscious or unconscious powers of the mind. While: "mind/body medicine" is a term used in this section of the encyclopedia to describe a growing field of study and practice in contemporary Western medicine, it is also used by others to describe ancient Eastern disciplines such as yoga, meditation, traditional Chinese medicine and subtle energy therapies. The variety of disciplines that comprise mind/body medicine in this encyclopedia combine a theory of the relationship between body and mind that has much in common with these ancient

---

[12] *Ibid.*, p. 141.

[13] Allison, Nancy, *The Illustrated Encyclopedia of Mind/Body Disciplines*, Rosen Pub. Group Inc. NY, (1999), p. 64.

Eastern disciplines with Western scientific models of biology and chemistry.[14]

The use of biofeedback started with therapists employing hypnosis-type therapies, and its use has extended into many health disciplines.

Third set of questions: What is the ultimate direction that the therapy is headed? Am I led toward Jesus Christ or away from Him? Do I still need Him as a Savior, or have I become my own savior? Biofeedback is considered to be the yoga of the West.[15] It is based on the same principles as *yoga* of the East. The basic principle is that within "SELF" lies all the wisdom of the universe. The body has all the intelligence and power to heal itself and also to grow into a higher consciousness called the Supreme Self.

The following quotation is from a letter from Dr. Elmer Green to Mr. Ihori, a Japanese businessman who wrote inquiring about the theory of biofeedback and if it would be applicable to his employees. The reply to Mr. Ihori is summarized as follows: deep within the unconscious mind of each person is hidden the *Source of Creativity*, which has the solution to all human problems. It is known by various names such as tao (the way) in China true self in Zen, Jiva in India, and in Tibet "lotus."

How does one bring out this hidden source of creativity? By putting the *body at complete rest*, the *emotions at peace*, and the *mind stilled* while conscious and ready to receive impressions from the creative center of the subconscious mind.

Biofeedback is an efficient, effective manner of bringing out this "source" by having the person place him/herself in the theta brain-wave status. This is demonstrated through the electroencephalographic (EEG) feedback wherein an electrode is applied to the left occipital area of the scalp, over the visual part of the brain. The final remark in Dr. Green's letter to Mr. Ihori states:

> In my view theta training is a form of *accelerated meditation*— and the benefits to students are incalculable.[16]

Richard Willis, in his book *Holistic Health, Holistic Hoax*, tells of the experience that Drs. Malcolm and Vera Carruthers had in their autogenic training classes conducted in England. They reported that everyone that became completely relaxed wanted to "go further." The doctors realized

---

[14] *Ibid.*, p. 64.
[15] Green, op. cit., p. 76.
[16] *Ibid.*, preface xiv.

that the Western approach, such as autogenic training or biofeedback, brought a level of treatment that meshed with the traditional spiritual practices of the East, similar to Eastern meditation. They then moved from autogenic training to the practice of yoga and meditation. The Carruthers felt that autogenic training is the best way to develop inner awareness, and this led them to seek the best Eastern meditation practices.[17] Willis tells us that

> the most popular form of Eastern meditation practiced by millions in the West is Transcendental Meditation (TM) which originated with Maharishi Mahesh Yogi.[18]

In this form of meditation, a mantra word or phrase is given to the student by the instructor. This *secret mantra* is repeated over and over in the mind as one rests in a comfortable position. The mantra is to facilitate bringing the mind into a "passive" attitude. The student is advised to meditate twice a day for twenty minutes. By using this style of meditation, physiologic changes occur. Herbert Benson, MD, writes in his book *The Relaxation Response* that a hypo-metabolic state would occur within three minutes of starting transcendental meditation, and the oxygen consumption of the mediator would be reduced by 20 percent, signifying a profound relaxation response.

The words given to be repeated, the mantra, are actually names of Hindu gods, and one is calling on those gods to possess oneself. I made mention of this fact at a seminar I was conducting on the subjects of this book in the state of Massachusetts where there is a large ashram for training people in transcendental meditation. A young gentleman came to me afterward with a puzzled expression on his face. He asked me:

> How did you know that the names given in the secret mantra were names of Hindu Gods? I worked at the Transcendental ashram and became a member. When I was initiated I knelt before an altar with idols of pagan gods and was given their names for my mantra.

---

[17] Willis, Richard J.B., *Holistic Health Holistic Hoax?*, Pensive Publications, 10 Holland Gardens, Watford Hertfordshire, England WD2 6JW, (1997), p. 223.

[18] *Ibid.*, p. 223.

In this belief system for health and healing, there is no room for a Creator God. There is no room for understanding the forces of darkness—of Satan and his angels—no place to understand that Satan has been allowed great power to influence man, and no room to understand that Satan has been allowed power over electrical forces.

Those who deny the existence of evil spirits, demons, fallen angels in spite of ample testimony from scripture that such does exist will be easy prey for the deceiver. When we are ignorant of the devil's wiles and depend upon our own wisdom, we are in at his non-mercy.

Fourth set of questions: Does the treatment method follow known laws of physiology? Does it teach and direct the patient to seek to know and follow God's laws of health?

Hypnosis, autogenic training, and biofeedback do not operate by any known laws of physiology. However, there are physiological changes that do occur through the autonomic nervous system in an individual. The explanation is that the body knows how to heal itself when it is told to do so. The practitioner's use of these modalities seldom gives appropriate attention to the underlining causes of disease.

The treatment methods spoken of in this book, and many more that have not been mentioned, have no basis in known laws of physics or chemistry. All have come about as a result of a theory based on pagan religious beliefs and a false understanding of the origin of the universe and man. For one hundred years, proponents of these methods have tried their best to reconcile these methods with known science. They have failed. Dr. Green mentions in his book that he took postgraduate studies in physics at UCLA so as to be able to demonstrate a scientific connection between his beliefs and experiences in Eastern mysticism and the physical laws that modern science recognizes.[19]

Eastern mysticism declares that all substances of the cosmos, earth, and man originate from universal energy and are said to be divided into seven levels (frequencies), or densities of energy. The question arises: why is it not possible for science, with its delicate instruments, to detect this energy force? These energy levels are labeled by author Green E-1 through E-7. E-1 refers to the transformation of energy into the physical universe, including the human body. The higher levels (frequencies) of energy that are written about have to do with the mind and consciousness—that is, "higher consciousness." Science has no instruments to detect these supposed higher levels of energy, and Green tells us why they are not measurable by science:

---

[19] Green, op. cit., p. 296.

Alternative & Mystical Healing Therapies

Humans have all the parts and can therefore detect a greater spectrum of energies. Instruments are made of minerals, and lack the transducer components needed for detection of E-2 through E-7 energies. In other words, living beings are coupled to the cosmos better than scientific devices, which are, after all, quite limited tools.[20]

In contrast to the above is God's way. We follow His spiritual and physical laws to maintain health. We look to God for the power to heal. He is our Creator and Sustainer and Redeemer.

Many will receive miraculous healing as wonders from God. Are we prepared to test every miracle, every statement by the word of God? Faith in God's word, prayerfully studied and practically applied, must be our shield from deception.

Fifth set of questions: Who receives the credit for healing, God the Creator or Satan the created? Dr. Green states the following:

> Why did biofeedback prove helpful in the treatment of so many and varied disorders? Suddenly I realized that it isn't biofeedback that is the "panacea"—*it is the power within the human being to self-regulate, self-heal, re-balance.* Biofeedback does nothing to the person; it is a tool for releasing that potential.[21]

Jesus never taught the above-stated philosophy; he did not direct man's mind to power within himself. He was always directing them to God His Father, the Creator of the universe, as the source of their strength and wisdom.

Five sets of questions show positive answers for identifying spiritualism in biofeedback. I no longer wonder why it has been listed as such in Christian books that have been written to expose the devil's wiles. The special report by the Biblical Research Committee included biofeedback as a procedure that we should shun. You will have to decide for yourself if biofeedback is a procedure you would choose to use. My goal is to present enough documented information in order for you to make an intelligent decision.

You may have noticed that the testimonies of people, as to the value of different treatment methods, or the personal experience of individuals who experienced relief and apparent healing from use of various alternative healing modalities have not been included as testing criteria. This book does not present the idea that these methods do not work. The purpose

---

[20] *Ibid.*, p. 304.
[21] Green, op. cit., p. 116.

of the book is to help us in answering the questions Who makes it work? What power is behind it?

I would like to present one additional bit of information to help you in making your decision about whether biofeedback is good, rational treatment or if it falls into the domain of the mystical. Dr. Green, in his book *Beyond Biofeedback* has an entire chapter on the use of "*volition*" in biofeedback therapy. Synonyms for volition are "the will" or "to choose." A person must first *choose* to participate in biofeedback, for without this willingness, the treatment will be ineffective. The following is from the book *Beyond Biofeedback*:

> Fundamental among (man's) inner powers, and the one to which priority should be given, is the *will's* central position in man's personality and its intimate connection with the core of his being—his very self.[22]

Dr. Green also states:

> Volition (will) is at the heart of the mind-body problem.[23]

> Attitude is a critical feature in biofeedback training, because volition (will) is influenced by what one believes.[24]

Elmer and Alyce Green are correct in their assessment of the power of the will. It is vital in deciding which power will control us. With the proper use of the will, the power of choice, changes can be made in our lives. By yielding to the will of Christ, we align ourselves with divine power. A life of victory over habits and passions is possible to all who will unite his weak human will to the omnipotent unwavering will of God.

The will is a governing power in man; it brings all other faculties under control. It is the decision-making aspect of the mind, which in the children of God brings obedience.

> Choose for yourselves this day whom you will serve. . . . But as for me and my house, we will serve the Lord. (Josh. 24:15)

---

[22] 26. *Ibid.*, p. 58.
[23] *Ibid.*, p. 59.
[24] *Ibid.*, p. 66.

20

A Critique Of Vibrational Medicine: The Handbook Of Subtle-Energy Therapies, Third Edition

RICHARD GERBER, MD

The motto of a Christian University School of Medicine, "To Make Man Whole," refers to man as a physical/mental/spiritual being. In the past thirty or more years the term *holistic medicine* has become a common expression. It too refers to a body/mind/spirit relationship. However, there is a difference between the two expressions. We need to look at the teachings as to the origin of man to understand this difference.

The biblical story of man's creation tells us of a living being, God, the source of life, who formed man from dust of the earth and breathed into him the breath of life.

> By the word of the Lord the heavens were made and all the host of them by the breath of His mouth. For He spoke, and it was done; He commanded, and it stood fast. (Ps. 33:6, 9)

To make man *whole* is to direct man to live in harmony with God's physical laws, as well as His spiritual laws.

A Critique Of Vibrational Medicine:
The Handbook Of Subtle-Energy Therapies, Third Edition

The word *holistic* refers to being in harmony with the world of nature, including the god of pantheism. In chapter 3 of *this book*, the pagan's view of creation is presented in brief. That theory tells us in very simplistic terms that the creation of man and the universe came about through evolution of a "god-force." This allowed every entity of the universe to be a part of each other, as each is a part of this "god-force" (also known as vital force, chi, prana, universal energy, and a hundred other terms). The theory contends that all matter is made up of *primordial* energy and/or light and that *material substance* is "frozen light."[1] This *vital energy* is said to be of contrasting divisions, positive/negative, masculine/feminine, yang/yin, and is also considered to possess *vibrational (frequency) energy characteristics*. Each substance, animate and inanimate, is supposed to emit an electromagnetic vibrational frequency peculiar to it alone.[2]

Holistic medicine refers to the teaching of and/or use of various treatment methods for illnesses that form healing methods based on this theory. This concept has its origin and propagation from Eastern religions and Western occultism's theosophy and has not been verified by present-day science.

The basis of vibrational energetics as a method of diagnosing and treating disease along with use of acupuncture, qi gong exercises, pulse diagnosis, etc., is a result of an attempt to connect and blend pantheistic healing methods with modern science.

Richard Gerber, MD, is recognized as a prominent advocate of this movement. In 2001 he published his third edition of *Vibrational Medicine: The #1 Handbook of Subtle-Energy Therapies*. The prior editions had sold more than 125,000 copies. The purpose of his book is to foster the belief that the ancient paganistic systems of healing are nothing more than, *when understood*, extensions of present-day scientific methods. Dr. Gerber and other authors of similar texts readily acknowledge that their hypotheses and theories are not in harmony with the present understanding of the sciences of medicine, physics, and chemistry. The goal of Dr. Gerber is to close this gap in understanding.

Dr. Gerber is to be lauded for aspiring to more natural methods in health and healing that will depend less on pharmaceuticals and more on our own systems to correct disorders. He is highly trained in internal medicine and states that he still finds it necessary to use the knowledge and methods for treatment from his specialty training. However, his book leads in a direction that a Christian must ponder and question. As I read the preface to this six-hundred-page book, I am impressed that Dr. Gerber has a deep belief in Eastern mysticism and his writing's purpose to convince the reader that it is truth.

---

[1] Gerber, Richard, M.D., *Vibrational Medicine, The #1 Handbook of Subtle-Energy Therapies,* Bear & Company, Rochester, Vermont, 2001, p. 59

[2] *Ibid.,* p. 171.

During his medical school days, Dr. Gerber enrolled in a class called *A Course in Miracles*, which changed his spiritual viewpoint. He tells us that as he went further in the course, he began to awaken psychic abilities within himself. The comment is made that he understood that

> the Course in Miracles had been *dictated* via a psychic or by telepathic means to a psychologist from a "high spiritual source."[3]

As a result of his study of The Course in Miracles and from other readings, two concepts developed in his mind. First, humans are more than just physical beings: they are also spiritual beings with consciousness on higher planes than recognized in this life, and that this higher mental state continues after death. Secondly:

> there are those "in Spirit" who seek to communicate with individuals still in physical incarnation.[4]

These communications are said to be twofold in nature: (1) to make us aware of *life after death* and (2) to relay information that pertains to

> healing, soul growth, and personal spiritual evolution.[5]

Curiosity had been awakened in him by this new knowledge, and he sought a deeper understanding of "technical channeled information" from spirit-channeled sources. Dr. Gerber shares with us the fact that he and his wife are clairvoyant. He states:

> I would like to point out to the readers of *Vibrational Medicine* that I believe this book is the result of cooperation between healers and researchers on the physical plane and beings who exist on the higher spiritual planes. This cooperation has made possible the transmission of a wealth of information that is needed on the planet at this time. Many of the sections of this book are actually "messages from spirit" channeled through various sources.[6]

---

[3] *Ibid.*, p. 29.

[4] *Ibid.*, p. 31.

[5] *Ibid.*

[6] *Ibid.*, p. 37.

Vibrational medicine does not arise from research in science that reveals the human system to have focalized areas of electromagnetic energy (chakras) that in turn produces an aura outside of the body. Nor does research find specialized channels (acupuncture meridian system) throughout the body that carries a non-measurable, non-demonstrable energy (ch'i, qi) that can be manipulated by pressure or needling particular points on the body. There has been no reporting of energy faster than light. Yet these beliefs, which are a result of messages from *spirits* by channeled sources and from ancient pagan religious dogma, form the basic principles of vibrational medicine. Much of this theory has already been presented in this book. My purpose for this chapter is to show that *by accepting even fragments* of this teaching as true, it can initiate change in our world view (concepts of our origin and destiny) and to which power we place our allegiance. Dr. Gerber, in chapter 3 of his book, uses the title "The Birth of Vibrational Medicine." Herein is presented the prediction that conventional medical/surgical medicine will experience a revolution and electromagnetic healing will take its place. This will occur, as physicians understand,

> that the human organism is a series of interacting multidimensional energy fields.[7]

A presentation and illustration of the proclaimed seven different frequency levels of universal energy is given in chapter 4. Frequency level 1 refers to all matter (substance) in the universe; second level, etheric and astral bodies; third level, mental and causal bodies; and progresses upward to level seven. This level has several names such as Supreme Self, Jewel, etc. (the level of *godhood*). These different frequency levels are said to make connection with the different levels of chakras, the higher frequency level of energy which are said to connect with the respective higher chakra.

Dr. Gerber explains this relationship as follows: the chakras act as *transformers*, converting energy (hypothesized to be) traveling at a far greater speed than light to a slower speed; the top chakra receives, then converts the highest energy frequency, level seven, to the next lower chakra; and again the frequency is reduced by that chakra.[8] This reduction of frequency may continue downward, strengthening each chakra until the energy frequency is converted to the speed of light, which is level 1 (the materialized physical body). These chakras (*transformers*) are said to also

---

[7] *Ibid.*, p. 91.

[8] *Ibid.*, p. 171.

act in the opposite direction, transforming energy frequency upward via the chakras. This is accomplished through meditation. By many lifetimes of meditation, the seventh frequency level may be perfected, resulting in "godhood."

Remember, the lowest level of energy is that of which all material substance is said to consist of. The next level, ethereal, is believed to be an electromagnetic template of the physical body and guides growth and restoration. Changes or influences on the etheric body or energy supposedly precedes and effects changes either positively or negatively in the physical body.[9] At these etheric and higher levels of frequencies, the belief is that outside electromagnetic fields influence a person's *electromagnetic bodies*. Such influences are said to restore balance to the etheric and other bodies and, in turn, health to the physical body. Dr. Gerber quotes a psychic source:

> There is a direct link between the nervous, circulatory, and meridian systems (acupuncture pathways) partly because ages ago, the meridians were originally used to create these two parts of the physical body. Consequently, anything that influences one of these systems has a direct impact on the other two areas. The meridians use the passageway between the nervous and circulatory systems to feed the life force into the body, almost extending directly to the molecular level. *The meridians are the interface or doorway between the physical and ethereal properties of the body.*[10] (italics added by Dr. Gerber)

From the book *Vibrational Medicine*, I read:

> All matter, both physical and subtle [etheric, astral bodies, etc.] has frequency. Matter of different frequencies can coexist in the same space, just as energies of different frequencies (i.e., radio and TV) can exist nondestructively in the same space.[11]

---

[9] Karagulla, S., Energy Fields and Medical Diagnosis, in *The Human Aura*, ed. N. Regush (New York: Berkeley Publishing, 1974); Reported in Richard Gerber M.D., *Vibrational Medicine 3rd Ed*, Bear and Company, Rochester, Vermont, (2001), p. 126.

[10] Gurudas, *Flower Essences and Vibrational Healing*, channeled by Kevin Ryerson (Albuquerque, NM: Brotherhood of Life, Inc., 1983), p. 29; Reported in, Richard Gerber M.D.; *Vibrational Medicine 3rd Ed.*, (2001), p. 126.

[11] Gerber, op. cit., p. 171.

From this concept, various alternative healing methods claim to affect health by their vibrational properties, such as flower essences, aromatherapy, gem elixirs, color therapy, sound therapy, homeopathy, and subtle energies from plant food. The concept is that subtle vibrational frequencies (faster than light energy) of plants, gems, colors etc., can be transferred to chakras. Through homeopathy, vibrations are claimed to be transferred via the water or diluent used in dilution for preparing the homeopathic remedy, even if there are no molecules of the original substance left in the solution due to dilution.[12] Flower essences are purported to have high frequency level vibration and influence upper chakras and, in turn, influence consciousness; gem elixirs (solution containing ground up gemstones), are believed to influence the middle and lower chakras. Homeopathic remedies are said to affect the Chinese meridian system and so connect the subtle (faster than light) energies of the cosmos with the physical body. None of these concepts are found in science.[13]

Vibrational Medicine chapter 8, "The Phenomenon of Psychic Healing," presents the history of the origin of therapeutic touch. It is believed to exist on the hypothesis that subtle energy is sensed by and/or passed through hands to another person even without actual physical contact. The explanation for psychic healing is that the mind of the therapist can pass healing vibrational frequencies of subtle energy from him/herself to another person over distance.[14]

Another common practice in alternative medicine is the use of machines or instruments that are purported to measure and/or correct subtle energy frequencies within the body. There are two different instruments that are used to measure the energy of acupuncture meridians and their points. One is called "AMI machine," which is supposed to reveal an imbalance (yin-yang) in the acupuncture meridian system; and the other machine is referred to as the VOL machine (electroacupuncture according to Voll), which measures subtle energy of individual meridian channels and/or acupuncture points. The operators of this machine claim it is able to reveal the energy status of specific organs, even to the ability of an organ, such as the pancreas, to form its specific digestive enzymes, lipase, protease, etc.[15] The VOL machine goes beyond diagnosing energy imbalance. It is said to be capable of finding the cause of imbalance as well as possible cures.[16]

---

[12] *Ibid.*, pp. 88–89.

[13] *Ibid.*, p. 272.

[14] *Ibid.*, p. 287.

[15] *Ibid.*, p. 207.

[16] *Ibid.*, pp. 206–208.

An additional style of instrument frequently used in alternative medicine since the early 1900s is referred to as a radionic black box. Such a machine is said to accurately diagnose various subtle energy-level dysfunctions. The successful use of these instruments depends upon the "psychic ability," known as radiesthesia, of the radionic practitioner. A substance referred to as a witness from the patient, such as hair, a spot of blood on paper, a picture of the patient, some object handled by the person, etc., will be placed in the instrument for analysis of the body's energy balance. Also, a substance, "a witness," can be sent long distances for analysis without loss of accuracy. If a spot of blood were to be sent for examination, that blood spot could continue to reflect the current energy status of that person without need for fresh samples. The substance sent for inspection provides a two-way link with the practitioner and patient so that not only the subtle (faster than light) energy status of the patient is revealed over distance, but the practitioner is able to return healing energies with the proper frequency to bring healing.[17]

There are other instruments that may be encountered that operate on the vibrational hypothesis such as the Homo-Vibra Ray and Rife beam ray machines. Both of these are promoted as capable of making a diagnosis by analysis of frequencies and provide treatment by correcting the same. It is interesting that Dr. Gerber considers these various instruments as *"electronic pendulums."*

Dr. Gerber looks to a Dr. William Tiller, a retired former professor at Stanford University and former chairman of the Department of Materials Science at Stanford:

as perhaps the leading theorist in the subtle energetic field.[18]

He credits him for the hypothesis of energy frequency faster than light (10^{10-20} times the speed of light for astral travel). Dr. Tiller has coined a new word to describe subtle energy, "magnetoelectric energy," which is just another synonym for universal energy.

Astral travel, out-of-body experiences, near-death experience, life after death, reincarnation, higher consciousness, Supreme Self, "godhood" are all explained on the hypothesis of *universal energy* and its supposed various frequency levels. The ultimate deception of what this mode of thought leads to is best illustrated by the following quote from Dr. Gerber.

---

[17] *Ibid.*, p. 235.
[18] *Ibid.*, pp. 151, 155–171.

> People through the centuries have accepted Jesus as the one true son of God. This is, in fact, a *misinterpretation*. What Jesus came to teach us is that we are all the children of God.... We who are the evolving souls or fragments of God's consciousness are *divine* brainchildren.[19]

That's it, the end of the journey, from partaking of the fruit from the tree to "godhood."

> For God knows that in the day ye eat of it your eyes will be opened, and you will be like God, knowing good and evil. (Gen. 3:5).

> For we do not wrestle against flesh and blood, but against principalities, against powers, against the rulers of the darkness of this age, against spiritual hosts of wickedness in heavenly places. (Eph. 6:12)

Is it possible that we could be accepting these spiritualistic teachings by participating in the healing modalities built upon this premise? We cannot serve two masters. We must make a choice. We have been blessed with heaven-sent directions for health and healing. Time and science have verified that it is the correct way, so why look to "Baalzebub, god of Ekron" to seek guidance? It seems appropriate to use again the words of Joshua as he addressed the children of Israel and challenged them with the following words:

> And if it seem evil unto you to serve the LORD, choose you this day whom ye will serve; whether the gods which your fathers served that were on the other side of the flood, or the gods of the Amorites, in whose land ye dwell: but as for me and my house, we will serve the LORD. (Josh. 29:15)

---

[19] *Ibid.*, pp. 493–494.

21

Babylonian Spiritualistic Mysteries: Compatible With The Atonement?

Atonement means "at-one-ment" with God. Salvation is the act of God in restoring man to be in harmony with his Creator. The seventeenth chapter of John records the great prayer of Jesus just before He started His night in the Garden of Gethsemane. We read His prayer in John 17:21:

> That they all (His disciples) may be one; as you Father, are in me, and I in You, that they also may be one in Us: that the world may believe that You have sent Me.

In heaven, a great battle for the loyalty of the angels occurred between God and Lucifer who desired to be in the place of the Son of God. That battle spread to this earth when man sinned (Rev. 12). Sin separated God from man so that there could be no direct communication, no salvation while in the separated state. Only by the *atonement* of the Son of God at the Cross could there be a restoration of communication, blessings, salvation for man. Satan became the "Prince" of this world when man believed Satan and distrusted God. This controversy, which started in heaven, based on the Satan's lies continues on earth today. God's defense is truth, righteousness, and love. He expects the same defense from His followers.

From the very start, all of Lucifer's accusations against God were based in falsehood, deceit, and self-glorification. These same principles he has taught his followers to utilize. The name "tree of knowledge of good and evil" contains much of the secret of Satan's methods. He has been able to convince man that within himself (man) exists all the knowledge of the universe and all man has to do is to learn how to bring it out.

The first *supplement* to attaining a higher level of consciousness and health and becoming wise like God was the fruit offered to Eve. Eve already had all that the serpent was offering except godhood, and she knew that was impossible; but on the *testimony of one, the serpent,* and without any evidence that it was so, she distrusted God and believed the lie.

The devil wishes to take the place of the Creator God in the minds of men. To do so, he must deceive mankind as to who their Creator is. He devised a story for the origin of man, which portrayed man as being formed by the balancing of a great (imaginary) two-part opposing energy (chi = yin-yang) or force that is presumed to be throughout the universe. When the balance of these two parts was perfect, then the universe, earth, and man were said to be formed. God the living Being Creator, who has power and life within Himself, is left out of this story. And so Lucifer, in truth, takes the credit for creation. These are *Babylonian mysteries*—that is, secrets of astrological concepts of origins. If we choose to utilize the modalities for health and healing that are based on this false premise, after we have been exposed to the truth about these false teachings, we are actually accepting this theory as the truth.

Immortality was promised to Adam and Eve on the condition of obedience. If they sinned, they would lose eternal life. Satan's lie that "you will not die" had to be explained to man because man did die. To cover this obvious untruth, the doctrine of immortal soul and reincarnation was formed.

God has allowed man to choose whom he will serve. This book has been written to help us see clearly that at times when we feel we are following God and using His methods, we may actually be deceived and be partaking of a counterfeit. The consequences are eternal.

How can I determine whether the method of *natural healing* that I am being offered is or is not of Satan's origin? After all, I seem to have improved with the method and others swear by it. The most frequent comment I hear is:

"It helped me" or "My friend was helped by it" or "It works."

The criteria as to whether a method is of Satan or not does not include whether or not an individual was benefited. People do get better and apparently receive healing at times. The issue is whose power brought healing? Another comment often heard is:

> Well, I just take the good out of it.

Any technique distinctly connected to the occult cannot be considered neutral. Participating in these methods may be the first step to altering our concept of our origin and the beginning of the changing of our world view. When a technique has its origin in pantheistic concepts and astrological beliefs, just accepting that it may do something desirable is actually unconsciously accepting this belief.

At times, a mixture of scientific medicine is combined with "holistic" methodology so as to stimulate the question, is it good or not? I would ask you to search out the answers to the following questions and make a determination. These questions were first printed in *Mystical Medicine* by Warren Peters, MD.

1. What and where are its roots?
2. What company (other healing modalities) does it keep in clinical use and in the books and literature describing it?
3. Does the method claim to activate the *innate powers within myself*, or does it direct me to recognize the *power of the Creator God* in healing?
4. Is its method of action in harmony with the known laws of physics and science?
5. Does it claim to balance, polarize, manipulate, unblock, and correct energies, electromagnetic frequencies, or vibrations?
6. Is it a technique that involves altering my consciousness or rational thought process so as to impede control of my mind and whose power controls me?

The most powerful deterrent to becoming bewitched by Satan's deceptions in health and healing is to know God's methods so well that it becomes easy to detect the counterfeit. One Christian writer on health defined sickness as an effort of nature to free the system from the effects of violating the laws of health.

God's remedies involve the use of pure air, sunlight, temperate use of good substances, avoidance of the injurious, rest, exercise, proper diet, the use of water inside and outside the body, and trust in divine power. Trust involves being obedient to the Creator's physical and spiritual laws.

The rapid spread of neo-paganism across the world, and especially here in America, has been, to a great extent, related to the dogma and modalities involved in health and healing practices of the so-called alternative healing methods. The devil has used these methods as the *right arm of his missionary message*. Satan presents his health and healing program so that it appears *natural* and that it is the same method God has given us. The difference can be ascertained by looking for the explanation of the source of the power for healing. If it is from some *energy* within us, and if we are doing some act to balance that power from within, then it is of the counterfeit.

We too believe that the health message is the right arm of the gospel. There is a difference, however. The difference is that we trust in a living God as our Creator and that His power sustains and restores us to health when we choose to place ourselves in harmony with His physical and spiritual laws and ask Him to bless our efforts.

The history of medicine should help give us the answers we need in making a correct choice in methods of health and healing. Wherever the system of medicine has been built upon the *energy* concept, the health of that country remained primitive. Over millennia those nations using such methods saw no improvement in health and healing. As soon as the scientific method, based upon the laws of physics, chemistry, and hygiene—God's physical laws—are instituted in the approach to health and healing, quick and great improvements occur. Keep in mind the change China experienced when they made changes directed by scientific understanding of disease and its cause. The traditional Chinese medicine had been available and used in medical treatment for the people for around four thousand years. With just a little use of scientific methods (cleanliness of water, body, and environment), the lifespan doubled in fifty years.

We have a written history of medical systems of several past and present civilizations, and the story is the same in all of them. When an approach to health and healing based on God's physical laws and methods is utilized, we see profound improvement. If we remember that systems like that of Ayurveda were designed by men on the basis of intuition, contact with spirit guides, and astrological concepts of origins, it should be easier to make the right choice in the selection of our health and healing methods.

For some years there has been coming into Christianity spiritualistic teachings that undermine the saving faith in Jesus Christ the divine Son of God of those who give heed to them. The theory that God is an essence, an actuating energy pervading all nature, is one of Satan's most subtle devices. It misrepresents God and is a dishonor to His greatness and majesty. Christ's death on the cross met the conditions of the *atonement* (Isa. 53:12; 1 Pet. 1:18,19). His work on earth was accomplished, and He won the kingdom (Rom. 5). Following Christ's resurrection, He ascended to the heavenly courts to hear from God the Father that His atonement for men's sins was sufficient.

Christ returned to earth for forty days, after which he returned to heaven, and there entered the heavenly sanctuary to be our High Priest, having finished the atonement. He is preparing His people to abide the day of His coming. The application of the atonement made on the cross for each of us is now taking place in heaven (Heb. 7, 8, 9). If we believe on the divine Son of God and have *no other gods before us*, He will, at the time of our judgment, present His life to the Father in place of our sinful lives. Let us guard carefully so that we do not allow *other gods before us* by becoming entangled in Satan's deceptions in health and healing.

Such spiritualistic theories concerning God make His grace ineffectual. If God is an essence, an actuating energy, pervading all nature, then we possess divinity within; therefore, He dwells in all men. Holiness then is attained in works by man developing the supposed power within.

As to the answer to the original question "Are the Babylonian mysteries of health and healing compatible with the atonement?" such theories, followed to their logical conclusion, wipe away the whole Christian foundation. They eliminate the need for atonement, and man becomes his own savior, and His (Christ's) word becomes of no effect.

That should answer the question.

Glossary

A.

A.A.—abbreviation for Alcoholics Anonymous, at times AA
Abrams's Black box— an electrical mechanical box used in divining
absent healing—healing a patient from a long distance
aconite—very poisonous plant used as a remedy in homeopathy
Acupuncture according to Voll—a special method of doing acupuncture by using electrical contacts on supposed acupuncture points, also known as EAV
acupuncture points—localized places on skin said to give access to movement of chi in meridians, supposedly channels for carrying chi
Acupuncture Watch—an Internet website that reports on and critiques or exposes acupuncture (www.acuwatch.org)
acupuncture—placing needles in skin on acupuncture points for therapy
Adonai—term used in Freemasonry to apply to Jesus Christ and considered to be the God of darkness and evil
Agni—fire in the body, actually normal metabolism, also a Hindu deity
Ahaziah—son of Ahab, king of Israel following death of Ahab
aikido—one form of martial art
alchemical—refers to a pre-chemistry discipline of medieval times, attempt by chemical changes to bring transformation of one thing into another; example, base metal into gold; mortality into immortality
alchemist—person practicing alchemy, looking for secret of life
alchemy—forerunner of chemistry; however, an alchemist was attempting to change one substance into another by physical means and change the soul from mortal to immortal (spiritual alchemy)

Glossary

Alice Bailey—author of twenty-four books directing the growth of New Age movement; all were messages channeled from a spirit guide, "the Tibetan master" or "Djwhal Khul"

allergen—substance that stimulates our immune system to produce antibodies

Allison, Nancy—author of *The Illustrated Encyclopedia of Body/Mind Disciplines*

alpha—first

alpha-omega—first and last

altered state of consciousness—referring to a change of mental state from the active mind

alternative—non-evidence-based, non-conventional therapy; refers to acupuncture, reflexology, etc., any treatment not shown to be scientifically evidence based

aluminum—mineral of the earth, found in some gems

Alzheimer's disease—mental disorder, memory fades causing senility

ama—imaginary white sticky substance in colon said to be spread through the cells of the body, called a toxin, term from Hinduism's Ayurveda concepts. Has never been seen or isolated

amber—petrified pitch, usually from pine tree

American Medical Society—society of American physicians organized to promote their interest, does not have any legal control over individual physicians

amulets—objects, artifacts, symbols, etc., worn to ward off bad luck or harm and illness, believed to possess supernatural powers

anatomist—person who is instructor or has special knowledge of anatomy

ancient wisdom—pagan religion of ancient Babylon and mystery schools' secret doctrine, man is God

anesthesiologist—medical doctor, specialist in giving anesthesia

animal magnetism—same as universal energy, vital force, etc.

animate—living substance

animism—attribution of conscious life to nature as a whole or to inanimate objects, same as paganism and basic same beliefs but more specific to Africa and some Far Eastern peoples. Belief in a universal energy, nature worship

Ankerberg, John—minister and coauthor of *Can You Trust Your Doctor?*

anthroposophy—knowledge concerning man: similar to theosophy but stresses the spiritual path as outlined by Rudolf Steiner, who had been member of Theosophy Society but left it to establish his own following

antibodies—usually a protein made by an animal to fight foreign invaders, germs, viruses, etc.

antidote—solution for a problem, often referred to a potion to cure some ailment

aphrodisiac—a substance felt to stimulate sexual powers

Apollo—Greek god in mythology

apothecary—pharmacy

applied kinesiology—mystical testing of muscles to determine weak internal organ, allergies, etc.

Arhat—an enlightened one

Aries—ram of the zodiac

aromatherapy—using fragrances and aromas from plants in medical treatment

asanas—postures of yoga, some postures named after Hindu gods

ascended masters—deceased individuals who supposedly have become immortal spirits and communicate with the living, actually fallen angels of Satan

Asclepius—Greek god of healing

assessment—a process of running the palms of the hands above a body to feel the energy pattern said to be present

astral body—one of several imaginary energy bodies or levels of universal energy above the material body. From this energy body, astral travel is said to occur, i.e., out-of-body experiences, etc. At death, this body is said to leave the material body and exist in an astral plane.

astrologer—one practicing astrology

astrologic medicine—medical therapy practiced by using information obtained from the zodiac

astrological concepts—beliefs in sun, moon, and stars having strong influence and association with man and the earth

astrology—belief that the gods live in the planets and that the sun, moon, and stars guide the destiny of man

atheistic—denies existence of God

atonement—at-one-ment with God achieved through Jesus Christ

attuned—initiated into being a Reiki practitioner, occultic/ spiritistic

aura—presumed body of energy arising out the chakras and radiating ten to twelve inches from the body, supposedly in colors of the rainbow; cannot be scientifically demonstrated; a Hindu concept

auricular therapy—using the external ear for acupuncture/acupressure instead of the body, supposedly represents the whole body

autogenic training—self-hypnosis, no external monitoring

Ayurvedic system—ancient Indian healing tradition; involves believing in universal energy called prana, energy that is believed to travel through the body via chakras

Aztecs—civilization in Mexico prior to the Spaniards' arrival

B

Baalzebub—idol god of city of Ekron in Bible days
Babylon—city in ancient times and now in ruins, in country of Iraq
Babylonian mysteries—religious secret initiatory rites and ceremonies originating from the ancient city of Babylon, consisted of the principles of pagan religions and promoting the "deity of man"
Bach flower remedies—thirty-eight flower essences originated by Dr. Bach, an English physician. Flowers are placed in water, and the sun is allowed to shine on them, believed to impart vital energy. Water then used as medicinal.
Bach, Edward, MD—originator of flower essences, English physician
baguazhang—a particular martial art
Baiame—name of supreme spirit god of Australian Aborigines
Baker, Douglas—author of *Esoteric Healing* and occultist
baua—one form of martial art
Bauman, Rudolf—wrote summary of effectiveness of acupuncture for Academy of Sciences of the German Democratic Republic, 1981
Bavarian Academy of Science—organization of scientists of Bavaria
Beatles—British musical group
Benson, C. Irving—minister who was an Oxford Group member
Benson, Herbert, MD—professor at Harvard School of Medicine and author of book *The Relaxation Response: Your Maximum Mind*; on the faculty of Harvard Medical School and who has had influence in the field of mental health treatment. He advocates the relaxation response, which is similar to autogenic training and/or Eastern meditation, teachings similar to Buddhism
Bergson, Anika—coauthor of *Zone Therapy*
Bernard, Theos—an American author and practitioner of yoga and Buddhism
Besant, Annie (a.k.a. Bessant)—directed the Theosophy Society after death of Blavatsky, also vice president of the French Co-Masonry
bewitched—attracted with pleasure to something
biblical world view—belief in the origin of life as described by the Bible, the purpose of life, the future and after life, as presented by the Bible
biochemical—chemicals involved with cellular chemistry, activity of chemicals in bio-systems
bioelectric energy—electricity formed within a biological system

biofeedback—autogenic training (self-hypnosis) using an electrical measuring device to observe temperature, blood pressure, brain-wave patterns, etc., while placing oneself into theta brain-wave status and self-hypnosis

bioplasma—universal energy, the name that Russians use

biopsy—to take tissue from the body for microscopic exam and analysis

bioresonance—referring to sound resonance as ascertained by voice analysis

Bird, Christopher—author of *The Divining Hand*

black magic—sorcery, to cause to happen something bad or destructive

Blavatsky, Helena—one of the originators of the Theosophy Society, 1875, spiritualist and by channeling wrote foundational books for the Theosophy Society and New Age

blue book—refers to the official book *Alcoholics Anonymous* used in fellowship meetings

bobbing—a form of water divining by use of a straight wire extending from the knee when in the sitting position. A reaction is when the end of the wire that has been curled and a lightbulb placed in it rises and falls, indicating the distance by increments to water. Each rise and fall indicates a certain distance as pre-chosen by the diviner.

Bodhidharma—Buddhist monk from India who went to China's *Shaolin temple* and known as the father of martial arts

body therapy—various types of body treatments such as massage, Rolfing, etc.

body/mind/spirit—a whole person with equal influence of each part

Brahman—chief god of Hinduism, creator god of pantheism

breastplate—rectangular heavy cloth with three rows of four gemstones worn on chest of high priests of Israel

breath of life—power involved in craniosacral therapy, same as chi, prana, vital force, etc.; power that Dr. Upledger attributes to healing in craniosacral therapy

Brint, Armand—astrologer and iridologist

Buchwald, Dedra, MD—faculty member of University of Washington, Seattle, Washington; wrote article appearing in the *Annals in Internal Medicine*, reporting study on acupuncture for fibromyalgia

Buddhism—religion of Buddha's philosophy, a religion split-off from Hinduism

C

Cabbala (Cabala, Kabalah, Kabbalah, Kabbala)—Jewish secret society

cachora—an Indian shaman of the Yaqui tribe

caduceus—a symbol of a rod with wings at the top and with two snakes ascending it, ancient symbol of medicine

calcium—mineral of earth and found in some stone formations

calomel—mercury chloride preparation used as medicine

cantharides—an extremely irritative substance made from Spanish fly

Carruthers, Malcolm, MD—author of *Meditation of the Heart* in *Yoga Today*

Carruthers—husband-and-wife team of physicians performing biofeedback sessions

causal body—body of mystical energy at higher plane or frequency than etheric or astral and is involved with reincarnation concepts, is supposed to be able to remember past life experiences and future life experiences

cell com system—a machine that is supposed to increase cell intercommunications and so brings health and healing from all types of disease

Celts—ethnic group of people found in the British Isles

centering—meditation

ch'i, chi, qi, ki—universal energy, Chinese, Korean, and Japanese names for such

chakra balancing—using any method that is believed to affect the chakras and so balance the proclaimed energy within

chakra—a supposed focal area of concentrated universal energy in the body. The body is said to have seven chakras, which are claimed to be in color. Each chakra will be one of seven colors of rainbow.

Chan Buddhism—a form of revised Hinduism, in short Buddhism

channeled—refers to receiving messages from spirits

channeler—a person who is able to contact spirits and communicate with them

charmer—a person who can affect by a magic spell

chelation—chelation therapy is wherein chemicals are placed within the body that will remove substances that the body cannot remove on its own. Lead in the body can only be removed by using a chelating agent. Usually intravenous administration.

chi kung—a martial art

ching—conduit

ching-mo—conduit vessel

chiromancy—palm reading, palmistry

chiropractor—type of medical practitioner trained in the philosophy of "chiropractic," the belief in an innate energy traversing the body via spinal nerves and that by manipulation movement of the back this vital energy may be unclogged or moved to clear congestion

Cho, Paul Yungi—author of *Solving Life's Problems*

choleric—angry, easily irritated, irate

Christ consciousness—term used in New Age jargon to refer to divinity within

Christian science—a religious body with pantheistic concepts, believes that all healing can be done with prayer

Circe—personality in Greek mythology

Cirlot—author of *Dictionary of Symbols*

clairvoyance—discerning or seeing objects or thoughts not observed by others

clairvoyant—having power of discerning objects not present to the senses, occultic power

coccyx—anatomical spot on the body, often referred to a tailbone

colonic cleansing—repeated enemas or use of machine that gives continuous cycling of water through large bowel, also use of herbs to cleanse bowel

color therapy—use of color to affect the chakra's energy balance

co-masonry—Masonic order for females in France

complementary—usually referring to non-conventional style of medical therapy

concepts—beliefs

Confucius—a Chinese who was a renowned ancient philosopher

Constance Cumby—a lawyer who also authored the book *The Hidden Dangers of the Rainbow*

contemplation—concentration in thought or study

controls—a term used to describe a spirit talking through someone; it may materialize at times

correspondence—synonym of association and/or sympathy

cosmic energy—universal energy of the cosmos

cosmological correspondence—refers to the belief in close association and relationship among cosmos, earth, and man

cosmology—science or subject of the cosmos, or suns and planets of the universe and their relationship to one another and to earth

cosmos—the sun, moon, stars, and the heavens

counterfeit—fake, false, fraud, phony, deceptive, imitative (see appendix J)

Cousens, Gabriel, MD—a popular physician who promotes integrative medicine

Craig, Winston, PhD, RD—author of book *Nutrition and Wellness: A Vegetarian Way to Better Health*, chair of Department of Nutrition, Andrews University

cranio-sacral (cranial-sacral, craniosacral)—one style of body therapy wherein very light massage or touch is applied to the base of the neck and back side of the skull and at times over the sacrum. This particular discipline claims that the bones of the skull are not in proper position and the massage is to reposition them. However, these bones are fused solid and cannot be manipulated. The fluid of the brain and spinal canal are supposed to be manipulated as well by the placing of hands about the head region.

creative energy—often referred to as prana, chi, life force, etc.

creative principle—synonym of universal energy, supreme self, One, god, etc.; referring to highest level of mystical energy

creative visualization—an act where in a person attempts to create by the power of his mind a happening, attitude, change, circumstance, etc.

crystal healers—healing by use of crystals that are supposed to influence universal energy of the body

crystal—stone with formation of internal structure of repetitive molecular formations

Cummings, Stephen—co-author of *Science of Homeopathy*

Cush—son of Ham but also had mythological names of Mercury, Thoth, Hermes

D

Dark Ages—period of history in Europe from between AD 500 AD and AD 1600

dan—level of attainment in martial arts ladder

dan-tien—refers to supposed concentration of chi in a local area. There are said to be three such centers in the body.

decubiti ulcer—an ulcer of the skin that forms usually from continuous pressure on the skin, which causes loss of circulation and death to the cells in that location

deification—making something god, such as a person made god

deists—belief that God created the earth and then went off and left it without divine influence to control and manage the earth

Deleuze, Phillippe Jean—author of several books and coined the term *animal magnetism*

Dolores Krieger—instructor in nursing profession and promoter of therapeutic touch therapy

deluge—flood

detoxification—the breakdown of a toxin or toxins and removal by various methods

Di Mina, Alfonso—biophysicist of United States

diuretic—substance that causes increased flow of urine and loss of water from the body

divination—act of divining to obtain information by occult method

divine mind—a term used by Christian science; also, it is a synonym of universal mind, universal intelligence, energy, etc.

diviner—one who divines

divine—the act to obtain information by an occult method, The word may be referring to the divinity of God

divining rod—stick or physical object used to divine

dogma—a doctrine or body of doctrines or beliefs

dojo—a location of martial arts practice and training

doshas—refers to three divisions of prana energy in Ayurveda medicine, similar to the two divisions in Chinese medicine, yin and yang

dowse—to divine, usually by pendulum

dowsing—using a pendulum of any type to divine

dualism—concept of opposing forces within universe; expressed as positive-negative, or negative-positive, dark-light, cold-hot, yin-yang, etc.

E

Eastern religions—religions based on pantheism: Hindu, Taoism, Buddhism, Shintoism, Shikh, etc.

East-West—combination of Eastern mysticism with Western occultism

eclectic—eclectic physician is one that uses many medicinals but in small doses, something for every symptom

ego—psychology term referring to the mental status of pride or self-worth

Egyptian mysteries—Egyptian religion came originally from Babylon and was formed out of the same basics, sun worship, nature worship, life after death, man having divine spark

Ekron—Philistine city on Mediterranean coast in country of Israel

electrocardiogram—a tracing on paper of the electrical activity of the heart muscle

electroencephalogram—a tracing on paper of the electrical activity of the brain revealing the frequency of electrical brain waves

electrolysis—movement of ions through a solution powered by electrical force to cause precipitation of the ion onto an electrode or some metal object

electromagnetic bodies—Hindu concept that there are additional bodies to our physical bodies and are composed of electrical forces, not recognized by modern science

electromagnetism—electrically induced magnetism

Elijah—prophet of God in Israel

Elixir of Life—life force, substance that sustains life

Emily Rose—nine-year-old girl who exposed therapeutic touch by her school project

empathy—the capacity to experience another's feeling as if it were one's own; emphasis is on spirit power for healing, known to use spirit power of animals in therapy

Emperor Fu Xi—developed the circle of harmony, pa kua, in 2900 BC

Emperor Hwang Ti—wrote the *Nei Ching* medical text near 2600 BC

Emperor Shen Nung—in 2800 BC compiled a text *Pen-tsao* on herbs

enchanter—one who influences by charms

enchantment—to be in a state of charm

enchant—to influence by charm

encyclopedists—refers to the movement and people of at the time of the Enlightenment late 1780s–90s. At that time, the encyclopedia was written and printed.

Endor—a village location near Mount Tabor in a large plain east of Nazareth and west of sea of Galilee

energy cyst—hypothesis of energy bound up in muscle, ligament, etc., where it has continued over the years; not connected with science or reality

energy medicine—medical therapy by balancing universal energy

Enlightenment—a period of late eighteenth century where reason was worshiped and religion put down; also refers to having reached the state of godhood, one with the universe, etc.

Ephesians—people living in Ephesus in Asia Minor, now Western Turkey

ephod—a special chest cloak worn by Jewish high priests in Bible

Epler Jr., D. C.—author of *Bloodletting in Early Chinese Medicine and Its Relation to the Origin of Acupuncture*

esoteric Christianity—refers to Christianity that practices mysticism

esoteric—occult or hidden

essence—having the qualities of the original; when referring to God, it refers to His very person or presence being in something. It may refer to a substance taken or extracted from something for application to something else. Universal energy is sometimes called essence; a fundamental nature or quality

essential oils—aromatic oils taken from plants that are supposed to contain universal energy

etheric body—this refers to an imaginary body said to be made of energy, and some authors describe it as having frequencies of a faster speed than light. It is said to act like a template for our bodies. Energy disturbance at that level is said to later show up in man as disease.

Ethiopia—country in Africa

ethnopharmacology—science of the study of plants for medicinal values relative to various ethnic groups

etiology—source or cause of illness or disorder

evidence based—"evidence based" means there is an accepted body of peer-reviewed, statistically significant evidence that raises probability of effectiveness to a scientifically convincing level.

Ezekiel—a prophet in Israel of Old Testament times and a name of a book written by him which is in the Bible

F

familiar spirit—demon spirit

fascia—connective tissue in animal and man: ligaments, tendons, etc.

falun gong—Chinese martial art

fibromyalgia—medical disorder consisting of painful muscles, joints, and points of insertion of tendons on bones; cause unknown

Finke, Ronald A.—author of *Creative Imagery*

fire walk—pertains to walking or running through hot bed of coals

Fitzgerald, Robert, SJ—Jesuit priest, author of book *The Soul of Sponsorship*, member of same order of Jesuits as Ed Dowling, the close friend of Bill W.

Fitzgerald, William, MD—originator of zone therapy later called reflexology

five ancestors—refers to five planets in astrology dogma that are supposed to be intricately related to creation

flower essences—mystical energy removed from blossoms of flowers and placed in water to be used for therapy

forbidden ground—a term used to refer to locations, instances or influences, subjects, etc., where the power of Satan will be manifest. Has reference to area of the Tree of Knowledge of Good and Evil in the Garden of Eden. Adam and Eve were advised to not go near it.

Free Masonry (Freemasonry or Freemason)—secret fraternal society, often called masonry

G

Galen (AD 129–200)—a physician who lived in Pergamum (now Turkey) and was instructor of medicine. He was a brilliant writer of medicine, and his opinions were the basis of medicine for more than 1,500 years.

Galyean, Beverly (now deceased)—author of article on psychology and consultant for the Los Angeles school system in psychology, promoted New Age doctrine

games of chance—gambling games

Garrison, Fielding, MD—author of *History of Medicine*

Gassner—Catholic priest who healed by use of hands only, lived at the time of Mesmer, an exorcist

gemstone—stones of beauty and of value

geomancy—divination by figures formed when a handful of dirt is thrown on ground or by lines randomly drawn; gems used as divination by throwing out many gems on a cloth with locations marked, signifying certain pre-assigned meanings

geometry—science of measuring angular areas, areas not always rectangular or square

Gerber, Richard, MD—medical doctor, believer in energy medicine and author of *Vibrational Medicine*

Gerome, Stan—wrote an article about synchronicity and craniosacral subject, instructor in craniosacral therapy at Upledger Institute

Gnosticism—secret society in early Christianity time, "a *thorn*" to Christianity; a mixture of Cabala, Judaism, and Zoroastrianism from Persia; believing in hidden spiritual knowledge; emphasis on knowledge instead of faith

God Calling—name of book written by two ladies that called themselves Two Listeners

Gods of the New Age **video**—a two-hour video illustrating the movement into the West the Hindu teachings of the East; produced by Jeremiah Films

grandmaster—top level of attainment in martial art, tenth dan

Grand Orient Lodge of France—Masonic lodges in and around France in mid-1700s and later, approximately 150 of such lodges

Grand Orient Lodge—Masonic lodges of Paris, France in mid- to later 1700s

great reality—term referring to universal energy, Higher Self, chi, prana, higher consciousness, etc.

Green, Elmer and Alyce—coauthors of the book *Beyond Biofeedback*, researchers in biofeedback

guided imagery (mental imagery, visualization)—using imagination to conjure an image in the mind, such as an animal or bird, which in turn becomes one's guide; actually a demon in disguise.

Gumpert, Martin—author of *Hahnemann: The Adventurous Career of an Adventurous Rebel*

Gurudas—a.k.a. Ronald Lee Garman, author of *Flower Essences and Vibrational Healing*

H

Hahnemann, Samuel, MD—originator of homeopathy discipline (1755-1843)

Hall, Manly—author of many books for the Masonic Lodge, *The Secret Teaching of All Ages*

hallucinogen—substance that will cause hallucinations

Hardinge, Mervyn, MD—author of book *A Physician Explains Drugs, Herbs and Natural Remedies*; professor of pharmacology, founder of School of Health, Loma Linda University

Harner, Michael—a shaman, teacher of shamans, and author of *The Way of the Shaman*

hatha yoga—type of yoga wherein the sun's energy is breathed in through the right nostril and the moon energy through the left, ha = sun, tha = moon, joining of sun and moon energies by use of yoga

Henry Mason—author of text *The Seven Secrets of Crystal Talisman*

herbal medicine—using herbs for medicinal use, often for their occult energies

herbalism—using herbs for health and healing

herbalist—one who practices the art of healing by use of herbs

herbs—plants used as special sources of nutritional substances and in the field of Eastern mysticism, yin-yang, hot-cold, status

Hermes—Thoth to the Egyptians, Hermes to the Greeks; mythical god figure; originator of alchemy; originally referred to Cush, son of Ham, son of Noah

hermetic tradition—following after the lore of Hermes Trismegistus, magical, alchemical, esoteric, etc.

Hester, Ben—author of *Dowsing: An Exposé of Hidden Occult Forces*

hieroglyph—a drawing or carving depicting a message or information

higher consciousness—refers to higher planes of the seven levels of universal energy, up to state of godhood

higher power—in Eastern thought refers to the subconscious that is at a higher level than your conscious thought process and near to godhood level. In Alcoholics Anonymous, it can refer to any entity that one may choose to be his "higher power" or "god."

Higher Self—mystical concept of being a god, having godhood

Hill, Ann—author of *A Visual Encyclopedia of Unconventional Medicine*

Hippocrates—famous physician around 400 BC and a great medical writer; recognized that lifestyle was connected to disease, a new concept at his time

Hitching, J. Francis—author of *Earth Magic*

Hoizey, Dominique and Marie-Joseph—authors of *A History of Chinese Medicine*

holistic health—health of body/mind/spirit as a result of a proper balance with nature

holistic—term used by New Age (neo-pagan) world view relevant to subject of health, emphasizing the interconnection of body, mind, and spirit

hologram—a small localized area or substance that is a template of a greater area, such as the cell of the body, as a template of the universe; often refers to a small localized area on the body considered to represent the entire body; not accepted in science

homeopathy—alternative medical style of practice with therapy consisting of using minute (at times no original molecules of the substance left in the solution) doses of substances as medicinals

Homer—ancient Greek poet who wrote about mythology

Homo-Vibra Ray—machine that claims to detect electromagnetic disturbances in an individual, sending them back into the body's electromagnetic frequencies to correct the supposed imbalance and thus effect healing

Hopp, H. J.—author of *Homeopathy*

house party—a gathering of members of the Oxford Group for two or more days of fellowship

Howard, Michael—author of the book *The Occult Conspiracy: Secret Societies—Their Influence and Power in World History*

Hsing-yi—a form of martial art

Huang Ti *Nei Ching* text—most important Chinese text at end of first century

Hubbard, Reuben—author of *Historical Perspectives of Health*

human potential—generally used in reference to a belief that man has divinity within and it can be raised to a higher level, a pantheistic concept

humanism—doctrine coming forth at time of Enlightenment (mid- and late 1700s); man is center of all and Self reigns supreme, divine within etc., self-sufficiency of man, does not derive assistance from a God

humanistic—life centered on man himself as the ultimate; God is left out.

humors—fluids, referring to the supposed four humors of the body, concept for the last 2,500 years until scientific medicine revealed its fallacy

Hunt, Dave—author and evangelical minster, coauthor of *America: The Sorcerer's New Apprentice—The Rise of New Age Shamanism*

hydrotherapy—treatment using water in many different ways

hypnosis—being in a state of mind alteration so that another person can control you, can be to a point of full trance or unconscious state

hypnotism—mind therapy wherein one submits his mind to the control of another

I

I AM—Name God called Himself; however, it is commonly used in neo-paganism to refer to the believed vital force said to be within man

I Ching sticks—stick of wood used in divination acts, Chinese in origin

Ignatius Loyola—established the Jesuit Order in early 1500s

illuminist—one belonging to Illuminati secret society. The Illuminati led by Adam Weishaupt infiltrated the Masonic lodges of France starting around 1776 and was an influence leading to the French Revolution of 1789.

immortality—life never ending

inanimate—nonliving substance, such as metal, rock, mineral, etc.

incantation—chanting some phrase or word

Ingham, Eunice—advanced the therapy of reflexology after Dr. Fitzgerald passed on

innate—name given to universal energy by chiropractors, the flow of which is said to be facilitated by manipulation of "subluxations" of vertebrae in the spine

inner self—similar to Higher Self, the subconscious that functions at higher level than conscious thought and has access to wisdom of the universe

integrative—blending or mixing of conventional and non-conventional medical practices

intuition—an ability to receive extrasensory intelligence and/or directions from a source not of the conscious mind but from the unconscious and/or possible spirit source

iridology chart—chart of the iris with ninety different divisions to it; each section is believed to relate to some specific part or organ of man.
iridology—alternative medicine discipline used to divine from iris of the eye, past, present, and future disease and its location in the body
iron—mineral of the earth, common substance used in hundreds of manufactured products, made into steel by adding carbon
irrational—no cause-and-effect consideration; in medical treatment, often referring to mystical considerations
Isis—mythical Egyptian goddess

J

Jaggi, O. P., PhD, MD—surgeon and author of the book *Yogic and Tantra Medicine*
Jensen, Bernard, DC—author of *The Science and Practice of Iridology*, New Age healer
John—John, an Apostle of Christ and wrote the Bible books of John and Revelation
Johnston, Dale, PT—physical therapist in La Grande, Oregon, author of *Underground Oasis*
judo—Japanese form of martial art
jiu-jitsu—Japanese form of martial art

K

Kabbala, Kabalah, Caballa, Cabala—secret society of Israel, considered "grandfather" of secret societies
Kah, Gary—author of *En Route to Global Occupation*
Kamiya, Joe, MD—San Francisco physician who coined the word *biofeedback* in his research on "autogenic training"
kapha—third division made up of a combination of the other two divisions (doshas) of prana energy
Karagulian, S.—author of *Energy Fields and Medical Diagnosis: The Human Aura*
karate—form of martial art
kata—physical movements in martial arts
Keating, Thomas—Catholic priest promoting Emergent Church movement
Kellogg, John, MD—physician from the mid-1800s until late 1940s, director of Battle Creek Sanitarium and author of many books, known

as a great leader in healthful living, also originator of breakfast cereals and other health food products
kenpo—form of martial art
Kent, James Tyler—author of *Lectures on Homeopathic Philosophy* (1979), reprint from original published in 1900
Khalsa, Dharma Singh, MD—author of *Meditation as Medicine*
kinesiology—true science of the action of muscles
ki—synonym for universal energy
kia—word shouted when practicing martial arts, to move "chi" throughout
Knights Templar—Catholic organization that went to the Holy Land to protect Crusaders but became involved in secret organizations of the Arabs and came back to Europe where eventually the king of France subdued them, evolved into many other secret orders over time
Koch, Kurt—a German Lutheran pastor who is known for his wisdom in counseling people and authoring articles connected with the occult
Krieger, Dolores, RN—nurse that promoted and made popular therapeutic touch therapy.
kundalini—"serpent power" supposed to be latent energy lying in the bottom chakra
kung fu—martial art of origin
Kunz, Dora—author of therapeutic touch discipline and past president of Theosophical Society and a spiritualist
Kurtz, Ron—Buddhist psychologist

L

Laban—nephew of Abraham of Bible history
lactic acid—a chemical produced by muscles when exercised. When builds up to high concentrations, pain occurs in the muscle; and at very high levels, action of muscle may cease.
Lanagan, John—author of *Worldview Times* website
laparoscope—instrument used to view inside of the abdomen, used in surgical procedures called laparoscopy
laser puncture—using laser than needle to puncture skin, as in acupuncture
latent forces—mystical forces supposedly stored in human mind or elsewhere in the body until liberated by various occult methods
lattice—formation of molecules arranging themselves in a repetitive physical position, creating a crystal
leukemia—cancer of white blood cells
levitation—raising objects by power of occult

Leviton, Richard—author of article in *East-West Journal of Natural Health and Living*

Levy, Robert—coauthor of *Shamanic Reiki*

ley lines—power lines of energy said to travel through the ground and is said to emanate increased power at points where the lines cross; universal energy power is believed to be accessed by humans where lines intersect one another (example, stone circles)

Li Xiao Ming—qi gong master from Beijing College of Traditional Chinese Medicine

life force energy—synonym for universal energy and all other synonyms

life force—synonym to universal energy, vital force, prana, chi, etc.

Lilly, Simon—crystal healer and author of *The Complete Illustrated Guide to Crystal Healing*

Linder, Rosa—author of article in *JAMA*, *Lancet*, and *British Medical Journal* exposing therapeutic touch

Living Temple, The—book written by John Kellogg containing pantheistic sentiments

Lockie, Andrew—author of *Natural Health: An Encyclopedia of Homeopathy*

lodestone—naturally magnetized piece of mineral magnetite that draws iron particles to it

logos—Greek term for universal energy

lotus—term referring to having reached godhood

LSD—lysergic acid diethylamide, a chemical used to bring mind-changing experiences to the person taking the substance, often induced a hallucinating mind change; at one time, it was legal to use.

Luciferian occultism—hidden knowledge and/or activities directed by Lucifer or Satan and used to promote worship of Satan

Lucifer—Satan, when he was an unfallen angel, means *light bearer*

Luthe, Wolfgang, MD—German doctor and student of Johannes Schultz, MD, and a leading exponent of autogenic training following Schultz's death

lymphatic—non-blood vascular system in animal and man that drains fluids from the body into the blood system

M

MacArthur, John—author of *The Truth War*

macrocosm—refers to sun, moon, stars, and the cosmos

magenta—an added color to the seven colors of the rainbow, deep purplish red

magic arts—sorcery, various paranormal acts or practices usually for healing, synonym with sorcery

magician—one skilled in magic, one involved in occult practices

magnesium—a mineral

magnetic energy—energy produced by magnets, such as electricity when magnets are moved against one another; also used in holistic health to refer to universal energy, etc.

magnetic field therapy—giving therapy by altering a magnetic field about someone

magnetic fluid—synonym for universal energy

magnetic healer—one who claims to heal by using magnets or electromagnetic energy frequencies

magnetic therapy—therapy given by use of magnet or magnets, may be by pulsating magnets or use of static magnet

magnetism—a true physical force found in the earth and seen in iron and some other substances having positive and negative poles

magnetoelectric energy—a synonym for universal energy. The term is coined by William Tiller, retired physics instructor of Stanford University.

magnets—iron that has been magnetized

Magus, Simon—a biblical character (Acts 8) who was a magical healer in the day of the Apostles. He asked of Peter to buy the power of laying on of hands to pass on the power of performing miracles. He was the originator of the Gnostic movement in early Christianity, which opposed Christianity.

mana—synonym for universal energy; name used in Polynesia for universal energy

mandala—in Sanskrit, it means circle; artwork of various designs placed in a circle to depict the theology of paganism; depicts the universe and the power of the gods

Manichaeism—secret order and movement that followed Gnosticism in the AD second and third centuries; had its doctrine out of Cabala, Gnosticism, and Zoroastrianism of Persia

mantra—word, phrase, sentence, or even Bible verse repeated over and over

Marcy, E. E.—author of *The Homeopathic Theory and Practice of Medicine*

marma points—localized position on the body where universal energy is said to flow through the connective tissue and where channel junctions of flow occur; points on the body where pressure is said to unblock congested flow of universal energy, similar to acupuncture points in traditional Chinese medicine, originates from Ayurvedic medicine

martial arts—physical type of exercise or movements used as a form of meditation and for defense through balance; many variations developed, such as judo, tai chi, etc.
massage, Swedish—massage given to facilitate blood and lymph circulation of the body
massage, trigger points (marma points)—massage given to particular points believed by Ayurvedic medicine to move universal energy when blocked
Ma-wang-tui graves—Chinese graves discovered in 1970s and contained writings of all medical treatment types in third and second century BC.
Ma-wang-tui—text from ancient Chinese graves (168 BC)
Maxwell, Jessica—author of "What Your Eyes Tell You about Your Health," an iridology article (in *Esquire* magazine)
McCarty, Michael—author of article in the *Lancet* exposing therapeutic touch
McMahon, T. A.—coauthor of *The Seduction of Christianity*
McNamara, Sheila—author of the text *Traditional Chinese Medicine*
meditation—placing the mind in a neutral state (detached awareness) or concentrating on only one thing so as to turn the thoughts inward
medium—a person who connects between earth and the spirit world
mediumistic trances—altered state of consciousness facilitated by a medium
mediumistic—being a spiritualistic medium
melancholic—depressed, sad
Menninger Foundation—psychiatric research institution in Topeka, Kansas
mental imagery (guided imagery)—forming in the mind a picture of what one may desire to have or create to change things, does not refer to regular thought and planning or creative ideas
Mercadante, Linda—author of *Victims and Sinners*
mercury—fluid-like metal, silver in color (quicksilver), comes from cinnabar ore, very toxic to living creatures, used for millennia as a medicinal
Mercury—mythological figure in Greek, same as Hermes in Egyptian mythology, synonym for Cush
meridian—an imaginary channel in the body claimed to transport energy
Mermet, Alexis—priest who felt he was first to use pendulum to diagnose medical abnormalities
Mesmer, Franz, MD—known for making hypnotism popular, and the use of hypnotism was called mesmerism (late 1700s into 1800s).
mesmerism—hypnotism

Mesopotamian civilization—past civilization that existed in present-day Iraq

meta analysis—combining the data of many different similar studies and analyzing them as one study

metabolism—normal internal chemical process of living creatures

metaphysics—physical phenomenon unexplained by conventional science of physics, has to do with paranormal-occult

microcosm—refers to man as the microcosm of the universe

Miller, Edith—author of *Occult Theocracy*

mind sciences—pertaining to various disciplines relating to explaining workings of the mind and related therapies

mind-set—belief system of an individual (example: creationist mind-set or understanding of origin in contrast to evolutionists' beliefs)

modality—method

monism—belief that all substances of the universe are parts of one basic energy, one is all and all is one, pagan concept of association of all substances of the universe

Moonies—individuals following cult leader Reverend Moon from Korea

Morgana—feminine for sun god of Celts

mother tincture—base substance from which dilutions of homeopathy remedies have their origin

moxibustion—burning of small cones of plants on the skin to effect localized heat, ancient Chinese custom, same effect as acupuncture

MRI (magnetic resonance imaging machine)—uses magnets and computers to image the interior of individuals, works by laws of physical science

mumio—mixture of medicinals popular in Russia, contains around fifty different substances

myography or electromyography—tracing graphs made of electrical activity of muscle action

mystical medicine—medical therapies that are actually using spiritualistic power in an attempt to promote health and healing

mysticism—the act of seeking union with the godhead. Noah Webster dictionary of 1828—The doctrine of the Mystics, who profess a pure, sublime and perfect devotion, wholly disinterested, and maintain that they hold immediate intercourse with the divine Spirit

mystic—one who through meditation or self-surrender seeks union with the godhead and one who believes in universal wisdom, cosmic consciousness; may believe that he holds direct communication with God

mystics—*Noah Webster Dictionary* (1828), a religious sect who professes to have direct intercourse with the Spirit of God

N

nature worship—worship of the *creation* rather than the *Creator*

naturopathy—medical discipline, promotes the concept of existence of toxins in the system, which must be removed by colon irrigation or special herbs to cleanse the colon. There is no scientific information to back up these claims.

Navajo—Native Americans found in Southwest USA

Nebuchadnezzar—king of Babylon, 600 BC

necromancer—one who practices the art of conferring with the spirits of the dead (a channeler)

Nei Ching—most celebrated text of Chinese medicine, written in 2600 BC

Nei-gong—martial art

neo-paganism—a return in beliefs to old nature worship, doctrine of pagans brought into modern-day setting packaged in new terms and made to appear as a new and great improvement in philosophy and religion

neutral—this word is used in reference to whether a method of therapy that had a long history of use in the occult could be taken out of that context for use in Christian setting and be spiritually safe

New Age movement—name given to a large number of groups and organizations and many people not in organizations who have a common philosophy, trend is toward nature worship in philosophy

new thought movement—supposedly a Christian renewal movement arising in 1800s and attempting to infiltrate other religious organizations with their teachings, pantheistic in nature but hidden

Newhouse, Sandy—coauthor of *Native American Healing*

ninjutsu—form of martial art

nirvana—land of paradise for the pagan, Buddhist, similar concept as heaven to the Christians

nitrosamine—chemical that has carcinogenic properties

noetic sciences—paranormal, mystical

Norse—early people of Norway

Nuga Best—table-type machine that has rollers that massage and infrared lamps that produce heat

numerics—determining meanings from a word or object by use of numbers, mystical application of numbers

O

oasis—a place in the desert with water and vegetation that gave *refuge* and rest to the traveler of the harsh desert environment. Underground oasis used in this text refers to a place of refuge for the weary soul in addiction.

observer of times—astrologer, horoscope user, etc.

Occident—Western civilization

occult—hidden, obscure, secret, connected with spirit world

occultist—one using occult theory or practice

odic force—synonym for universal energy

Odyssey—Homer's Greek mythological epic chronicling Odysseus

Olcott, Henry—co-originator of the Theosophy Society in New York, 1875

omega—last, at the end

omen—a sign or warning of a future event, situation, or condition

One—term used in pagan theology to refer to the highest level of the universal energy, godhood, Supreme Self, etc.

Oneness— a. to be in total accord (Christian use—Accord with God); b. duality of vital force/universal energy brought into "one" (Pagan definition)

Ophiel (a.k.a. Edward C. Peach)—author of a book on creative visualization, become one with the universe, to arrive at the state of dissolution of the duality into a single force, immortality, godhood

optometrist—doctor of optometry, non-medical doctor of vision care

orenda—universal energy name used by a certain Indian tribe. Each tribe had its own name for such.

organon energy—synonym for universal energy, associated with homeopathy

origins—explanation of origin of cosmos, earth, and man

Oschman, James—scientist and author of *Energy Medicine: The Scientific Basis*

oscilloscope—instrument that is used in physics to demonstrate electromagnetic waves of energy in visible form (television screen, for example)

osteopathy—discipline of medicine, originally practiced by manipulation of joints as treatment for disease but now same as mainstream scientific medicine practice

Ouija board—instrument of divination with alphabet and numbers and yes-and-no words. Questions asked of the board are answered by a pointer going to the different numbers, letters, or words on the board.

oxygen—gas of the atmosphere, may combine with certain minerals and form various stones

P

pa kua—Chinese circle of harmony
pagan—one who is not a Christian, Jew, or Moslem; is a nature worshiper, lunar goddess worshiper, dedicated to establishing "old religion"
palmistry—using the palm of the hand to divine the future
pantheism—a doctrine that equates God with the forces and laws of the universe, universal energy, god in everything and everything god
pantheistic world view—belief in the origin of life as described by *pagan religions* (created out of a two-sided energy by the perfect balancing of the two parts); the future is nirvana in the spirit world but only after many lives by reincarnation.
Paracelsus—very famous sixteenth-century physician who believed in universal energy, also an astrologer and believed in vital energy and dualism
passive mind—a mind that has been brought to the state of non-thinking
peer review—scientific articles reviewed by other scientists before publishing to make certain that the study has followed proper methods of investigation, thereby giving the study greater probability of accuracy in its results
Pegasus—producers of flower essences
Pelletier, Kenneth, MD—author quoted in an article written by Biblical Research Committee of SDA, General Conference of SDAs (1987). Pelletier is a believer in New Age concepts.
pendulum—divining instrument, usually an object hanging from a string swinging independently so as to give answers to questions by predetermined parameters
Pen-ts'ao—text on 365 herbs, earliest text on herbs written
Pergamos—city in Western Turkey or Asia Minor in biblical days
Pergamum—city in Asia Minor or nowadays country of Turkey (same as Pergamos)
peyote—cactus that has hallucinatory properties when ingested
Pfeiffer, Samuel, MD—author of *Healing at Any Price*
phallic symbol—symbol of the male sex organ
Philistines—people or small nation next to Old Testament Israel and occupied territory on south part of the coast
phlegmatic—showing steady temperament

phrenology—pseudoscience with belief that the shape of the head determined personality and character. These were believed to be changed by applying pressure on the head in specific locations.

physiology—normal function of living creatures

piezoelectric effect—electrical charge generated from a crystal when crystal is compressed

Pike, Albert—in mid-1800s, he was the grandmaster of the Masonic Order and authored the book *Morals and Dogma of the Ancient and Accepted Scottish Rite of Freemasonry.*

Piper, Mrs. L. E.—spiritualist with whom William James joined in séances for over twenty-five years

Pisces—zodiac symbol of the fish

pitta—second division of prana energy

Pittman, Bill—author of *AA: The Way It Began*

polarity—term applied to a "non-recognized" condition of one side of the body being of positive polarity and the other side the negative

potassium—a mineral

potentizing—making more potent or adding strength by thumping the mixture

potion—a substance to be taken internally that would have some magic effect on the creature that took it

power object—an object used by a shaman in his treatment of the ill or injured, often a quartz crystal

power of the will—power of choice

prana—air, breath, and said to carry universal energy into body with the breath

pre-Christian mystery tradition—Babylonian mysteries and/or pagan religion

precepts—doctrine, teaching, law of, etc.

Priessnitz, Vincent—initiated hydrotherapy clinic in Austria

primordial—original, first created or developed state, first evolution story and theory

prognosticator—one who foretells from signs or symptoms

Prophet, Elizabeth Clare—authored the book *Intermediate Studies of the Human Aura*, as received dictation by the spirit Djwal Khul

psora—Samuel Hahnemann, MD, determined to his satisfaction that all diseases, apart from surgical maladies and syphilis, originated from a basic infectious disease he called psora. All acute and chronic disorders he believed originated from this. He states in his book *Organon* (p. 78) that it took him twelve years to discover this fact. Such a basic infectious disorder—the source of all other disease—is not recognized by science.

psychedelic—referring to a chemical, when ingested, causes mind-altering changes

psychic healing—healing another by the power of one's mind

psychic therapy—directing by mind, supernatural forces to effect therapy

psychic—effect or status of mental state, refers to sensitivity of a person to supernatural forces or one that uses such

psychology—science of the mind and behavior, or science of the soul in the word's early meaning

psychometry—diagnostic technique of determining the characteristics of people who are not present by means of objects that have been in their possession. The practitioner might use a personal object such as a watch, a ring, or other jewelry, and hold the object with the eyes closed in order to receive psychic impressions of its owner.

psychoneuroimmunology—science or study of the influence on the immune system by mental activity and the thoughts

psychophysiology—study of function of the brain processes

psychotronic radionics—use of electronics and machines combined with mental activity to divine and/or treat

pulse diagnosis—using the nature of the pulse to diagnose disorders in the human body, has its origin in Chinese traditional medicine

purer consciousness—synonym for One, Supreme Self, god, etc.

pyruvic acid—one of the chemical metabolites of body metabolism, a chemical

Q

qi gong (ki gong)—most fundamental of Chinese martial arts, meditation in action or without motion to effect balance of chi

quartz—crystalline form of silica

Queen's Work—Catholic magazine published by Jesuit Society in St. Louis, Missouri.

R

radiesthesia—ability of a person to perform as a medium in divining information by use of pendulums or machine pendulums, ability depends upon degree of connection with occult powers

radionics—use of electrical machines for divination for diagnosis and at times treatment

Ragon—Masonic author of *Maconnerie Occulte*
Ramacharaka—yogi, pseudonym for William Atkinson
Raman, R. V.—sage of astrology in India
Rand, William Lee—author of *The Nature of Reiki Energy*
Raphael, Matthew J.—author of *Bill W. and Mr. Wilson*
Raso, Jack—author of *Expanded Dictionary of Metaphysical Health Care*
Raso, MD, RD—author of *Mystical Diets*
rational therapies—therapies given that are based on cause-and-effect relationship
Ray, Barbara, PhD—author of *Reiki Factor*
Raynaud's disease—disorder of spasms of arterioles of hands and feet causing reduction of blood flow to the anatomical part and may result in pain, sometimes death to tissue
reflexology—alternative treatment method, rubbing the palms of the hands or the bottom of the feet to effect healing of various areas of the body
rei—ghost, spirit, soul, etc.
Reiki guide—a spirit that assists in Reiki healing; often embodied; occultic, spiritistic
Reiki master—one who has reached the third level in training and practice of Reiki healing
Reiki—a form of body therapy from Japan and is closer to psychic therapy than to soma therapy; uses, if any, very light touch for therapy
reincarnation—the doctrine of re-birth and many lives
Reisser, Paul C., MD—medical practitioner and coauthor of *New Age Medicine*
relaxation response—title to program of yoga-like actions taught by Dr. Herbert Benson. This technique made yoga acceptable to medical profession.
religion of nature—paganism, Wicca
re-pattern—to reform a pattern of action or appearance
Reuter's Health Information—Internet website that gives daily review of new science reporting on medicine
Rife machine—machine that is supposed to measure the frequencies of electromagnetic waves said to be coming from infectious agents (fungus, bacteria, viruses) within our bodies. The machine is said to send corrective waves of proper frequencies back into our bodies to rid the body of these agents. This is said to cure infectious disease and sometimes cancer since its founder believed that all cancer is a result of virus infection.

Ritter, Johann Wilhelm—German scientist member of Bavarian Academy of Science in early 1800s
Roberts, Lynn—coauthor of *Shamanic Reiki*
Rodriquez, Cardinal Caro—bishop of Santiago, Chile, who recognized that the Theosophy Society was supported by the Masonic Lodge in that city
Roeckelein, Jon E.—author of *Imagery in Psychology*
Rogers, Carl—leader in secular humanistic psychology
Rohr, Richard—Catholic priest promoting Emergent Church movement
Rolf, Pauline—originator of Rolfing massage, correcting the flow of universal energy
rolfing—heavy, painful massage therapy to point of bruising the tissues
Rosicrucian—one of the prominent secret societies existing for past several centuries
rune dice—special dice used in divination
Russian parapsychology—psychology involved with the use of supernatural forces

S

sage—Hindu holy man
Sampson, Wallace, MD—wrote a critique on the report on acupuncture put out by the National Institutes of Health
sanguine—cheerful, hopeful
sanitarium—treatment facility usually involving the use of more "natural" treatment methods; use of exercise, rest, sunshine, diet, physical therapy, etc., as main treatment methods; this word was first used by John H. Kellogg, MD, at Battle Creek, Michigan.
Sanskrit—ancient Indian language that the Vedas were written in
Satan's ground—at the Garden of Eden, the immediate area around the Tree of Knowledge of Good and Evil would be considered Satan's ground. God had directed Adam and Eve to not go near it. If they placed themselves in an area where the devil had influence, they would be more susceptible to his wiles. E. G. White uses the expression "Satan's ground" to refer to not only locations but to associations, reading material and author's works, therapies, attitudes, etc., that when utilized or we become exposed to we are on Satan's ground and our protecting angel is hindered in his work for us.
Satanism—Satan worship or following of
Schultz, Johannes, MD—neurologist in Berlin who continued Oskar Vogt's work on autohypnosis

sciences—a term referring to physics, chemistry, engineering, medicine, dentistry, nursing, etc.

scientific medicine—medical care based on known laws of physics, chemistry, and physiology as learned by demonstration and testing through scientific methods

scrying—crystal ball gazing, divination act

Seal of Solomon—same as Star of David

sensei—director of dojo, instructor in martial arts (twice born/reincarnated)

sensitive—one who has special psychic powers or special senses in the occult

Shaolin Temple—Buddhism temple in China that was a place of origin of martial arts

shaman—name given to native "medicine man," a witch doctor

shiatsu—body therapy of specific type from Japan, very gentle

Shi-Chi text—acupuncture first found in these Chinese writings of 90 BC

Shing Moon—Oriental name for female sun god

Shiva—Hindu god

Siberia—Northeastern part of Russia with natives similar to American Indian

signature—refers to association "like cures like" where a substance may influence another due to its similar appearance

silicon—a mineral of the earth, one-seventh of the earth's surface (sand is silicon dioxide)

Smith, Anne—wife of Dr. Bob Smith, co-founder of AA

sodium—a mineral

solidified light—claim made by shaman of Australia that light can turn into a quartz crystal

Sol—sun and name referring to sun god

soma body work (somatics)—physical treatment to the body by various massage-type methods

Somatoemotional release—act of the "inner physician," bringing healing by releasing bound-up energy in "energy cyst"

sonopuncture—use of ultrasound to affect acupuncture points instead of using needles

soothsayer—one that foretells events

sorcerer—one who uses witchcraft or occult forces, one who by enchantments or charms persuades another to make decisions that are detrimental to his eternal well-being

sorceries—all forms of witchcraft and their acts, all actions that persuade or influence an individual so as to cause a decision to be made that ill effects his eternal destiny

sound therapy—application of sound or music to affect the chakras to effect electromagnetic balance

spirit guides—Satan's angels, demons acting as if a beneficial guide to a human

spirit—intelligent entity of the unseen world, Satan's angels

Spiritual Counterfeits Journal—a journal exposing spiritualism in New Age, holistic healings

Spiritual exercises of Ignatius Loyola—principles applied in the training of a Jesuit priest to bring the person to total surrender and loyalty to the Jesuit Order

spiritualism—belief that spirits of the dead communicate with the living; any act or belief that connects us to the power of Satan; any precept that entertains progression to godhood, divinity within

spiritualist—one who uses spiritual powers

spurious healings—false or counterfeit

Sri Aurobindo—a yogi

Stalker, Douglas—author of *Examining Holistic Medicine*

Star of David—a symbol of one triangle placed over another so as to form six points in the star

Star Wars—Hollywood movie that featured "universal energy" under the name "The Force"

stargazer—astrologer

statistically significant—results of a test reach a level that is likely to indicate significant relationship

Stein, Diane—author of *Essential Reiki*

Stewart, David PhD—author of *Essential Oils of the Bible*

subluxation—supposed congestion or obstructive focus of *innate energy* (universal energy) flow along the spinal column and outward to the periphery of the body. This does not refer to "out of place" vertebrae as many believe. Spinal manipulation is believed to unclog the energy congestion. This teaching is the basis upon which chiropractic medicine was founded. Subluxations have not been demonstrated by science.

subtle energy medicine—using universal energy to effect healing, producing an effect upon etheric body

subtle energy—same as universal energy

subtle teachings—doctrine of universal energy or pantheism

successed—homeopathic remedy that in its preparation has been shaken hard or "thumped" in the mixing

Sufis—secret society of the Islamic peoples

Sumerian—ancient civilization of Babylon or from the land of Mesopotamia (Iraq), same as Mesopotamian

sun worship—to worship the sun as a deity
Sunna—feminine name for sun god
super soul—synonym for reaching godhood
Supreme Self—synonym for godhood, the divine within raised to its zenith of development so that it connects with the cosmic intelligence and power of the universe
supreme ultimate—synonym for One, Supreme Self, god, highest level of theoretical universal energy
Sutherland, William, DO—osteopathic physician considered originator of craniosacral therapy
Swain, Bruce—author of article in *East-West Journal*
sway test—method of divination wherein an object is held near the chest and questions asked will be answered by one's body being pushed forward by a yes answer and pushed backward by a negative answer (described as a standup Ouija board)
Swedenborg, Emanuel—very influential writer and spiritualist of late eighteenth and early nineteenth century
sympathetic remedy—remedy founded upon the doctrine of association, sympathy, and/or correspondence
sympathetic—showing relationship such as correspondence
synchronicity—a hypothesis of Carl Jung wherein release of a physical distress relieves a mental condition
Szurko—ex-mystic

T

taekwondo—form of martial art
tai chi chuan—Chinese exercise, form of qi gong, meditation in motion, a form of martial art
Takata, Hawayo—Japanese woman that came to the United States and popularized Reiki
talisman—an object thought to act as a charm, may be of letters, numbers or sentences, may be a gemstone worn on the body as a charm or for protection, then called an amulet
Taoism—Chinese religion meaning "the way" based in astrological beliefs, man is a microcosm of the cosmos (macrocosm)
Taoist—believer in Chinese religion based out of mystic philosophy and Buddhist religion
tarter emetic—an old-style medicine used to cause vomiting (contains antimony)
template—a mold or pattern used to form some other object

The Force—universal energy.

theology—study of God, doctrines of

Theosophical Research Center—an organization and center within Theosophical Society dedicated to experimentation with mystical methods

theosophy—divine wisdom, term used to describe esoteric and mystical beliefs that describe the relationship of human beings to the universe and the godhead. These belief systems may describe emanations from the "Supreme God" who reveals different aspects of transcendent reality through various intermediary deities, spirits, or intelligences.

therapeutic imagery and dialogue—name given additional acts in craniosacral therapy; patient uses imagination to visualize "inner physician"; therapist dialogues with inner physician as a part of healing therapy; occultic, spiritistic in nature

therapeutic release and dialogue—a contribution of Dr. Upledger to therapy of craniosacral, spiritistic in nature

therapeutic touch—healing therapy by using the hands to balance energy. No real touching is done. Hands are held a few inches from the body.

therapeutic—a remedy for disease

Theriac—prime medicinal of Galen, formed of more than 70 substances grew to 230 substances through the centuries, considered the universal antidote

theta—a specific frequency of brain wave that correlates with neutral state of thought process; same frequency of brain wave that biofeedback takes place in and at times the same wave frequency that occurs with yoga meditation; alpha wave may also occur with yoga.

theurgic—magical, miracle, supernatural intervention, white magic

Thomsen, Robert—author of biography *Bill W.*

Thoth—same as Mercury, Hermes or Cush

Three ABN—television network, Christian

times—used in the Bible referring to prognostication to times of events determined by astrology

Tisserand, Robert—author of *The Art of Aromatherapy*

Tower of Babel—biblical story of tower built by Nimrod and place where God confounded languages

Towns Hospital—alcoholic rehab hospital in New York operated by William Silkworth, MD

Trachtenberg, Dr. Alan—arranged for summit on acupuncture for National Institute for Drug Abuse of the National Institutes of Health

transcendental meditation—basis is same as Eastern meditation (relaxation and use of mantra to obtain passivity of mind) with minor changes to make it acceptable in the West. The mantra consists of a secret word or phrase. It's a popular form of meditation in the United States, England, Australia, New Zealand and popularized in West by Maharishi Mahesh Yogi.

Trojan horse—refers to ancient story of city of Troy where a large wooden horse filled with soldiers was left outside the city as the surrounding army left. The horse was pulled into the city, and the gates were opened in the night by these soldiers, and the besieging army returned and entered the city to conquer.

Tuchak, Vladimir—coauthor of *Zone Therapy*

U

Ullman, Dana—coauthor of *Science of Homeopathy*
unified energy field—synonym for universal energy
universal energy—one of one hundred terms to describe an unmeasured, unproven, mystical force said to permeate the universe and from which all things are made. Popular terms are vital force, vitalism, universal intelligence, etc.
universal intelligence—refers to universal energy, chi, prana, etc. All the knowledge of the universe is supposed to be in the composition of universal energy, prana, chi, etc.
universal magnetic fluid—synonym for universal energy
unruffling—a movement of the hands sweeping across a body supposedly to smooth out the energy pattern of the body
Unschuld, P. U.—author of *Medicine in China: A History of Ideas*, and *Nan-ching: The Classic of Difficult Issues*
Upledger, John, DO—osteopathic doctor who has continued the craniosacral therapy technique and popularized it, developing the Upledger Institute to promote the technique
Usui, Mikao (1865–1926)—known as the originator of Reiki, Japanese
usurp—to take possession of something from someone or power

V

vata—one division of prana
Vedas—writings or books in Sanskrit language of ancient Indian times
vibrational medicine—synonym of energy medicine; focus is on electromagnetic wave frequency concept.
vibrational therapies—reference to special attention to treatment methods claiming to alter or correct electromagnetic vibrations

viscera—internal organs
visualization—making a picture in one's mind with the belief that the picture that is formed will come about, more relevant to situations and attitudes than to material substance
Vita Florum—flower essences brand
vital energy—synonym for universal energy, a non-entity but believed to permeate the cosmos, the creative principle
vital essence—synonym for vital force or universal energy
Voegeli, Dr. Adolf—famous homeopathic doctor
Vogel, Marcel—author of *The Science of the Mind: The Healing Magic of Crystals*
Vogt, Oscar, MD—brain physiologist in Berlin who used hypnotism to his patients, developed autohypnotism
volition—the will of a person, the power of choice
von Peczely, Ignaz—founder of iridology concepts
von Reichenbach, Baron—student of Mesmer and is credited with forming the Ouija board
von Schelling, Friedrich Wilhelm Joseph—German philosopher

W

Walters, Dale, PhD—co-researcher on biofeedback with Drs. Greens in Menninger Clinic, Topeka, Kansas
wand—a rod, often referring to staff or stick of a diviner; it may be a precious stone ground to a length and diameter to simulate a pencil or small stick
Warrier, Gopi—coauthor of *The Complete Illustrated Guide to Ayurveda*
water witching—searching for water with various divining techniques
Weil, Andrew, MD—medical doctor with Hindu-type beliefs, has become somewhat of a guru in influencing people in alternative medical beliefs and practices
Weldon, John—coauthor of *Can You Trust Your Doctor?*
Western occultism—same doctrine as paganism but coming from the West
wholistic health—proper balance of body/mind/spirit as taught by the *Bible*
Wicca—organization of witches
Wikipedia—encyclopedia on the Internet
Willis, Richard, MD—author of *Holistic Health, Holistic Hoax*
Wilson, Lois—wife of Bill Wilson

Winemiller, Mark, MD—author and researcher on magnet use for Achilles' tendonitis

witch—a person believed to have magic power

witchcraft—the practices of a witch (sorcery), an irresistible impulse or attraction

witch doctor—medicine man, shaman, native healer usually connected with the spirit world

witness—some object having been worn, touched, or from a person and supposed to conduct vibrational patterns said to be specific to the person it came from; used in Radionics and not found to be science based.

Witt, Claudia, MD—author of article on acupuncture, faculty of Charité University Medical Centre in Berlin

wizard—diviner

Woodstock—name of the location of a festival held for young people in 1969. Five hundred thousand people were estimated in attendance. The name is commonly used to refer to that particular festival.

world view—a person's understanding and orientation to the question of one's origin, purpose, and future

Worwood, Valerie Ann—author of *Aromatherapy for the Soul* and other aromatherapy books

Y

yang—positive energy force, Chinese

yin—negative energy force, Chinese

yoga exercises—various types of snake-like physical movements and/or postures with the purpose of moving kundalini (serpent energy) up through the chakras to reach the crown chakra and become "one with the universe"

yoga-meditation—to yoke, involves practice of maintaining different postures (asanas) for extended time; objective is to move out of the reincarnation cycle and enter the bliss of the spirit world with the ascended masters; purpose is to yoke up with the spirit world.

yogi—practitioner of yoga, teacher

Yungen, Ray—minister, author of *A Time of Departing*

Yuman—tribe of American Indians in southern California

Z

zapping machine—a small handheld battery-operated electrical instrument that is supposed to kill a specific type of parasite to live in the intestines, which, when it moves to organs, causes all types of diseases, especially cancer. The person making and selling the machine is the only one who makes such claims.

zodiac—pathway of the planets in the cosmos, represented by a round circle illustrating the pathway, twelve houses, thirty-six rooms to the zodiac

zone therapy—reflexology of hand and foot massage to correct energy imbalance

Zoroastrianism—pagan religion of ancient Persia prior conversion

INDEX

A

Abrams's Box, 271
absent healing, 31, 240, 276
aconite, 251, 253
acupuncture, vii–viii, 1–3, 27, 30–31, 105, 113–14, 116–18, 120, 122, 126–45, 175–76, 179, 185–86, 272–74, 320–22
acupuncture according to Voll, 272, 274
acupuncture points, 129, 132, 134–35, 137, 144, 175, 179, 272–73, 322
Acupuncture Watch, 128–29, 133
Adolph, 43
Adolph, Franke, 43
Adonay, 47–48
Aesculapius, 266
agate, 224
agni, 98
Ahaziah, 13, 264, 292
aikido, 126
alchemist, 285, 287–88
alchemy, 19, 27, 51, 162, 205, 284–88, 310
aldehydes, 210
Alexander, 19, 286
allergen, 251–52
Allison, Nancy, 311
alpha, 153, 301
altered state of consciousness, 64, 68, 70, 77, 85, 152, 228, 301, 307, 309
alternative, 2–3, 30, 32–33, 60–61, 68, 89–90, 113, 140–41, 198, 254, 261, 265, 272–73, 306, 322–23
alternative medicine, 41, 52, 68, 103, 127, 165, 245, 254, 258, 261, 306, 322–23
Aluminum, 228
Alzheimer's disease, 179–80
ama, 98
amber, 187, 225
American Indian, 27, 35, 365
American Medical Society, 135
amethyst, 224–25
AMI machine, 322
amulets, 224, 232
Analytical Concordance of the Bible (Young), 284
anatomist, 98
Ancient Wisdom, 51
animal magnetism, 35, 188, 212, 245–46, 299
animate, 27, 56, 60, 318
animism, 74, 228, 246
Ankerberg, John, 150, 241
anthroposophy, 248
aphrodisiac, 119

Index

Aphrodite (Greek goddess), 54
Apollo (Greek god), 231, 266
apothecary, 205
applied kinesiology, 2, 167, 177–79, 209, 236, 239
Ares (Greek god), 54
Arhat, 124
aromatherapy, 2, 31, 97, 108, 118, 184, 204, 206–7, 210–11, 213–19, 276, 322, 365
asanas, 82, 86, 91, 93–94, 110–11, 126–27, 365
ascended masters, 181, 365
assessment, 139–41, 181, 202, 316
association, 20, 23–25, 28, 30, 36, 50, 56, 80, 107–9, 117–19, 165–67, 174–75, 182, 217, 300
astral body, 38, 247
astrologer, 60
astrological concepts, 144–45, 309, 326, 328
astrologic medicine, 265
astrology, 19–20, 23, 25, 29, 32, 43, 51, 53–54, 99, 106, 111–12, 117, 127, 226–27, 284–85
atheistic, 11, 48
atonement, 34, 325–26, 328–29
attuned, 126, 194–95, 197
aura, 36, 39, 56–62, 102–5, 107, 149, 165, 208, 218, 233–34, 242, 272, 276, 320–21
auricular therapy, 172
autogenic training, 12, 308–9, 312–14
autohypnosis, 155, 307–9
Ayurveda, 26, 29, 32, 36, 52–54, 56, 61, 63–64, 94, 97–100, 107–8, 111–13, 205, 210, 214
Aztecs, 231

B

Baalzebub, 13, 264–65, 324
Babylon, 19, 25, 42–43, 46–47, 231, 265
Babylonian mysteries, 42–43, 47, 326, 329
Bach (doctor), 208–10, 276
Bach Flower Remedies, 208
Bahti, 27
Baiame (supreme god in Australia and Southeast Asia), 227
Bailey, Alice, 50, 149
Basser, Stephen, 127–32
Bauman, Rudolph, 132
Bavarian Academy of Sciences, 267
Baylay, Doreen, 169
Beatles, 2, 65–66, 85
beliefs in origins Influences concepts of cause of disease, 12, 33, 39
Benson, Herbert, 68–70, 313
Bernard Jensen, 190–91
beryl, 224–25
Besant, Annie, 48–49
Bessy, Maurice, 23
Beverly Galyean, 163
bewitched, 327
Biblical Research Committee, 306–7, 315
Biblical world view, 220
biochemical, 97, 119, 204–6, 208, 211, 215, 245, 287–88
bioelectric energy, 168
bioelectromagnetics, 61, 168, 185, 273–74
bioenergy, 273–74
biofeedback, ix, 12, 31, 39, 62, 151, 156, 161, 296, 301, 303, 305–16
bioplasma, 35, 212
biopsy, 260
bioresonance, 273–75
black box, 271, 273, 323

black magic, 284
Blavatsky, Helena, 48–49
bobbing, 270–71
Bodhidharma (Buddhist monk), 121
body/mind/spirit, 317
body therapy, 167
Bopp, H. J., 246, 249–50
Boyatzis and McKee, 75
Brahman, 63, 66, 82, 93–94, 110–11, 311
breath of Life, 5, 116, 176, 199–200, 317
Brint, Armand, 192
Buchwald, Dedra, 137
Buddhism, 2, 54, 76, 121
Buddhist, 22, 25–26, 65, 76–78, 80, 93, 97, 110, 121, 125–26, 159, 162, 193, 201
Burke, Abbot George, 262

C

Cabalists, 45, 285
Caballa (Cabala), 43, 45, 159
Cachora (Indian Shaman), 207
caduceus, 287
calcium, 170, 228
calomel, 205
cantharides, 251
carbuncle, 224
Carcinosin, 253
Carruthers (doctors), 312–13
Carter (doctor), 190
causal body, 38
cell com system, 273–74
Celts, 231
centered, 64, 118, 121, 233, 240
centering, 71, 73–74, 126, 181, 233
cerebrospinal, 177, 198–200
cerebrospinal fluid, 198–200
chakra balancing, 31, 235–36

chakras (aura), 36, 56–59, 61–63, 66, 86–87, 92, 320–22
chalcedony, 225
chamomile, 249
Chan Buddhism, 121
channeled, 50, 149, 160, 197, 209, 214, 292, 319–21
channeling, 31, 80, 106, 149–50, 160, 220, 232, 241–42, 276, 278
charmer, 291
Cherkin, Daniel, 141
chi/ki/qi, 126
chi kung, 119
Chinese physiology, 127, 130
ching, 114, 128, 130, 216
ching-mo, 128
chiromancy, 166
chiropractic, 35, 185, 195, 254, 265
Chopra, Deepak, 107
Chou En-lai (premier), 1
Christopher Bird, 268
chrysolite, 225
chrysoprasus, 225
church of new Jerusalem, 33, 225
Circe, 282
circle of harmony, 25, 30, 114, 288
Cirlot, J. E., 24–25, 285
clairvoyance, 106, 159, 218, 299
clairvoyant, 160, 230, 319
cleansing, 63–64, 81–82, 84, 86, 88, 90, 92, 94, 96, 98–102, 104, 106, 108, 110, 112
coccyx, 56, 59, 87, 233
Cochrane Collaboration, 139, 143
colonic cleansing, 98, 101
color therapy, 31, 60, 265, 276, 322
Co-Masonry, 48–49
complementary, xv, 105, 107, 211, 290, 300, 306
concepts, xiv, 11–12, 19, 29–30, 32, 42, 47, 51–52, 125–26, 143–45,

151–52, 220, 292–93, 319–20, 326–28
Confucius (philosopher), 246–47
consciousness, xiii, 18, 39, 70–72, 77–79, 85, 149–50, 160–61, 174, 212–13, 292–93, 307–10, 314, 323–24, 326–27
contemplation, 64, 72
contemplative prayer, 72
controls, 46, 134, 137–38, 327
convents, 197
coral, 225
correspondence, 20, 23–25, 28, 36, 116–18, 130, 165–67, 169, 174–75, 217, 289
correspondence, association, sympathy, 23
cosmic, 63, 73, 97, 111, 116, 165–67, 173, 177, 198, 205, 208, 213, 218, 248, 288
cosmological correspondences, 130
cosmology, 55
cosmos, 21, 23–24, 37–38, 54, 58, 63, 66, 83, 94, 116, 130, 157, 165–66, 172–75, 314–15
counterfeit, xiv–xv, 3, 11, 16–17, 24, 33, 40, 47, 63–64, 92–93, 101, 116, 206, 215–16, 326–28
Cousens, Gabriel, 60, 292
Craig, Winston, 204, 208
creation, temptation, fall, deluge, 18
creative principle, 53–54, 64
creative visualization, 71, 148, 152–56, 158–59
crystal healers, 233, 235, 242
crystals, ix, 27, 31, 65, 122, 151, 161, 170, 216, 224–30, 232–37, 239–42, 263, 276–78
Cumbey, Constance, 50
Cummings, 251
Cush (son of Ham), 19–20, 286

D

dark ages, 54
decubiti ulcers, 180
deification, 45
deists, 48
Deleuze, Jean Philippe Francois, 299
deluge, 18–19
DeRuvo, Judy, 218
Desert Fathers, 72
detoxification, 108
diamond, 224
Di Mino, Alfonso, 122
disease treatment methods, 118
diuretic, 205
divination, ix, 27, 54, 85, 135, 177, 179, 188, 239–40, 262–66, 268–72, 274, 276–78, 280–81, 284
divine, xiv–xv, 4–5, 47, 64, 106, 164, 193, 212, 218, 220
diviner, 237–39, 268–69, 281
Djwal Khul, 39, 50, 107, 149
Does it work? 144, 296
dogma, 45–46, 285–86
Dominique and Marie-Joseph Hoizey, 145
doshas, 55–56, 98, 210, 214, 228
dowse, 60, 268
dowsing, 216, 236, 240–41, 265–68, 271, 279–81
dowsing rods, 216
dragon, 10
dreams, xiii, 22, 156, 249
dream therapy, 12, 150
Drmatron, 274
dualism, 19–20, 22, 27–28, 33, 42–43, 54, 56, 115, 214, 288

E

Eastern religions, 2, 11, 36, 39, 126, 310, 318
East–West, 47, 51–52

East-West Journal, 47, 50–52, 165, 168, 172
eclectic, 113, 250
Eden, 6, 14, 16–17, 21, 197, 204, 224, 284, 288
Edith, 46
ego, 149
Ekron, 13, 264, 324
electroacupuncture according to Voll, 276
electrocardiograms, 306
electroencephalogram, 306
electromagnetic bodies, 321
electromyography, 61, 102, 306
Elijah (prophet), 13–14, 264–65, 292
elixir, 90, 204, 214, 287, 322
emerald, 224–25
empathy, 213, 299
enchanter, 177, 291
enchantments, 284, 311
encyclopedists, 48
energy cyst, 201
energy medicine, 103, 105–6, 131, 181, 254, 258, 272–73, 275–76
Ephesians, 3, 125, 281
Ernst, Edzard, 139, 255
Esdaile, James, 299
esoteric, 46, 48, 51, 105–7, 124, 163, 208, 246, 258
esoteric Christianity, 51
essences, 31, 105, 207, 209, 212, 214–15, 321–22
essential oils, 2, 31, 94, 96–97, 207, 210–11, 213, 215, 217–23
esters, 210
etheric body, 38, 247, 321
evidence-based, 140, 256, 261
evolutionary theory, 4
Ezekiel (prophet), 8, 224–25, 263

F

falun gong, 179
familiar spirits, 291
fascia, 167, 173–74
fibromyalgia, 136–37, 187
Fielding, 19, 166, 299
fire walk, 291
first-degree reiki, 194–95
Fitzgerald, William, 167–69
flower therapy, ix, 206, 208, 276
Force, 35
Foster, Richard, 74
frankincense, 217–18
Freemason, 45–47, 51, 245, 285–86
Freud, Sigmund, 202
Fu Hsi (emperor), 114

G

Galen (physician), 287, 289
Gall, Franz Joseph, 300
games of chance, 19
Garden of Gethsemane, 325
gems, 59, 224, 226, 229, 233, 235, 240, 322
gemstone, 227, 229, 232, 240
geomancy, 51, 239
geometry, 19, 229
Gerber, Richard, 37, 39, 59, 63, 105–6, 160, 209, 214, 220, 230–31, 241–42, 317–21, 323
Gerome, Stan, 201–2
Gerson, Scott, 26
Ginseng root, 119
Gnosticism, 45–46, 51
Gnostics, 45
Gopi, 53, 82
grand master, 123–24
Grand Orient lodges, 47–48, 50
great wisdom from the East, 52
Greek, 46, 266, 282–84, 286, 288, 290, 310

Green, Alyce, 156, 301–2, 308–9, 316
grounded, 218, 233, 240
guided imagery, 31, 65, 146–48, 150, 152, 154, 156, 158–60, 162–64, 233, 290, 311
Gumpert, 245
Gurudas, 321

H

Hahnemann, Samuel, 243–47, 249, 252
Hakomi, 78
Hall, Manley, 286, 289
Hardinge, Mervyn, 208
Hare Krishna, 2
Harner, Michael, 149, 226, 301
Has homeopathy been verified? 254
hatha yoga, 68, 82–83, 87–91, 181
herbalism, 206–8
herbal medicine, 108, 211, 214, 265
herbs, 26–27, 54, 63–65, 97, 99, 114, 117–19, 130, 143, 178, 188, 204–8, 216–17, 262, 288–90
herbs and minerals, 97, 204
Hermes (messenger of the gods), 54, 266, 282, 286, 310
Hermetic Tradition, 51
Hester, Ben, 279
hieroglyph, 168
higher consciousness, 210, 213, 293, 312, 314, 323
higher power, 153
Higher Self, 210, 212
Hindu, 2, 25–26, 29–30, 53–55, 62–64, 66–67, 74–75, 81, 84, 88–93, 100–101, 110, 181, 218, 313
Hinduism, 2, 29–30, 54, 63, 66–67, 81–82, 84–85, 87, 91–94, 107, 112, 121, 131, 149, 151
Hippocrates, 29, 288–90

holistic, 30, 51, 86, 131, 149–51, 158, 163, 167, 176, 192, 211, 214, 228, 312, 317–18
hologram, 167
homeopathy, ix, 31, 35, 105, 113, 211, 214, 220, 243–44, 246–48, 250–52, 254–58, 261, 265, 322
  laws of, 248
Homer (Greek epic poet), 266
Homoeopathy, 246, 251
Homo-Vibra Ray, 261, 323
horoscope, 25
Horus (Egyptian god), 231
Howard, Michael, 51
Huang-ti nei-ching text, 128
Hubbard, 259
humanism, 48
humanistic, 162–63, 304
human potential, 157, 163, 231, 309
humors, 117, 288
Hunt, Dave, 66–67, 82–83, 85, 150, 161–63, 250, 310
Hwang Ti (emperor), 114
hydrotherapy, 173
hypnotism, 80, 134, 144, 158, 187, 262, 297–304, 306

I

I AM, 35
I Ching sticks, 216
ida, 90
Ignatius Loyola, 72, 121
Ihori (Japanese businessman), 312
illuminists, 48
immortality, 8, 14, 18, 39, 63–64, 66, 92, 107, 126, 149, 285, 287, 293, 326
imprint, 214, 251–52
inanimate, 27, 56, 60, 272, 318
Ingham, Eunice, 169
innate, 35, 160, 212, 239, 327

inner self, 29, 126, 156, 218
integrative, 108, 141, 290, 292
intuition, 106, 207, 236, 240, 328
iridology, 2, 31, 188–92, 262, 265
iron, 228, 299
Isis (Egyptian goddess), 262
Islam, 65, 74, 292

J

Jaggi, 36, 90, 92
jasper, 224–25
Joan, 26
Johnstone, Peter, 138–39
judo, 125
Jung, C. G., 13, 83, 201–2
Jupiter, 26, 54

K

Kabalah (Kabbala), 43, 46
Kabat-Zinn, Jon, 76
Kah, Gary, iv, 51
Kamiya, Joe, 308
kapha, 210, 228
karate, 12, 121, 125–26
kata, 124, 126
Keating, Thomas, 73
ketones, 210
Khalsa, Dharma Singh, 64–66, 68, 83
ki, 35, 126, 176, 193
Kinesiology, 2, 167, 177–79, 209, 236, 239
Knights Templars, 46
Krieger, Delores, 181
kundalini, 87, 109
kung fu, 125
Kunz, Dora, 181

L

laparoscope, 260
laserpuncture, 31, 276
latent forces, 87, 89, 91, 108, 149

lattice, 229, 232, 235, 264
LAWS of HOMEOPATHY, 248
Leeds, Robert, 122
lemon oil, 210
leukemia, 271–72
Levi, Jerome Meyer, 226
Life Force, 230–31
life force energy, 37, 101, 165, 179, 183, 193, 206, 231, 237
ligure, 224
Lilly, Simon, 226
Li Xiao Ming, 122
Lockie, Andrew, 252
lodestone, 187
logos, 19–20, 35, 150, 212
lotus, 39, 63, 86, 312
LSD (lysergic acid diethylamide), 68, 85
Lucas, George, 35
Lucifer, 8, 18, 47–48, 325–26
Luciferian Occultism, 46
Luthe, Wolfgang, 308
lymphatic, 177
Lyons, Albert, 29–30, 53, 55, 114, 286, 288

M

macrocosm, 24, 36
magenta, 59
magic arts, 108, 282–84, 294
magician, 45–46, 237–38
magnesium, 228
magnetic energy, 57, 102
magnetic field therapy, 273
magnetic fluid, 188, 298
magnetic healer, 186
magnetic therapy, 104, 187, 262, 299
magnetism, viii, 27, 35, 187–88, 212, 245–46, 297–99
magnetoelectric energy, 323

magnets, 31, 103, 105, 144, 186–88, 267, 298–99
Maharishi Mahesh Yogi, 2, 65–66, 313
mana, 35, 116, 131, 193, 212
mandala, 24, 192
Manichaeism, 46
mantra, 65–66, 68–70, 72, 307–9, 313
Marcel, 241
Marcy, 250
marma point, 31
Mars, 26, 54
martial arts, 3, 31, 65, 118–21, 123–27, 130, 167, 181, 278
Mason, Henry, 230–31
massage, 3, 31, 94, 96, 108, 167, 170, 173–76, 179, 182, 184–86, 193, 196–97, 300, 305
  Swedish, 168, 182
  trigger points (marma points), 94–95
Ma-wang-tui graves, 128
Maxwell, Jessica, 189
maya, 310
McMahon, T. A., 85, 150, 161–63, 310
McNamara, Sheila, 116, 122
MD Anderson Cancer Center, 138
medical care, early reforms in, 3–4
meditation, 12, 29–31, 52–54, 62–72, 75–78, 83–86, 90–94, 110–11, 126–27, 130, 149–50, 152–55, 162–63, 293–94, 311–13
medium, 8–9, 73, 214, 240, 245, 250, 262
mediumistic, 57, 85, 299, 301
mediumistic trances, 299
memories, 79, 216, 235
Menninger Foundation, 308
mental imagery, 310
mercury, 26, 54, 205, 253, 266, 286
meridians, 106, 116, 118, 123, 127–28, 130, 132, 142, 165, 179, 185, 233, 321–22

meridian therapy, 31, 276
Mermet, Alexis, 266
Mesmer, Franz Anton, 35, 103, 144, 187–88, 245, 262, 277, 298–99
mesmerism, 144, 246, 262, 276, 298–300
Mesopotamia, 204, 286
Mesopotamian civilization, 19
meta-analysis, 143, 187, 255
metabolism, 97–98
metaphysics, 88, 106, 310
microcosm, 22–24, 36, 54, 86, 90, 115–17, 145, 166, 173, 175, 188, 192, 267, 285, 298
Miller, 46, 48, 241
mindfulness meditation, 75–78, 80
mind-set, 115, 157, 287, 289
Mitchell, William, 138
mo, 128, 219
modality, 158, 174, 179, 196, 200, 299
monism, 36, 212
Morals and Dogma (Pike), 45–46, 285
Mora machine, 261, 274–75
Morgana (feminine sun god), 231
mother tincture, 235, 243, 251–52
moxibustion, 27, 31, 113, 118, 130, 185, 276
MRI (magnetic resonance imaging), 103, 142, 188
mumio, 289
myrrh, 217
mysteries, 16, 41–42, 46, 50, 93, 110, 126, 213, 281, 325
mystical medicine, 17, 41–42, 45, 50, 307, 327

N

nature worship, 3, 5, 19, 34, 42, 45, 47, 228, 280
naturopath, 190
Navaho, 231

Nebuchadnezzar (king), 265
necromancer, 291
Nei Ching, 114
neo-paganism, 11
neuro-optic reflex, 189–90
neutral, 64, 97, 151, 163, 241, 309, 327
New Age Movement, 2–3, 11–12, 36, 47–48, 51, 149, 306
nirvana, 4, 39, 63–64, 90, 100–101, 149, 154, 293
Norman, 90
Norse, 231
numerics, 19

O

observer of times, 177, 291
Occident, 46
occult, xi, xiv–xv, 32, 45–46, 51–52, 54, 67, 135, 208, 245, 247–48, 258, 271–72, 276–77, 279–80
occultism, iv, 2, 11, 20, 39, 46–47, 82, 137, 158, 162, 181, 202, 228, 263, 284
occultist, 208, 285
ODIC FORCE, 35, 212
Odysseus (king of Ithaca), 282
Office of Public Policy, 139, 203
oil of peppermint, 211
Olcott, Henry, 48
omega, 274
omen, 166, 240, 262–63
One, 53, 64
oneness, 18, 20, 22, 82–83, 90, 126, 212
onyx, 224–25
Ophiel (Edward C. Peach), 152, 159
orange oil, 210
orenda, 35, 212
origins, 2, 42, 116, 222, 326, 328
orthomolecular medicine, 276
Oschman, James, 103, 254, 258

oscilloscope, 305–6
osteopath, 200
osteopathy, 113, 200
Ouija board, 216, 263, 277–78
oxygen, 69, 228, 313

P

paganism, 11, 19, 25, 36, 39, 42, 47, 54, 92–93, 110, 112, 131, 228, 328
pagan religious theology, 4, 11, 19, 25, 54, 84, 86, 107, 150, 212, 216, 285, 314, 320, 366
pa kua, 30, 114
Palmistry, 166
panchakarma (cleansing/purification), 98, 100
pantheism, xi, 27, 36, 40, 45, 47, 72, 77, 165, 205, 219, 246, 318
Pantheist's explanation for cause of disease, 39
Paracelsus (physician), 187–88, 245, 298
parapsychology, 296, 310
passive mind, 64, 68, 72, 77, 151, 313
passivity of mind, 84
past life regression, 31
pearl, 225
Peczely, Ignaz von, 189
Pegasus, 209, 214
pendulum, 31, 60, 209, 215, 236, 239–40, 250, 261–62, 265–69, 271, 276–79, 294, 323
pen-tsao, 114
Pergamum, 287
Peter (apostle), 45
Petrucelli, R. Joseph, 29, 53, 114, 286, 288
peyote, 85, 283
phallic symbol, 119
Philistines, 264

philosophy, xiv, 9, 16, 20, 22, 32, 42, 47–48, 92, 97, 106, 126, 206–7, 247–48, 300
phrenology, 176, 198–99, 300
physiology, 34, 38, 52, 54, 61, 69, 100, 127, 130, 132, 142, 200, 219, 254, 314
piezoelectric, 229
Pike, Albert, 45, 47, 286
pingala, 90
Pisces, 28, 165
pitta, 210, 228
Plato (philosopher), 45
polarity, 31, 167, 176, 186, 233, 267, 276
Polynesian, 32
post-deluge Babylon (dispersion), 19
potentizing, 249
potion, 282, 287–88
power of the will, 156, 316
prana, 29, 31, 35, 58, 64, 83, 87, 89, 91, 94, 96–98, 106, 116–18, 131, 181
pranayama, 82–83, 86, 91, 94, 111
precepts, 37, 121
pre-Christian Mystery Tradition, 51
precious stones, 224–26, 230
preparation of remedies, 243, 247, 251–52, 288
primordial, 318
Prophet, Elizabeth Clare, 39, 107, 149
proposition, 32
psora, 248
psychedelic, 2, 65, 85, 283, 285, 293
psychiatry, xiii
psychic, 31–32, 40, 54, 67, 86, 104, 106, 109, 208–9, 248, 276, 301–2, 310–11, 319, 321–23
psychic healing, 245, 248, 250, 265, 276, 311, 322
psychic therapy, 31
psychoanalysis, 149, 228, 301

psychology, xiii, 68, 75–76, 83, 149, 152, 162–63, 201, 208, 266, 300–301, 304
psychometry, 277
psychophysiology, 308
psychotherapy, 27, 32, 78, 162
psychotronics, 271
pulse diagnosis, 118, 129, 318
purer consciousness, 35, 212

Q

qi, 35, 118–21, 123, 126–27, 131, 136, 193, 278, 293, 318, 320
qigong, 65, 119–22, 124, 127, 130, 144, 167, 179, 202, 278, 293, 318
qigong exercise, 293, 318
quartz, 225–27, 229, 241

R

radiesthesia, 60, 135, 271, 276, 323
radionic pendulum, 250
radionics, 31, 135, 248, 271–72, 276
Ragon (Freemason), 45
rajas, 53, 56, 97, 214
Ramacharaka, 89
Raman, R. V., 53
Rand, 196
Raso, 55, 60, 99
rational therapies, 316
reality, 77, 107, 150, 153, 156, 161, 184, 196, 220, 222, 303, 310–11
reflection, 209, 231
reflexology, viii, 31, 165–76, 178, 180, 182, 184, 186, 188, 190, 192, 222, 265, 366
Rei, 193
Reich, Wilhelm, 45, 174
Reichenbach, Baron von, x, 277
Reiki, 31, 109, 167, 176, 193–98, 200, 202, 292

reincarnation, 2, 4, 38, 62–63, 82, 86, 94, 106, 149, 163, 190, 293, 323, 326, 365
Reisser, 181–82
relaxation, 63, 65, 68–71, 79–80, 151, 153, 155, 158–60, 194, 307–10, 313
religion of nature, 207
remedies, 28, 118, 205, 208–9, 220, 244, 247–49, 251–52, 254–55, 257, 274, 278, 284, 327
Reuters Health Information, 134, 137, 187
Rife machine, 261, 273–74
Ritter, Johann Wilhelm, 266
rod, divining, 264, 269
Rodriquez, Caro, 49
Rolf, Ida Pauline, 173–74
Rolfing, 167, 174–75, 254
Roman Catholic, 72–74, 197–98
Ron Kurtz, 78–79
Rosa, Emily, 104, 182
Rosicrucians, 46, 285
rune dice, 216
Russian parapsychology, 35

S

samadhi, 86
Sampson, Wallace, 133
sandalwood, 218
Sanskrit, 24, 29, 53, 65, 76, 86, 91, 214
Santorelli, Saki, 76
sapphire, 224–25
sardius, 224–25
sardonyx, 225
Satan, 3–4, 8–14, 16–18, 21, 29–30, 34, 93–94, 157, 164, 214–16, 278, 280–81, 291–94, 314–15, 325–29
Satanism, 48, 283
Saturn, 26
Schelling, Friedrich Wilhelm Joseph von, 267
Schultz, Johannes, 307
sciences, xiii, 17, 34, 45, 60, 67, 100, 108, 131–32, 162, 214, 267, 284, 289, 300
scientific medicine, 4, 98, 108, 113, 133, 141, 145, 244, 261, 327
Seal of Solomon, 233
second-degree reiki, 195
secret societies, 43, 45, 47–51, 285
self, 155–58, 195, 210, 212, 312, 320, 323
self-realization, 83
sensitive, 57, 61–62, 102, 122, 267, 272, 276, 279
Sephat, 44
serpent, xv, 5, 8–9, 14, 16, 18, 59, 66, 87, 91, 149, 216, 227, 296–97, 326
shamanism, 149–50, 226, 228, 301
Shen Nung (emperor), 114
shiatzu, 175
Shiva, 149, 205
Siberia, 227
signature, 118, 240, 251–52
silicon, 228
Slack, Robert, Jr., 139–41
sodium, 228
Sol, 231
soma body work, 31
soma therapy, 167, 176
somato-emotional release, 200
sonopuncture, 31, 276
soothsayer, 240, 262
sorcerer, 45, 66, 68, 85, 109, 240, 262, 284, 310
sorceries, 283, 290, 294, 311
soul, 5, 50, 53, 63, 82, 86, 116, 153, 193, 201, 205, 210, 213, 247, 276
sound therapy, 31, 322

Spirit, 10, 34, 72, 82, 84, 101, 153, 164, 207, 212, 242, 281, 293, 297, 319
spirit guides, 85, 109, 150, 242, 250, 328
spirits, 10, 14–15, 17, 27–28, 54, 71, 124, 128, 138, 160, 207, 214–16, 220, 227–28, 277–79
spiritual exercises, 121
spiritualism, x–xi, xiv–xv, 10–11, 14, 48, 67, 80, 92, 112, 197, 200, 202, 237, 298, 306
spiritualist, 181, 202, 292, 299–300
Sri Aurobindo, 88
Stalker, 249
stargazers, 311
Star of David, 233
Star Wars, 35
statistically significant, 261
Steed, Earnest, 21, 32, 285
Stein, 197
Stewart, David, 219–23
subtle energy, 58, 66, 161, 187, 210, 233, 235, 241, 276, 311, 322–23
subtle energy medicine, 275
Sufis, 46
suggestion, 132, 298–99, 302
Sumerian, 166
Sunna, 231
sun worship, 20, 29, 112
supplements, 178, 236
Supreme Self, 312, 320, 323
supreme ultimate, 36, 212
Sutherland, William, 199–200
Swain, 180
Swedenborg, Emanuel, 168, 245, 292, 298
Swedish, 168, 182
sympathetic, 28, 118, 169, 173, 189, 245
sympathetic remedy, 173
sympathy, 20, 23, 25, 36, 118–19, 166, 174, 289
Szurko (ex-yogic master), 86, 88

T

tai chi chuan, 3, 12, 65, 120, 122–23, 125–26, 130, 162, 167
Takata, Hawayo, 194
talisman, 125, 232
tamas, 54, 56, 97–98, 214
Taoism, 115, 121, 131
Taoist, 25, 125–26, 287
tartar emetic, 251
telepathy, 202
temptation, xiv, 4–5, 7, 12, 18, 26–27, 54, 64–65, 115–16, 131, 212, 219–20, 224, 281, 317–18
terpenes, 210
theology, 2–3, 36, 47, 51, 93, 110, 146, 245, 276
Theosophical Research Center, 276
theosophy, 2–3, 12, 47–50, 135, 181, 276, 310, 318
therapeutic approaches, 31
therapeutic imagery, 200
therapeutic touch, 181, 276
Theriac, 289
theta brain-wave, 308–9, 312
third-degree reiki, 195
Thoth, 286, 310
three world centers of medical influence, 29
Tibetan, 26, 39, 50, 93, 110, 126, 149, 159, 181, 193, 201
tiger, 119
times, 291
tincture, 215, 235, 243, 251–52
Tisserand, Robert, 204, 210–12
Tonatiuh, 231
Toning, 31, 276
topaz, 224–25

touch for health, 31, 179
transcendental meditation, 65–66, 109, 276, 313
Trojan Horse, 161
tumor therapy, 273
turquoise, 59, 224, 227
Tyler, 247

U

Ullman, Dana, 251
unified energy field, 36, 54, 57, 64
universal energy, 29–31, 36–40, 56–58, 62–63, 89–92, 96–98, 101–2, 105–7, 153–54, 167–70, 183–84, 192–94, 205–6, 230, 247
Universal Intelligence, 35
universal magnetic fluid, 188, 298
Unruffling, 181
Unschuld, 129–30
Upledger, John, 200–201
Usui, Mikao, 193–94
usurp, 42

V

vascular, 129, 145, 177, 179, 307
vata, 210, 228
Vedas, 29, 53, 166
Venus, 26, 54
vibrational healing, 275, 321
vibrational medicine, 37, 105–6, 160, 209, 214, 220, 230, 318–22
vibrational therapies, 60, 275
video by Jeremiah Films, 30
viscera, 123
visualization, 31, 65, 71, 100, 121, 146, 148–64, 228, 233, 236, 301, 303, 307–11
visualize, 25, 60, 121, 147–49, 151, 161
Vita Florum, 208
vital energy, 35, 119, 165, 172, 181, 193, 244, 246, 278, 288, 318

vital essence, 120
Vitz, Paul, 162
Vladimir, 170, 175
Voegeli, A. (doctor), 250
Vogel, Marcel, 241
Vogt, Oscar, 307
volition, 151, 157, 309, 316
VOL machine, 322

W

Walters, Dale, 308
wand, 179, 237–39, 265–66, 273
Warrier, 53, 82, 99
Webster, Nesta, 43, 45, 47–48, 50
Webster's Collegiate Dictionary, 6
Weil, Andrew, 140, 245, 290
Weldon, John, 150, 241, 250
Western yoga, 309
Wicca, 283
Wikipedia, 148–49
WILHELM REICH, 174
Willis, Richard, 30, 82, 86, 88–89, 312–13
Wilson, 32, 67, 174, 277
Wilson, Lois, 364
Winds, 1, 3, 117, 128, 130, 266
Winemiller, Mark, 187, 365
wisdom of the East, 52, 111
witch, 125, 157, 177, 226–27, 268, 291
witchcraft, 163, 240, 262–63, 281, 283–84
witness, 127, 178, 240, 323
Witt, Claudia, 137
wizard, 163, 238, 284, 291
Wolfgang, 308
Woodstock, 2, 365
world view, 206, 220–21, 245, 320, 327, 365
Worwood, 207, 213, 365

379

Y

yang, 20, 25–27, 40, 54–55, 97–98, 114–19, 130–31, 142, 205, 211–12, 214, 228, 318, 322, 326
Yellow Emperor (Hwang Ti), 114
yin, 20, 25–27, 40, 54–55, 97–98, 114–19, 130–31, 136, 142, 205, 211–12, 214, 228, 318, 322
yoga, vii, xi, 2–3, 12, 29–31, 62–69, 81–94, 108–11, 121, 124–27, 162–63, 181, 293, 311–13, 365
yoga exercises, 3, 65, 81, 86, 88, 91–94, 110, 118, 293, 365
yoga meditation, 84, 88, 293
yogi, 66, 83, 86, 88–89, 93, 110, 126, 365
Yonggi Cho, Paul, 150
Youngen, 196–97
Yuman, 228, 365
Yungen, Ray, 71, 73–74

Z

zapping machine, 273–74, 366
Zeus (Greek god), 54
zodiac (meridians), 106, 116, 118, 123, 127–30, 132, 142, 165, 177, 179, 185, 233, 321–22
zone therapy, 167–70, 175–76, 366
Zoroastrianism, 43, 366